AF673607

RXpert SERIES Student's Companion

Pharmaceutical Formulation Development

Rxpert SERIES
Student's Companion

Pharmaceutical Formulation Development

Dulal Krishna Tripathi Ex-Director

Santosh Rungta Group of Institutions,

Bhilal, CG.

PharmaMed Press

An imprint of BSP Books Pvt. Ltd.

4-4-309/316, Giriraj Lane,

Sultan Bazar, Hyderabad - 500 095.

Pharmaceutical Formulation Development
by **Dulal Krishna Tripathi**

© 2025, *by Publisher*

All rights reserved. No part of this book or parts thereof may be reproduced, stored in a retrieval system or transmitted in any language or by any means, electronic, mechanical, photocopying, recording or otherwise without the prior written permission of the author.

Disclaimer: The authors and the publishers have taken due care to provide the authentic, reliable and up to date information related to the subject. However, neither the authors nor the publisher shall be responsible for any liability for any damage caused as a result of use of this book. The respective user must check the accuracy from other sources too.

Published by

PharmaMed Press
An imprint of BSP Books Pvt. Ltd.
4-4-309/316, Giriraj Lane, Sultan Bazar, Hyderabad - 500 095.
Phone: 040-23445688; Fax: 91+40-23445611
E-mail: info@pharmamedpress.net
www.bspbooks.net/www.pharmamedpress.net

ISBN: 978-93-48734-27-3 (Hardback)

RXpert SERIES
Student's Companion

Pharmaceutical Formulation Development

Dulal Krishna Tripathi Ex-Director
Santosh Rungta Group of Institutions,
Bhilai, CG.

PharmaMed Press
An imprint of BSP Books Pvt. Ltd.
4-4-309/316, Giriraj Lane,
Sultan Bazar, Hyderabad - 500 095.

…on Development

Pharmaceutic…

by Dulal Kris…

©2025, by P…

All rights reserved. No part of this book or parts thereof may be reproduced, stored in a retrieval system or transmitted in any language or by any means, electronic, mechanical, photocopying, recording or otherwise without the prior written permission of the author.

> **Disclaimer:** The authors and the publishers have taken due care to provide the authentic, reliable and up to date information related to the subject. However, neither the authors nor the publisher shall be responsible for any liability for any damage caused as a result of use of this book. The respective user must check the accuracy from other sources too.

Published by

PharmaMed Press

An imprint of BSP Books Pvt. Ltd.

4-4-309/316, Giriraj Lane, Sultan Bazar, Hyderabad - 500 095.

Phone: 040-23445688; Fax: 91+40-23445611

E-mail: info@pharmamedpress.net

www.bspbooks.net/www.pharmamedpress.net

ISBN: 978-93-48734-27-3 (Hardback)

Preface

Among the most research-intensive industries, pharmaceutical industry is one. Pharmaceutical industries are also extensively regulated by regulatory authorities. The research is conducted in various directions. Moreover, the industries are supposed to follow Good Manufacturing Practice as per ICH guidelines. Any formulation of a drug whether new or existing is supposed to carryout formulation development studies and the result must be reproducible, and permission must be accorded from the respective drug regulatory authority.

Thus, formulation development work is not small one, rather it is a complex afford. In fact, earlier to 2017 different educational institutions of this country affiliated various Universities had different syllabus for their respective M. Pharmacy courses. But, from the academic session 2017 – 2018, the Pharmacy Council of India have done a revolutionary work by according the permission from the Government of India and implementing across the country. Therefore, all the academic Institutions including their affiliating Universities are bound to implement the syllabus.

Therefore, this book, **Pharmaceutical Formulation Development** has been prepared as per the syllabus for M. Pharm course with specialization in Industrial Pharmacy, 1st semester. The contents have been prepared with as per as possible simple languages, so that the reader can understand easily. The book has five chapters in accordance with the syllabus. The five chapters are Preformulation, Formulation additives, Solubility, Dissolution and Product stability respectively. At the end of each chapter there are some model questions such as multiple-choice questions, short questions and long questions. There are some references also. During preparation of the book adequate care has been taken to avoid any mistake; however, if any mistake is found later kindly inform the publisher or the undersigned. So that, during subsequent printing error can be corrected.

Dulal Krishna Tripathi

Content

CHAPTER - 5

Product Stability

CHAPTER - 1

Preformulation Studies

Molecular optimization of APIs (drug substances), crystal morphology and variations, powder flow, structure modification, drug-excipient compatibility studies, methods of determination.

MOLECULAR OPTIMIZATION OF APIs (DRUG SUBSTANCES)

Since long the physical properties of optimized active pharmaceutical ingredients (API) such as bulk properties, surface/ interfacial properties, and mechanical properties are important for manufacturing of drug product. The APIs with these challenging properties can produce the issues, such as inconsistent powder feeding, de-mixing of blends, variable die-filling, and punch sticking. Ultimately these produce unacceptable final tablet quality attributes. Inefficient processes and high batch rejection rates also affects environmental impacts. Some of these effects may not be directly affect the patient. The processes can be costlier or can cause problems with the availability of the products. Such processes are not robust. These processes show high degree of rejections or are difficult to be scaled-up and their technology are difficult to be transferred, the ability to tailor the physical properties of APIs can have great possibility to cause various problems for manufacturing of drug products. This helps both the conventional batches and advanced continuous manufacturing processes. The second one, that is, the continuous manufacturing process has gained priority as an emerging technology. These are considered and promoted by the regulatory agenciies[1-3], and attracted the interest of academics, and research interests[4]. One way to manage the physical properties of an API is the selection of an appropriate crystal form. The physical or chemical stability and the morphology of the drug product depend mainly on the selection of an appropriate polymorph, hydrate or solvate, salt, or co-crystals of the API. However, this is not always true for the conventional, or targeted *in vivo* behavior. When the selection of an alternative solid form is not an option, by adjusting the process parameters of crystallization, such as rate of supersaturation, temperature, concentration, solvent system, mixing parameters, such as, wet-milling or seed size/quantity, mixing speed, etc., can produce the improved physical properties of the drug products. However, this is not a universal solution, and in certain cases may cause slightly positive results. There is another method of spherical crystallization. This technique involves intentional controlled agglomeration process during isolation/drying. Such process can greatly improve physical properties of drug product[5-10].

Emulsion based crystallization process can produce spherical agglomerations of the API[11,12,] this is another method. A recent study reveals that by using solvent diffusion, or by changing the pH, the quasi-emulsification can cause spherical crystallization[13]. In general, the spherical crystallization could not be commercially feasible because of the problems such as volumetric productivity, managing solubility in complex ternary solvent systems. Process complexity of developing and scaling multi-phase slurries, and the difficulty in maintaining intact particles during isolation and drying of powders.

Moreover, there is another class of pharmaceutical materials evolved which do not show the properties of well-defined crystalline materials. With ever-increasing knowledge of biological systems that provides novel biological targets, the pharmaceutical industry is developing new molecules with different modalities, such as, macrocycles, peptides, protein degradomers, RNA, siRNA[14]. In most cases, these do not comply with Lipinski's rule of five for drug-like properties[15]. New molecules today can frequently be large (>500 Da). New molecular entities today can be lipophilic (poorly-water solubles)[16,17] and show a lack of propensity for crystallization[18,19]. Properties of these classes of compounds render them difficult to be isolated and stabilised. Therefore, these become challenging, if not impossible, to formulate in conventional drug product processing routes.

An important and more universal route to optimise API properties (both crystalline materials, and non-crystalline materials or a poorly defined crystalline materials) is to incorporate the non-active components during formation of particles and/or subsequent isolation and drying to provide coprocessor API[20]. Many pharmaceutical companies agree that despite the promises posed by co-processed API, regulatory uncertainty for co-processed API inhibits commercial implementation.

Co-processed API can be defined as *a drug substance, manufactured in a drug manufacturing facility, that contains the API in addition to one or more non-covalently bonded, non-active component, and differs from salts, solvates and/or crystals.* Co-processed APIs differ from salts, solvates and crystals because API and non-active components do not exist in the same crystal lattice and do not always bear a defined stoichiometry. Non-active component is defined as *a component such as a carrier, additive, or other excipient that is non-covalently bonded with the API and is included in the co-processed API to improve the physical properties.* The non-active components commonly cited in the literature are compendial excipients, with a smaller subset of cited work involving GRAS materials, and an even smaller subset of novel excipients. In case of novel excipients, safety/toxicology information, the route of administration, dose and CMC information would require to be considered and provided in regulatory submission as appropriate.

The proposed definition of co-processed API is in the line with the ICH Q7 definition of an API or drug substance. This includes any substance or mixture of substances to be used in the manufacture of a drug product. When used in the production of a drug, becomes an active ingredient of the drug product[21]and the ICH Q7 Q & A clarifies that mixtures with "the addition of substances to an API to stabilise the API" can be classified in the regulatory filing as an API[22]. A co-processed API may improve the stability of the drug substance. If polymorphic. form is stabilised by the presence of the non-active components[23-25]. Moreover, it is suggested that an additional appropriate justification to include non-active components in a drug substance. It is for the purpose of optimization of physical properties of API. There are some examples of regulatory acceptance of inclusion of non-active components in a commercial drug substance with justification based on stabilisation of an amorphous form[26] or improvement of physical properties[27]. ICH Q7 recognises that in some cases physical properties such as particle size distribution, bulk density, and tap density, may be critical for a drug substance, further emphasising the importance of the optimization of API properties and potential benefits of co-processed APIs.

Usually, the co-processed API is a formulation-ready entity that can be appropriately characterized and reproducibly meet the required specifications for the drug substance critical quality attributes (CQAs). Co-processing at a drug manufacturing facility is beneficial with respect to the equipment and controls are necessary for solvent-based manufacturing such as damage limiting construction and utilises for operation under inert atmosphere, required to generate, isolate, and dry the co-processed API generally do not exist at drug product manufacturing facilities. In fact, for many co-processing methods, co-processed API can be produced 'in-the-flow 'of existing drug substance manufacturing. That is, before addition of non-active components the API do not require isolation and co-processing does not require any added unit operations or even extended time cycle. Moreover, the designing of co-processed API as a drug substance from a regulatory perspective allows the potential to support a rework/reprocessing procedure of the co-processed API. It suggests an approach for the API to expiry dating that assures quality. These allow greater supply chain flexibility and reducing a costly discard.

There have been appreciable developments in regulatory considerations for APIs with special circumstances, for example, regulatory agencies have been more receptive to introducing excipients during commercial drug substance processes where there are either physical or chemical stability challenges[28].

Moreover, the allowance to extend the hold-time of amorphous solid dispersions following an end-to-end (in-series) stability testing protocol is encouraging[29]. The FDA's recent cocrystal guidance states the reason for selecting a cocrystal in place of traditional crystalline API. That is, "co-crystals can be made to improve the bioavailability and stability of the drug product and to improve the processability of APIs during the manufacture of drug product[30]. This statement accepts that the processability of the APIs should be considered as an important factor along with bioavailability. The ability to use more complex multi-component materials isolated as drug substances can allow this goal to be realised.

These processes use typical drug manufacturing equipment, with limited logistical and technological hurdles for quick commercial implementation. The commercial application of the co-processing technologies requires similar regulatory treatment on the following topics:

1) The definition of co-processed API and proposal to manufacture co-processed APIs at a drug substance facility as per ICH Q7,
2) Primary stability and expiry dating expectations for a co-processed API,
3) Characterisation and release test expectations for a co-processed API.
4) It is desired that collaboration with global regulatory agencies will be required to fully capture the implications of pursuing co-processed APIs and identifying a route for the pharmaceutical industry to cater these innovative processes forward in development and commercialisation.

CRYSTAL MORPHOLOGY AND VARIATIONS

In 1669 when the Danish scientist Niels Steensen, studying in Florence the quartz and hematite crystals from Elba Island, suggested the first law of crystallography (the constancy of the dihedral angle) and mechanism of face growth (layer by layer). Thereafter the interest for crystal habit of minerals has been observed. H.J. Scheel[31] has described the history on this topic and crystallization with short account on crystal morphology. Crystal habit drew the attention of the great scientist like Kepler, Descartes, Hooke, Huygens. Since beginning of crystallography as science, crystal habit has become relevant scientifically. At the end of the 18th century the study of calcite crystals leads to formal stating of the first theory on crystal structure and discovery of the second law (rational indices). In the first part of 19th century the study of crystal habit led to the development of the concept of symmetry and derivation of the 32 crystal classes.

From about 1950 onwards, the interest for crystal growth becomes more and more increasing due to the role of crystals in all kind of industry and to the discovery of relevant properties of new crystalline compounds. The crystal habit has been receiving a growing attention due to theoretical interest and industrial needs. The Donnay-Harker principle is exclusively crystallography. Computer facilities have promoted tremendously in any kind of calculation, necessary in the different sectors of crystal growth, allowing progress in theoretical approach and sophisticated simulations. These are now a routine practice.

When equilibrium attains between a crystalline phase and its surroundings, the statistical amount of growth units exchanged between the two phases remains the same and does not change with time. This states that the crystallised volume remains constant, but nothing is specified about many important questions:

i) What is about the surface of the crystals, that is, how large is its extension and what are the (hkl) forms entering the equilibrium shape (E.S.) of the crystal?

ii) What is the difference, if any, between the stable E.S. of a crystal immersed either in a finite mother phase or in an infinite one and the unstable shape which obtains when the activation energy for nucleation is reached?

iii) How the E.S. does change when some adhesion sets up between the crystal and a solid substrate?

iv) How can be the solvent and the impurity concentration affect the E.S.?

Factors influencing the crystal habit:

The morphology, we mean the set of (hkl) crystal forms, occurs in a crystal independently on the surface areas. In many industrial sectors the crystal-habit change is necessary to

- Prevent crystal-caking,
- Filter crystal precipitates,
- Obtain more convenient crystal products (shape, size, size separation, purity, quality),
- Make easy storage and package, etc.

The procedures to study the crystal habit change are well established:

(1) Experimental crystal habits, and (2) growth in different solvents, are compared to the theoretical one, which may be obtained by calculations with different available methods (BFDH; PBC-attachment energy-connected nets); the analysis or by growing the crystal from the vapour phase, in which the fluid-solid and fluid-fluid interactions are negligible. As the crystal-solution interface is the critical site to face the growth and crystal habit, all the disposable devices are applied to the study of surface. They are usually classified into two main categories:

i) *Internal factors:* the crystal structure, on which the surface structures (i.e., the profiles) of the faces depend; the crystal defects;

ii) *External factors*, which act from the "outside" are: supersaturation, nature of solvent, solution composition, impurities, physical conditions (temperature, solution flow, electric and magnetic field, microgravity, ultrasound, etc.)

iii) There are also *mixed factors,* such as the free energy of crystal surfaces and edges, which depend both on crystal surface structure (an internal factor) and growth environment (external one).

Surface structure

Each crystal face has a specific surface structure, which controls its growth mechanism. The surface of a F face is not perfectly flat and smooth. The face is covered by steps and other features (hillocks), the growth rate of the face and its development. Indeed, layer growth is possible when the edge energy of a 2D nucleus is positive[32]. Surface features (dislocation activity, step bunching) and parameters (step speed, hillock slope) are sensitive to supersaturation, impurities and behave in different ways at low and high supersaturation, with linear and non-linear dependence[33]. Surface phenomena and morphology have been recently reviewed[34-36]. AFM has enormously enlarged the research field, as it allows to observe the surface features of the growing faces ex situ and in situ at a molecular level.

- **The α factor and the roughening transition**

  The concept of α factor was brought in as a measure of roughness of a surface and of its probable growth mechanism. Knowledge of α is mostly useful, however it may not be sufficient, as noticed for several alkanes. These show the same α in different solvents yet have different growth mechanisms[37] such as faces of succinic acid grown from water and isopropyl alcohol (IPA). Each face has the same α value in both solvents, nevertheless the growth rates are appreciably lower in IPA than in water, because of different efficiency of hydrogen bond in IPA and water molecules[38]. With increasing temperature, the α factor decreases and may reach values lower than 3.2. In that case the surface loses its flatness, becomes rough and grows by a continuous mechanism. The transition occurs at a definite roughening temperature which is characteristic for each face. Below the TR, the faces are straight, above it. They become round off even if supersaturation is very low[39].

- **Kinetic roughening**

  Beside thermal roughening, a surface may undergo a kinetic roughening. This occurs below the roughening temperature when supersaturation exceeds the critical value. In that case the sticking fraction on the surface is so high and critical two-dimensional nucleus so small that the surface becomes rough and grows through a continuous mechanism. This behaviour was observed on the faces of NaCl in aqueous solutions and in naphthalene crystals, which become fully rounded-off when σ attains 1.47%. in toluene solvent. The same does not occur with hexane, due to structural dissimilarity of hexane molecules with respect to naphthalene. Four criteria used to identify the beginning of kinetic roughening have been studied by Monte Carlo simulations on a Kossel surface, which lead to different values of the critical driving force[40].

- **Polar crystals**

In polar crystals a slice dhkl may present a dipole moment. In that case, a correction term, E_{corr}, should be brought into the expression of E_{att} to maintain constant the value:

$$E_{cr} = E_{att} + E_{slice} + E_{corr}$$

Where, Ecorr = 2 π μ 2 / V,

V = the volume of the primitive cell and

μ = the dipolar moment of the slice.

The surfaces of the two opposite faces (hkl) and (<u>hkl</u>), being structurally similar can interact in a selective way with the solvent and impurity molecules. The final result is a development of these faces, which may lead to the occurrence of only one form. In the case of water molecules, these faces are selectively adsorbed on the opposite faces since they have different surface distribution of sulphite ions. The structural differences can be so great that the two opposite faces may grow with different mechanism.

- **Surface with AFM (Atomic Force Microscopy)**

AFM has become a routine technique in laboratories where crystal-growth experiments are studied. Most experiments are carried out in static conditions, some in dynamic conditions. For example, besides proteins, one of the most studied compounds is calcite. The cleavage form grows via monomolecular steps, which are affected by anion and impurities present in calcite. AFM has been used to assess the stability of the faces of NaCl in pure and impure aqueous solutions and in the attempt to solve the problem of surface reconstruction. Through Atomic Force Microscopy (AFM) investigation of the faces of Potassium Dihydrogen Phosphate (KDP), the dependence of macro-steps and hillocks on β-form was measured and the new values of the step edge energy, kinetic coefficients and activation energies for the step motion were calculated, confirming the models of Chernov and van der Eerden and Müller-Krumbhaar[41]. In studying the influence of organic dyes on potassium sulphate the link between the surface features at the nanoscale level and the macroscopic habit change was proved. To sum up, the AFM analysis allows to seize local details of surface structure and their evolution in real time, brings a lot of information, but has the drawback as it does not permit to have a large-scale glance of the face, so it has to be integrated with other instrumental, optical or X-ray, techniques.

Crystal defects

Defects in crystals are easily and usually observed. It is not necessary to emphasize the role of screw dislocations in crystal growth. In case of edge dislocations, these could affect the growth rate since a strain energy is related to the Burgers vector and the growth rate increases. Combined research on the effect of dislocations on crystal growth with in-situ X-ray topography was done on Adenosine Dihydrogen Phosphate (ADP) crystal. Edge dislocations are proved to be inactive in step generation on the ADP face, whereas the screw dislocations are active. When a dislocation line emerges on a given (hkl) face, the face grows at higher rate than the other equivalent ones and therefore decreases its morphological importance with respect to the others. In the crystals of cubic symmetry, the habit may change from cube to tetragonal prism or square tablet. When a screw dislocation crosses an edge, it becomes inactive. On the other hand, currently it is stated that if the growth rate increases, the defect density, also increases; this is supported by Monte Carlo simulations. That is, the large crystals having a high degree of structural perfection can be obtained with the method of "rapid growth". This consists of overheating a supersaturated solution, inserting a seed conveniently shaped and strongly stirring the solution submitted to a temperature gradient. This method allows to prepare in short time very large crystals of technologically important compounds as KDP and Deuterated Potassium Phosphate (DKDP) up to 90 cm long and nearly free of dislocations. Crystals grown with the traditional method at low temperature are smaller, rich in striations and dislocations, originated by liquid inclusions. Large perfect crystals can be fast grown also from highly concentrated boiling water solutions. The method has been successfully applied to some compounds, as KDP, $Pb(NO_3)$, $K_2Cr_2O_7$. Due to the high growth rates and β-form of the crystal habit becomes equidimensional [42].

POWDER FLOW

Knowledge of the flow properties of a powder or a bulk solid is necessary to design silos and other bulk solid handling equipment so that no flow problems (flow obstructions, segregation, irregular flow, flooding, etc.) can occur. Furthermore, quantitative information regarding flowability of bulk products is required as a part of comparative tests (such as, the effect of flow agents or other additions on flow behaviour) and quality control. The flow properties depend on several parameters, such as

- Particle size distribution,

- Particle shape,
- Chemical composition of the particles,
- Moisture,
- Temperature.

On the basis of all of these parameters, it is not possible to determine theoretically the flow behaviour of bulk solids. This would have been possible, even the expense for the determination of all parameters of influence would be very high. Thus, it is necessary, and also simpler, to determine the flow properties in appropriate testing devices. All types of solids are called bulk solids, powders, or granulates. In the following the general expression "bulk solid" is used for all these products.

Stresses in bulk solids Figure 1.1 shows a bulk solid element in a container (assumptions: infinite filling height, frictionless internal walls). In the vertical direction, positive normal stress ($\sigma_v > 0$, compressive stress) is exerted on the bulk solid. If the bulk solid behaves like a Newtonian fluid, the stresses in the horizontal and vertical direction (and in all other directions) would be of equal magnitude. In reality the behaviour of a bulk solid is quite different from that of a fluid, so that the assumption of analogies is often misleading. Within the bulk solid (Figure 1.1) the horizontal stress, σ_h, is a result of the vertical stress, σ_v, the resulting horizontal stress is less than the vertical stress exerted on the bulk solid from the top. The ratio of horizontal stress to vertical stress is the stress ratio, K, known as λ.

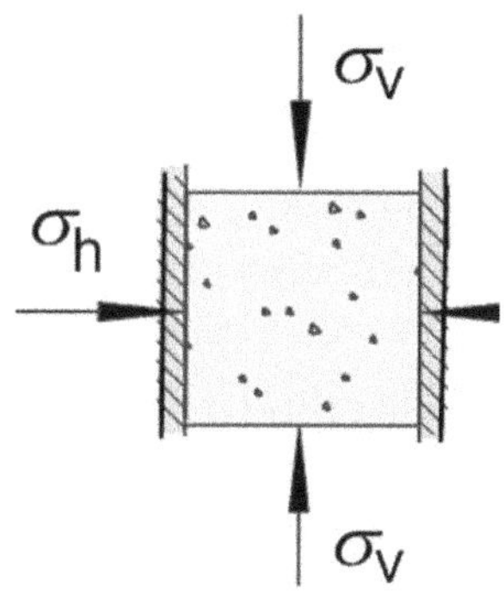

Fig.1.1 Element of bulk solid.

In analogy to solids– a bulk solid of different stresses can be found in different cutting planes. Stresses in cutting planes other than the vertical and the horizontal can be analysed using a simple equilibrium of forces. No shear stresses τ are exerted on the top or bottom surface of the bulk solid element in Figure 1.1; that is, the shear stresses in these planes are equal to zero. No shear stresses can act at the lateral walls, since the lateral walls were assumed as frictionless. Thus, only the normal stresses shown act on the bulk solid from outside. Using a simple equilibrium of forces at a volume element with triangular cross-section cut from the bulk solid element shown in Figure 1.1, the normal stress, $\sigma\alpha$, and the shear stress, $\tau\alpha$, acting on a plane inclined by an arbitrary angle α, can be calculated. After some mathematical transformations, which need not be considered here, it follows that:

$$\sigma_\alpha = \frac{\sigma_v+\sigma_h}{2} + \frac{\sigma_v-\sigma_h}{2}\cos(2\alpha) \qquad .....(1)$$

$$\tau_\alpha = \frac{\sigma_v - \sigma_h}{2}\sin(2\alpha) \qquad .....(2)$$

The pair of values, σ_α, τ_α, can be calculated according to equations (1) and (2) for all possible angles α, can be plotted in a σ,τ-diagram (normal stress, shear stress - diagram); If one joins all plotted pairs of values, a circle emerges; i.e., all calculated pairs of values form a circle in the σ,τ-diagram.

This circle is called "the Mohr stress circle". Its centre is located at,

$\sigma_m = (\sigma_v+\sigma_h)/2$ and $\tau_m = 0$.

The radius of the circle is $\sigma_r = (\sigma_v-\sigma_h)/2$.

The Mohr stress circle represents the stresses on all cutting planes at arbitrary inclination angles α, that is, in all possible cutting planes within a bulk solid element. Since the centre of the Mohr stress circle is always located on the σ-axis, each Mohr stress circle has two points of intersection with the σ-axis. The normal stresses defined through these points of intersection are called the principal stresses, whereby the larger principal stress, the major principal stress is designated as σ_1 and the smaller principal stress, the minor principal stress is designated as σ_2. If both principal stresses are given, the Mohr stress circle is well defined.

In the Fig 1.1 both the horizontal and the vertical plane are free from shear stresses (τ = 0) and are thus principal stress planes. In this case, the vertical st products are "poorly flowing"; stress, σ_v, which is greater than the horizontal stress, σ_h, is the major principal stress, σ_1, and the horizontal stress, σ_h, is the minor principal stress, σ_2.

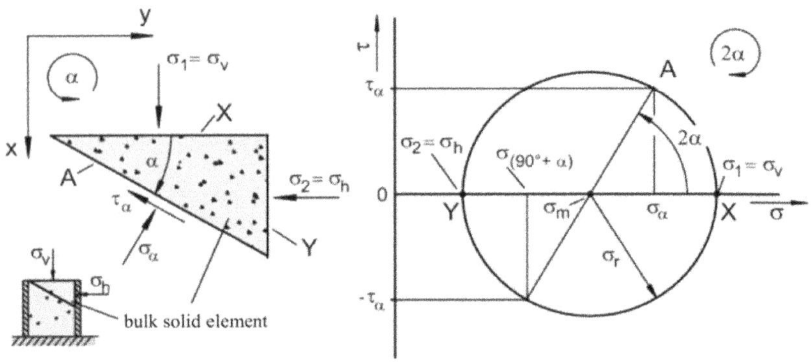

Fig.1.2 Force equilibrium on an element of bulk solid, the Mohr stress circle.

An important qualitative result of the above analysis is that shear stresses can occur in bulk solids at rest. This is impossible for a Newtonian fluid at rest (in contrast to Newtonian fluids, bulk solids can have sloped surfaces even at rest). Therefore, a representation of the stresses (fluids: pressures) in different cutting planes of a Newtonian fluid at rest in a σ, τ-diagram would yield a stress circle with the radius zero (equation (2) with $\sigma_h = \sigma_v$ yields $\tau_\alpha = 0$). From the explanation above it follows that the state of stress in a bulk solid cannot be completely described by only a single numerical value. On the basis of the actual load acting on a bulk solid element, the corresponding Mohr stress circle (Fig 1.2) can have a smaller or a larger radius, a centre at a lesser or greater normal stress, and hence also different principal stresses, σ_1 and σ_2. In principle, at a given major principal stress, σ_1, stress circles with different values for the lowest principal stress, σ_2 are imaginable. Therefore, a stress circle is defined clearly only if at least two numerical values are given, i.e., σ_1 and σ_2. In summary, the following can be stated with regard to the stresses acting in bulk solids:

- A bulk solid can transmit shear stresses even if it is at rest.
- In different cutting planes different stresses are acting.
- Stress conditions can be represented with Mohr stress circles[43-45].

Flowability

Uniaxial compression test

The phrase "good flow behaviour" commonly refers to that a bulk solid can flow easily. If they experience flow obstructions or consolidate during storage or transport, the products "poorly flows". In contrast to these qualitative statements, a quantitative statement on flowability is possible only when one can use an objective characteristic value. This considers those physical characteristics of the bulk solid that are responsible for its flow behaviour. "Flowing" means that a bulk solid is deformed plastically due to the loads acting on it. The magnitude of the load necessary for flow is a measure of flowability. This will be demonstrated first with the uniaxial compression test. Figure 1.3 shows a hollow cylinder filled with a fine-grained bulk solid (cross-sectional area A; internal wall of the hollow cylinder assumed as frictionless). The bulk solid is loaded by the stress σ_1, the consolidation stress, in the vertical direction.

The more the volume of the bulk solid specimen is reduced, the more compressible the bulk solid becomes. In addition to the increase in bulk density from consolidation stress, one will observe also an increase in strength of the bulk solid specimen. Hence, the bulk solid is both consolidated and compressed through the effect of the consolidation stress.

After consolidation, the bulk solid specimen is relieved of the consolidation stress, σ_1, and the hollow cylinder is removed. If subsequently the consolidated, the cylindrical bulk solid specimen is loaded with an increasing vertical compressive stress, the specimen will break (fail) at a certain stress. The stress causing this failure is called *compressive strength* or *unconfined yield strength*, σc (another common designation is f_c). In bulk solids technology one calls the failure "incipient flow", because at failure, the consolidated bulk solid specimen starts to flow. Thereby the bulk solid dilates somewhat in the region of the surface of the fracture, since the distances between individual particles increase. Therefore, incipient flow is plastic deformation with decrease of bulk density. Since the bulk solid fails only at a sufficiently large vertical stress, which is equal to the compressive strength, there must exist a material-specific yield limit for the bulk solid. When this yield limit is reached, the bulk solid starts to flow. The yield limits of many materials (e.g. metals) are material dependent. However, the yield limit of a bulk solid is dependent also on its stress history, i.e., previous consolidation: The greater the consolidation stress, σ_1, the greater the bulk density, ρ_b, and unconfined yield strength, σ_c. Uniaxial compression tests conducted at different consolidation stresses, σ_1, leads to different pairs of values (σ_c, σ_1) and (ρ_b, σ_1).

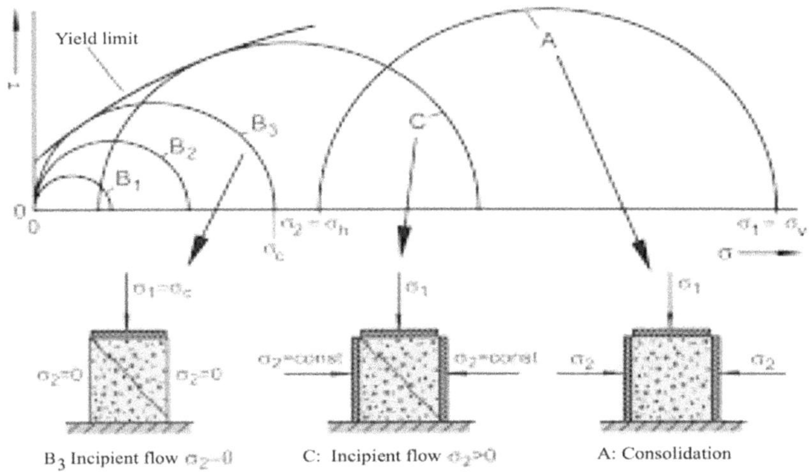

Fig.1.3 Measurement of unconfined yield strength in a σ, τ-diagram.

Time consolidation (caking)

Some bulk solids increase in strength if they are stored for a longer time at rest under a compressive stress (e.g. in a silo or an intermediate bulk container). This effect is called time consolidation or caking. Time consolidation can be determined with the test. For this one the loads the specimen with consolidation stress, σ1, not only for a short moment, but for a defined period of time, t_1. Then the unconfined yield strength is determined following the principle. This shows the flow function $\sigma_c(\sigma_1)$ of product A as previously (unconfined yield strength without influence of time consolidation, that is, for a storage period t = 0). This result is true for many bulk solids, but not for all. There are bulk solids which undergo no or only very slight consolidation over time, i.e., σ_c does not increase, or increases only very slightly with increasing storage period, t (e.g. dry quartz sand). Other bulk solids undergo a large increase in unconfined yield strength after storage periods of only a few hours, whereas after longer storage periods their unconfined yield strength does not increase further. These differences are due to the different physical, chemical, or biological effects that are the causes of consolidation over time, for example. chemical processes, crystallisations between the particles, enlargement of the contact areas through plastic deformation, capillary condensation, or biological processes such as fungal growth.

With measurement of time consolidation, a "time-lapse effect" is not realisable; that is, one must store a bulk solid specimen at the consolidation stress, σ_1, for exactly that period of time for which one would like to get data on time consolidation. Without such a test no quantitative statement can be made regarding time consolidation.

Practical determination of flow properties

The flow behaviour has been explained in a simplified way by using the uniaxial compression test as a model. The use of the uniaxial compression test with fine grained, cohesive bulk solids is problematic, because one obtains unconfined yield strength values that are too low[46], and preparation of the hollow cylinder to obtain frictionless walls is very time-consuming. In addition, further important parameters such as, internal friction and wall friction cannot be determined with this test. It is, however, an appropriate measurement technique for the measurement of the time consolidation of coarse-grained bulk solids. In order to measure the flow properties of fine-grained bulk solids, in advanced bulk solids technology so-called shear testers are used. In the following first the principle of shear testing is outlined. Afterwards, the translational shear tester introduced by Jenike around 1960[47-49] and the Schulze ring shear tester[50,51].

Shear test procedure (yield locus)

The goal of a shear test is to measure the yield limit of a consolidated bulk solid. The yield limit is called *yield locus* in bulk solids technology. For a shear test, a bulk solid specimen is loaded vertically by a normal stress, σ (Figure 1.4a). Then a shear deformation is applied on the specimen by moving the top plate with a constant velocity, v. This results in a horizontal shear stress, τ (Figure 1.4.b). With increasing shear stress the resultant force, F_R, acting on the bulk solid specimen, increases. When a point of a yield locus is measured, in analogy to the uniaxial compression test, two steps are necessary: (1) First the bulk solid specimen is consolidated, what is called "pre-shear". (2) Subsequently a point of the yield limit is measured. This step is called "shear" or "shear to failure".

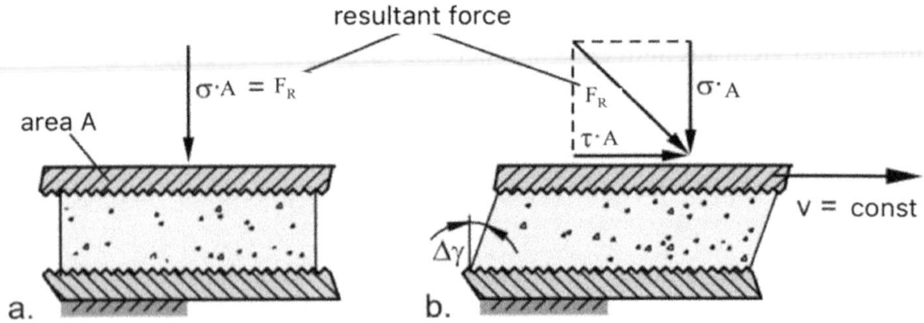

Fig.1.4 Bulk solid specimen: a. initial loading with normal stress σ; b. shear deformation (velocity v = const).

For pre-shear the bulk solid specimen is loaded in the vertical direction by a well-defined normal stress, $\sigma = \sigma_{pre}$. Then, the specimen is sheared. At the beginning of pre-shear, the shear stress τ increases with time as shown in the left diagram in Figure 1.4. With time the curve of shear stress vs. time becomes flatter, and finally the shear stress remains constant even though the specimen is sheared further. The constant shear stress is called τ_{pre}. After constant shear stress has been attained, neither shear resistance (and strength) nor bulk density increases further. Thus, the bulk solid specimen is sheared at constant normal stress, σ, constant shear stress, τ, and constant bulk density, ρ_b. The flow, or plastic deformation, occurs at constant bulk density. This type of flow, attained at pre-shear, is called steady-state flow. The state of the bulk solid after steady-state flow is attained is called "*critically consolidated with respect to normal stress, σ_{pre}*". The characteristic stress for this consolidation – the major principal stress σ_1 – will be considered later. The bulk density, ρ_b, and the shear stress, τ_{pre}, attained at steady-state flow are characteristic for the applied normal stress at pre-shear, σ_{pre}. In principle, an identical state of consolidation, characterised by the same bulk density, ρ_b, and the same shear stress, τ_{pre}, will be attained with other specimens of the same bulk solid pre-sheared under the same normal stress, σ_{pre}. After the bulk solid specimen has been consolidated by the pre-shear procedure, the shear deformation is reversed until the shear stress plot of shear stress vs. time; yield locus, τ, is reduced to zero. The pair of values of normal stress and shear stress at steady-state flow (σ_{pre}, τ_{pre}) is plotted in a normal stress - shear stress diagram (σ,τ-diagram, Figure 1.5 right). Point (σ_{pre}, τ_{pre}) is called the "pre-shear point"[52].

After pre-shear the bulk solid specimen in the shear cell is defined as a critically consolidated specimen.

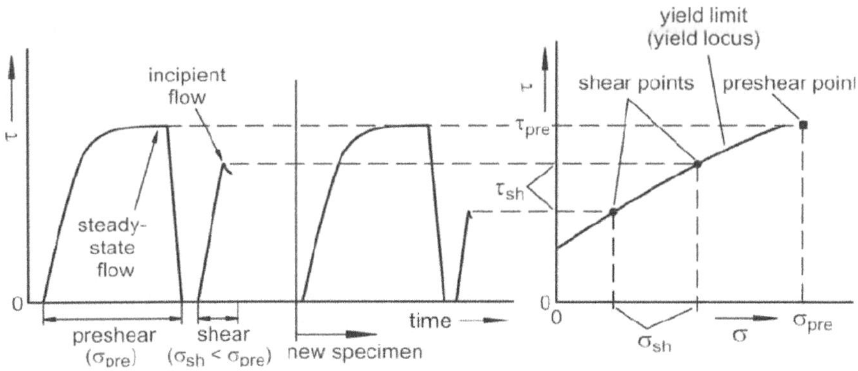

Fig 1.5 Plot of shear stress vs. time; yield locus.

The second step of the test procedure – shear or shear to failure – is discussed next. For shear to failure the normal stress acting on the specimen is decreased to a value σ_{sh}, which is less than the normal stress at pre-shear, σ_{pre}. Had the specimen been pre-sheared under the lower normal stress, σsh, and not under σpre, its bulk density and strength would have been less. Since the specimen was pre-sheared under the greater normal load, σ_{pre}, it was consolidated more than it would have been with the lower normal load, σsh. If the consolidated specimen is sheared under the normal stress σsh < σpre, it will start to flow (fail) when a sufficiently large shear force, or shear stress, is attained.

At that point particles start to move against each other. The material will start to dilate (decrease in bulk density) and shear resistance and thus shear stress will decrease. The maximum shear stress 15 characterizes incipient flow. The corresponding pair of values (σ_{sh}, τ_{sh}) is a point of the yield limit of the consolidated specimen in the σ,τ-diagram. Such a point is called a *shear point* or a *point of incipient flow*. To measure the course of the yield locus, several of the tests described above must be performed, where the specimens first must be consolidated at identical normal stress, σ_{pre} (pre-shear). Then, the specimens are sheared (failure) under different normal stresses, $\sigma_{sh} < \sigma_{pre.}$ As outlined above, by pre-shearing at identical normal stress, σ_{pre}, each specimen reaches the same state of consolidation. Each test yields the same pre-shear point (σ_{pre}, τ_{pre}), and one individual shear point (σ_{sh}, τ_{sh}) in accordance with the different normal stresses, σ_{sh}, applied at shear. The yield locus follows from a curve plotted through all measured shear points.

Yield locus

The parameters which describe the flow properties can be determined from the yield locus (Figure 1.6). The relevant consolidation stress σ_1 is equal to the major principal stress of the Mohr stress circle which is tangential to the yield locus and intersects at the point of steady state flow (σ_{pre}, τ_{pre}). This stress circle represents the stresses in the sample at the end of the consolidation procedure (stresses at steady state flow). It corresponds to the stress circle at the end of consolidation at the uniaxial compression test (Figure 1.6). The unconfined yield strength, σ_c, results from the stress circle which is tangential to the yield locus, and which runs through the origin (minor principal stress $\sigma_2 = 0$). This stress circle represents a similar stress state as the one which prevails in the second step of the uniaxial compression test. In contrast to the uniaxial compression test the unconfined yield strength, σ_c, has to be determined on the basis of yield locus and does not follow directly from the measurement. It may be noted that the analogy between the uniaxial compression test and the shear test is used here for the explanation of the yield locus. In reality, the stress circles at uniaxial compression and at steady state flow are not exactly the same, and a uniaxial compression test usually results in a smaller unconfined yield strength than a shear test[53]. A straight line through the origin of the σ,τ-diagram, tangent to the greater Mohr circle (steady-state flow), is the effective yield locus as defined by Jenike (broken line in Figure 1.6). It encloses the σ-axis with the angle φ_e (effective angle of internal friction). Because the largest Mohr stress circle indicates a state of steady-state flow, the angle φ_e can be regarded as 0, right).

A measure of the internal friction at steady-state flow. This angle is required for silo design according to Jenike's theory. If several yield loci are measured at different stress levels, that is, with different normal stresses at pre-shear, σ_{pre}, each yield locus represents another state of consolidation and another bulk density. The above-mentioned flow properties (unconfined yield strength, effective angle of internal friction) can be indicated as a function of the consolidation stress, σ_1, where bulk density and unconfined yield strength are plotted vs. the consolidation stress.

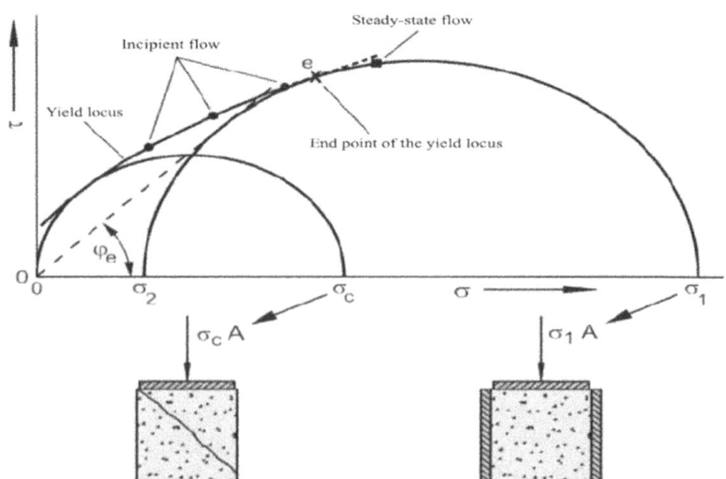

Fig.1.6 Yield locus, analogy to uniaxial compression test.

Time consolidation

Before time consolidation can be measured, a yield locus must be determined at the same consolidation stress. The time consolidation, which describes the increase of the unconfined yield strength with time during storage at rest, is measured with a shear tester similar to the measurement of a yield locus. First a bulk solid specimen is pre-sheared (consolidated). After pre-shear the specimen is stored for a period, t, under the vertically acting normal stress, σ, which is selected to be equal to the consolidation stress, σ1, of the corresponding yield locus. This ensures that during the consolidation period the same major principal stress = consolidation stress, σ_1 acts on the specimen as during steady-state flow at pre-shear.

After the time consolidation period t the specimen is sheared to failure. For this, a vertical normal load, σsh < σ1, is selected. As with shear without time consolidation (measurement of a point of a yield locus), so also after time consolidation will one observe a shear stress maximum. If consolidation time affects the bulk solid under consideration, after the consolidation period the shear stress maximum will be larger than it would have been without a consolidation period between pre-shear and shear.

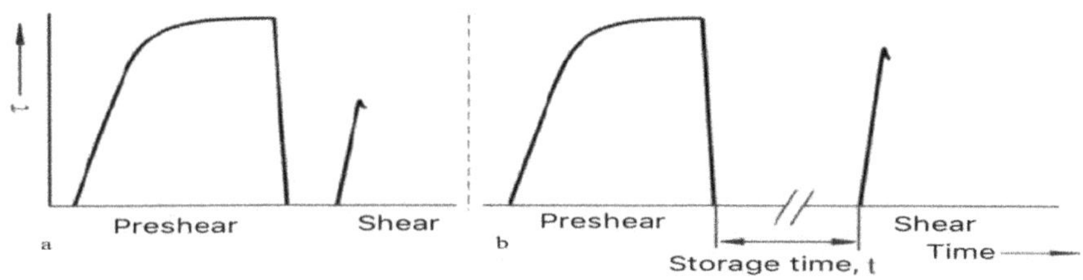

Fig.1.7 Shear stress vs. time at shear; with (a) and without (b) time consolidation.

The maximum shear stress, τ, is a point of a yield limit, which is valid for the applied storage period, t, and called a "time yield locus". Figure 1.7 shows a yield locus and two-time yield loci obtained for different consolidation periods, t_1 and t_2. The yield locus can also be regarded as a time yield locus for t = 0.

With the measured shear points, a time-yield locus can be approximated similarly to the approximation of a yield locus. Compared to the yield locus, the time yield locus is shifted towards greater shear stresses, τ (if the bulk solid shows an increase of strength with time). The unconfined yield strength, σc, is determined in the same way as for a yield locus by drawing a Mohr stress circle through the origin and tangent to the time yield locus. In Figure 1.7 the values of the unconfined yield strength for the consolidation periods, t_1 and t_2, are designated as $\sigma_c(t_1)$ and $\sigma_c(t_2)$. Time-yield loci can be determined for different storage periods (consolidation periods). Each time yield locus is valid for only one consolidation period and one consolidation stress. If the strength of the bulk solid increases over time, the time-yield loci will be shifted towards larger values of τ as the consolidation period, t, increases (Figure 1.7, $t_2 > t_1$).

Wall friction

Wall friction is the friction between a bulk solid and the surface of a solid, such as, the wall of a silo or a bin. The coefficient of wall friction or the wall friction angle is important for both silo design for flow and silo design for strength, but also for the design of chutes and other equipment, where the bulk solid will flow across a solid surface. Knowing the wall friction angle, it is possible to decide whether or not the polishing of the wall surface or the use of a liner would have advantages in the flow of the bulk solid. The principle of a wall friction test, where the kinematic angle of wall friction is determined, is shown in Figure 1.8. The bulk solid specimen is subjected to a vertical normal stress. The normal stress acting between bulk solid specimen and wall material is called the wall normal stress, σ_w.

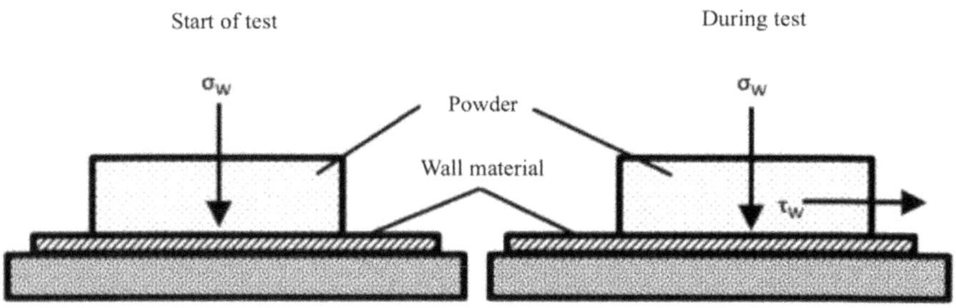

Fig.1.8 Principle of a wall friction test.

The bulk solid specimen is then shifted relative to the wall material surface with a constant velocity, v. This process is called shear (similar to the yield locus test). The shear stress acting between bulk solid specimen and wall material can be measured. It is usual to measure wall friction at incrementally decreasing wall normal stresses. Thus, one begins with the greatest wall normal stress, σ_{w1}. At the beginning of the shear process the wall shear stress, τ_w, increases. With time, the increase of the wall shear stress becomes less until finally a constant wall shear stress, τ_{w1}, is attained (steady-state shear stress). The constant wall shear stress, τ_{w1}, is characteristic for the applied wall normal stress, σ_{w1}. After the steady-state condition is attained, the normal load is reduced. With each decrease in wall normal stress, wall shear stress, τ_w, also decreases. After a certain time, a steady-state shear stress is again attained. In this way values of steady-state wall friction at several wall normal stresses are measured. The pair of values of wall normal stress and constant wall shear stress (σ_w, τ_w) describes the kinematic wall friction at the wall normal stress, σ_w, and is used for the evaluation of the test. All pairs of values of wall normal stress and steady-state wall shear stress are plotted in a σ_w, τ_w-diagram. The curve (or line) running through the measured points is called the wall yield locus.

The wall yield locus is a yield limit like the yield locus. The wall yield locus describes the wall shear stress, τ_w, necessary to shift a bulk solid continuously across a wall surface under a certain wall normal stress, σ_w. Since the wall yield locus is based on the shear stresses measured at steady-state conditions, it describes the kinematic friction of the bulk solid. Thus, the wall yield locus could more exactly be called a kinematic wall yield locus. To quantify wall friction, the wall friction angle, φ_x, or the coefficient of wall friction, μ, are used. The larger the wall friction angle or coefficient of wall friction, the greater is wall friction. The coefficient of wall friction, μ, is the ratio of wall shear stress, τ_w, to wall normal stress, σ_w. The wall friction angle, φx, is the slope of a line running through the origin of the σ_w, τ_w-diagram and a point of the wall yield locus. If the wall yield locus is a straight line running through the origin (Figure 1.9), the ratio of wall shear stress, τ_w, to wall normal stress, σ_w, has the same value for each point of the wall yield locus. Thus, one can obtain the identical wall friction coefficient, μ, and the identical wall friction angle, φ_x, for each point of the wall yield locus. In this case wall friction is independent of wall normal stress. The wall yield locus shown in Figure 1.9 is curved and does not run through the origin. In this case one finds a different wall friction coefficient and wall friction angle for each point of the wall yield locus. Thus, the wall friction coefficient and the wall friction angle are dependent on wall normal stress, σ_w. This can be seen by the wall friction angles, φ_{x1} and φ_{x2}, which follow for the wall normal stresses, σ_{w1} and σ_{w2}. A wall yield locus intersecting the τ-axis at $\tau_{ad} > 0$ is typical for materials tending to adhere at walls (e.g. like moist clay). The shear stress, τ_{ad}, at the point of intersection is called adhesion.

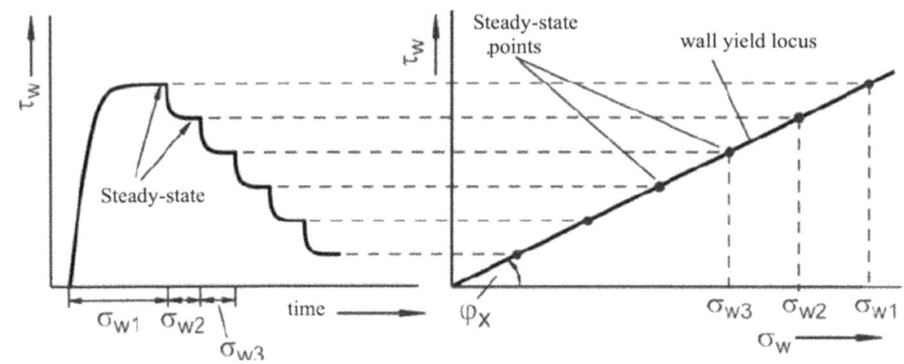

Fig.1.9 Course of wall shear stress in a wall friction test; wall yield locus.

Wall friction can be measured with the shear testers. The bottom ring of the shear cell is replaced by a sample of wall material (e.g. stainless steel, coated steel). The wall normal stress is then adjusted by the normal force, F_N, and the shear force, F_S, is measured following the procedure outlined above.

The setup of the wall friction shear cell of the Schulze ring shear tester. The annular bottom ring contains the sample of the wall material. On the top of the wall material sample is the bulk solid specimen, which is covered with the annular lid of the shear cell. The lid is connected to the crossbeam. Except for the geometry of bottom ring and lid, the setup is similar to the setup of the shear cell for flow properties testing. To measure wall friction the shear cell is rotated slowly in the direction of arrow ω, while the lid is prevented from rotating by the two tie rods. The forces acting on the tie rods, F_1 and F_2, are measured. The layer of bulk solid located between the lid and the surface of the wall material sample is prevented from rotating by the lid, which has a rough underside. Thus, the bulk solid is shifted across the surface of the wall material sample while it is subjected to the normal stress, σ_W. The wall shear stress, τw, is calculated from the F_1 and F_2.

STRUCTURE MODIFICATION

During the design of all mechanical structures, it is necessary to fulfil certain mechanical criteria. Any modification made onto a structure has an effect of changing the structural properties, such as, resonant frequencies, mode shapes and deformation distribution. When an aircraft is modified by attaching external payload to it, the dynamic behaviour of the aircraft changes. This change can be critical as it may cause serious vibration problems; hence, dynamic behaviour of the modified aircraft has to be predicted in the design stage. Molecular modification by nature has been going on since the beginning of life on this planet. In the relatively short time since chemistry has developed into a science, the chemists had learned well from nature the significance of small changes in chemical structures of drugs to the biological activity in living organisms. For example, opium, the sun-dried latex of the unripe fruit of *Papaver somniferum*, cultivated from early times for this drug, contains at least 23 alkaloids. Of the major alkaloids three—morphine, codeine, and thebaine—contain the morphinan ring system. Morphine for more than a century has been the most important agent for the relief of pain. Codeine, with its phenolic hydroxyl group protected by methyl, has about one tenth the analgesic activity of morphine. But as such has found its place in the relief of mild pain and as an antitussive agent. Thebaine differs from codeine by the addition of methylene groups and the removal of two hydrogen atoms, is neither an analgesic nor an antitussive. Instead, it resembles strychnine and brucine in its spinal convulsant properties. It is not used in medicine; it has utility, however, in the synthesis of codeinone derivatives, some of which are useful as analgesics. The chemist has identified the morphine-analgesic pattern and has gone far beyond nature in his quest for an analgesic with the powcr of morphine but without its liabilities.

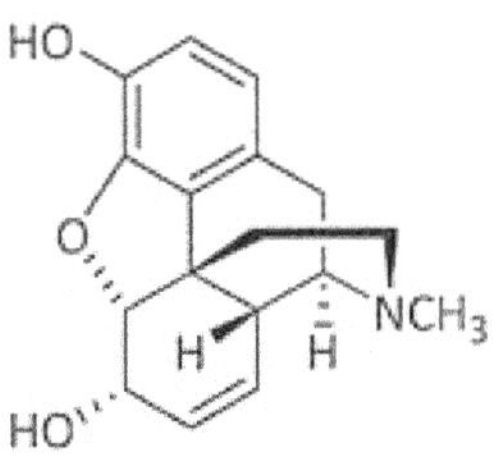

morphine

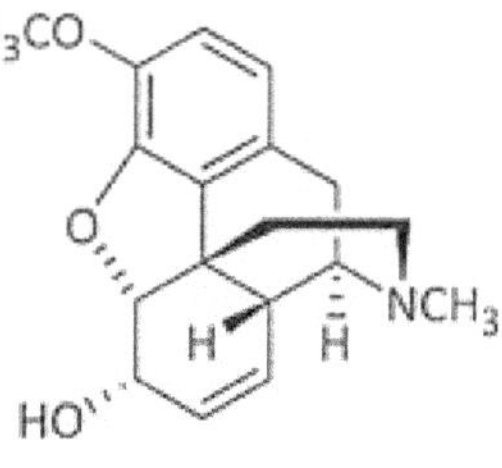

codeine

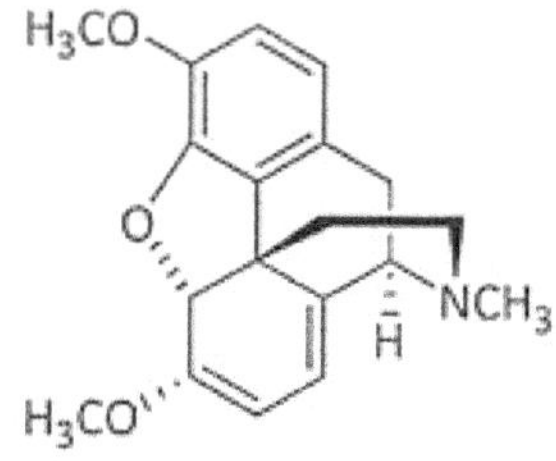

thebaine

The chemical structure affects the physicochemical properties of a molecule which in turn affects its drug-like properties. In a structural modification problem, the additional dynamic stiffness matrix due to structural modification is given by

$$[\Delta A] = [D] - [D_0] \qquad .....(1.1)$$

Where, [D] and [D_0] are the dynamic stiffness matrices of the modified and original structures, respectively. For lumped modifications [ΔD] corresponds directly to dynamic stiffness matrix of the modifying structure. For distributed modifications, it is calculated by using Eq. (1) which may not correspond to the dynamic stiffness matrix of the modifying structure. When the size of the bounded region which covers the modifying area is larger, the error introduced to [ΔD] will be smaller. In order to avoid such errors, a different approach for the application of the structural modification technique is used. If distributed modification is applied to an original structure in such a way that additional (degree of freedom) DOF is introduced, then it is not necessary to use Eq. (1) to calculate the additional dynamic stiffness matrix due to structural modification, as the problem will be a structural coupling problem. In that case, the additional dynamic stiffness matrix due to structural modification will be equal to the dynamic stiffness matrix of the modifying structure which can directly be used in the structural modification method.

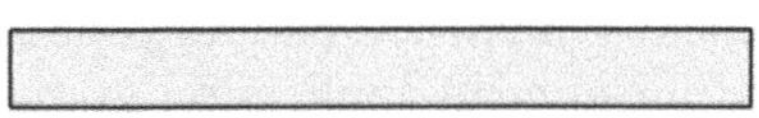

Fig.1.10 Original beam.

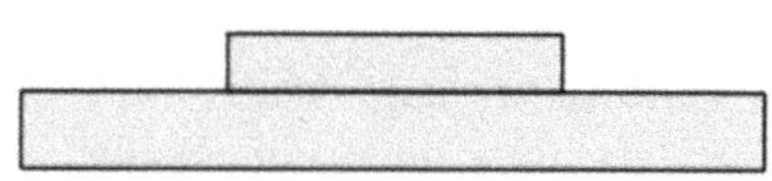

Fig.1.11 Modified beam.

For example, the dynamic stiffness matrices of the original and modifying structures for the modified beam in Figure 1.10 are given by

$$[D_0] = [K_0] - \omega^2[M_0] + i[H_0]$$

$$[D_{mod}] = [K_{mod}] - \omega^2[M_{mod}] + i[H_{mod}]$$

Where, [K_0], [M_0] and [H_0] are the stiffness mass and structural damping matrices of the original structure,

[K_{mod}], [M_{mod}] and [H_{mod}] are stiffness, mass and structural damping matrices of the structure

They all can be obtained directly from the (Finite Element model) FE models of the original and modifying beams. When additional DOF is introduced to the original structure, the dynamic stiffness matrix of the modified structure can be obtained by assembling the dynamic stiffness matrices of the original and modifying structures. Similarly, for distributed modifications, if additional DOF is introduced to the original structure, there is no need to use Eq. (1); instead, additional dynamic stiffness matrix due to structural modification can directly be obtained.

Historically, natural substances had been used as the main sources of medicine to treat a wide spectrum of human diseases. Although the total number of new chemical entities launched has declined in recent years, structurally diverse natural products (NPs) continue to be used as leads or main sources for novel drug discovery. Among the 112 drugs have been approved by the Food and Drug Administration (FDA) between 1999 and 2013, out of which 31 drugs (28%) were developed based on natural pharmacophores. Although NPs have a proven track record in drug discovery and uncontested unique structural diversity, there are still several problems associated with NPs. Typical restrictions for the development of novel drugs from NPs include their,

* Low solubility,
* Metabolic instability, and
* Unknown exact mechanisms of action,

which especially hamper the development of similar drugs. Additionally, many NPs are often structurally complex, and their 'heavy 'structures break Lipinski's rules and most likely will limit their absorption from the gut into the blood, thus impeding oral formulation[54]. Furthermore, the intellectual property situation is often ambiguous for unmodified NPs. Therefore, it is highly desirable to develop NPs through structural modification to achieve the final candidate drug. Many NPs and synthetically modified natural product derivatives have been successfully developed for clinical application to treat human diseases in almost all therapeutic areas. These involved well-known drugs such as penicillin (antibacterial), morphine (analgesic), artemisinin (antimalarial), paclitaxel (anticancer), etc. These efforts demonstrate that, despite many limitations of NPs, with reasonable modifications, sometimes even alteration of a single atom, may result in the discovery of a novel drug. For example, a change in the logP of NPs may increase their potency and efficacy against drug resistance cells. Removing unnecessary groups of NPs can truncate them to be analogues with more simple structure. On the other hand, introduction of water-soluble groups would help to improve the water solubility of NPs.

- NPs are vital sources of drug discovery; their various deficiencies or shortcomings limit their wide applications in drug development, and thus, structural modification of NPs is in urgent necessity to develop the novel entities with specific properties.
- Major changes may be required for the structural modification of NPs, but commonly they require fine tuning. In somecases, a single alteration can make a great difference.
- NPs embody inherent structural complexity and biological activity, and modification of NPs is a versatile approach to explore their mode of actions.
- Making logical and systematic changes to NPs is an effective way to increase their potency and activity spectrum and therefore counter resistance mechanisms.
- Biologically active NPs often have privileged scaffolds and diverse biological activities; sometimes, with proper modifications, they could be used for new treatments.
- Complex NPs often suffer from high molecular weights and poor oral bioavailability. Structural modification may provide structurally simpler compounds that retain bio-activities.
- Structural modifications that reduce the compound's binding affinity or reactivity at the labile site may increase metabolic stability.
- Low aqueous solubility is a common problem in developing NPs into drugs, but chemical modification is a powerful strategy that could be applied to enhance the water solubility of NPs.
- Because of their unique chemical properties and potential interactions with disease-associated proteins, natural products will remain a reliable source of lead compounds in drug discovery.

DRUG-EXCIPIENT COMPATIBILITY STUDIES

Drug-excipient incompatibility means that the drug is inactivated through either decomposition or loss of drug by its conversion to a drug-loss by its conversion to a less favourable physical or chemical form. It can affect the safety, therapeutic efficacy, appearance or elegance. When two or more drugs and/or excipients are mixed and if they are antagonistic and affect adversely the safety, therapeutic efficacy, appearance or elegance then they are called incompatible.

Importance of drug-excipient incompatibility study

Stability of a dosage form can be maximised. Any change in physical or chemical interaction between drug and excipient can affect the bioavailability of the drug. It can help to avoid the surprise problems. If the drug-excipient incompatibility test is performed, the possible reaction before formulating the final dosage form can be known. Drug discovery can bring only new chemical entity. After formulation and processing with suitable excipients, it becomes the drug product. With the help of drug-excipient compatibility study, suitable type of excipients can be selected. Drug-excipient compatibility study data is necessary for submission of investigational new drug to drug regulatory agency. Now it has become compulsory to submit these data to get approval of USFDA for any new formulation. To prepare a list of excipients that can be used to formulate any dosage forms, one would not consider using sucrose or lactose. If the drug substance under consideration is a primary amine. This system has the scope for interaction to form a coloured compound, this can be readily detected by a change in colour.

Types of incompatibility

There are three types of incompatibility between drug and excipient, such as:

1. ***Physical incompatibility:*** It involves the change in the physical state of the formulation, which means the change in colour, liquefaction, phase separation or immiscibility.
2. ***Chemical incompatibility:*** It involves undesirable change in formulation which is due to formation of new chemical compound with undesirable activity or our formulation undergoes hydrolysis, oxidation, reduction, precipitation, decarboxylation, racemizatoon.
3. ***Therapeutic incompatibility:*** It is one type of *in vivo* compatibility. This involves change in therapeutic response of the formulation which is undesirable to patient as well as physician.

Reasons for compatibility study

1. Identification of compatible excipients for a formulation.
2. Identification of stable storage conditions for drug in solid or liquid state.

Solid state reaction

Solid state reactions are much slower and more difficult to be interpreted than solution state reactions. Because there are reduced number of molecular contacts between the drug and excipient molecules and multiple phase reactions occur. Preformulation is the first step in the rational formulation of drug substance (API). It is an investigation on the physicochemical properties of the drug substance alone and also in combination with excipients. Investigation of the possible incompatibilities between the drug and various excipients is an important part of the preformulation. Sometimes, the formulation of a drug substance involves it after blending with different excipients to manufacture easily and administer the dose of a drug effectively. Excipients are known to

* Facilitate the administration, and
* Modulate the release of the active component, drug.

The excipients are used to stabilise the drug-product against degradation from the environment.

* Most of the excipients do not have any pharmacological action.
* They are used to exert some useful properties to the formulation.
* They can also give rise to inadvertent and/or unintended effects such as an increased degradation of the drug.

The physical and chemical interactions between the drugs and excipients can affect the chemical nature, the stability and bioavailability of the drug products, consequently their therapeutic efficacy and safety. Thus, the drug-excipient compatibility study plays an important role in identifying the possible duration of interaction between the excipients used in the formulation and the drug concerned. Commonly, for detection of physical-chemical investigation and detecting the possible interaction, the thermal analysis such as DSC, DTA, DTG, ITC, spectroscopic methods such as FT-IR, X-ray diffraction, NMR, and chromatographic methods such as LC, LC-MS/MS, dissolution tests etc., are performed. The most sensitive and appropriate methods for detection of possible interaction is thermal analysis. However, the method can be unspecific, and the results are difficult to interpret. Sometimes, the results are found to be false positive or false negative, and thus, difficult to be interpreted.

Differential Scanning Colorimetry (DSC) has been currently used in this area. The major advantage of DSC is its ability to quickly screen the potential excipients for incompatibilities derived from the appearance, shifts or disappearance of peaks and/or variations in the corresponding ΔH (enthalpy of transition). Other characteristics of this method is that the sample required is low. Although DSC is a valuable technique, the interpretation of the data is not straightforward. In this method, the sample is exposed to high temperature, up to 300°C or more. This high temperature is not experienced by the dosage form. Therefore, DSC results should be interpreted very carefully.

From this point of view, the IR spectroscopic methods are relatively less sensitive. This method is complementary for the thermal-analytical techniques, particularly due to detection of the atom groups involved in the excipient/API interaction and these allow the quantitative estimation of these interactions. The aim of study was to analyse by DSC and IR studies the compatibility of some excipients with potential use in binary or ternary mixtures, as vehicles for the preparation of mucoadhesive systems with antimicrobial (MZ, CD) or anti-inflammatory drug substances (IB).

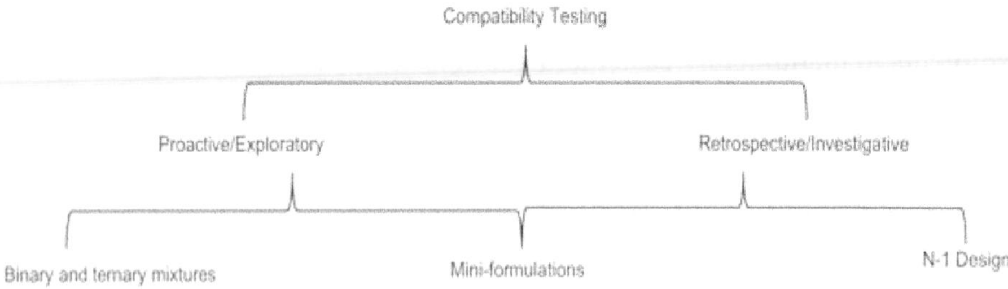

a

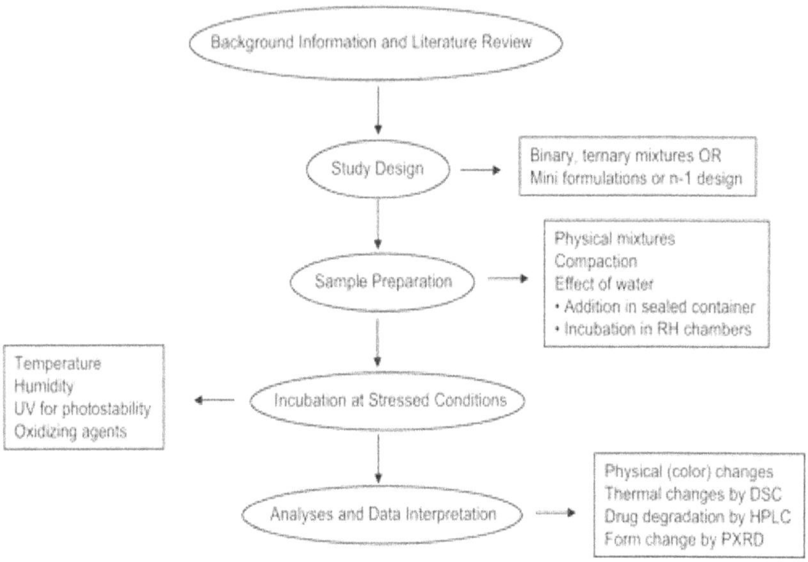

b

METHODS OF DETERMINATION OF DRUG-EXCIPIENT COMPATIBILITY

The drug-excipient compatibility studies are carried out for the purpose of identifying, quantifying and prediction of potential interactions (physical or chemical). Moreover, these impact of these interactions on the manufacturability, quality and performance of the final drug product. On the basis of previous knowledge about the physico-chemical properties and about the degradation mechanisms of the drugs and the excipients, these studies are finalised. In addition to evaluation of the direct interactions between the API and the excipients, the influence of factors such as water (moisture) and temperature is also explored in these studies. These factors are known to accelerate the possibility, and the extent of drug-excipient interactions either by altering the physico-chemical properties or rate of degradation of the drugs and/or excipients. These studies generally involve bringing the API and the excipient/s into intimate contact with each either as physical admixtures in a predetermined ratio, or as a preliminary dosage form; and subjecting them to various stress conditions. The physico-chemical and performance attributes of the API and the excipients are then evaluated using one or more analytical techniques.

The evaluation of drug-excipient compatibility includes a broad range of thermal and non-thermal analytical techniques. These techniques are diverse with respect to their-

* Principles of operation,
* Sample size,
* Duration of analysis,
* The type of stress i.e. thermal, mechanical etc.

Moreover, due to the wide variation in the chemical and physical nature of drugs and the excipients, and the complex nature of their interactions, there is a lack of universal standards in the methodology used in the evaluation of compatibility between the API and the excipients.

There has been a significant increase in the number of individual studies reporting the use of one or more methods for screening the API-excipient compatibility. The commonly reported methods include, thermo-analytical techniques such as differential scanning calorimetry (DSC), thermo-gravimetric analysis (TGA), differential thermal analysis (DTA), isothermal microcalorimetry (ITC), hot stage microscopy and non-thermal techniques such as x-ray diffraction (XRD), fourier transform infrared spectroscopy (FTIR), scanning electron microscopy (SEM), high performance liquid chromatography (HPLC), near infrared spectroscopy (NIR) and solid state nuclear magnetic resonance spectroscopy (ssNMR)[55]. Applications of these techniques as drug-excipient compatibility screening tools, along with their advantages and drawbacks are briefly discussed below.

Thermal techniques

Differential scanning calorimetry

Differential scanning calorimetry (DSC) is the most common thermal technique used for testing the excipient incompatibilities. This technique usually requires a small size of sample, and the results are obtained relatively rapidly. The thermogravimetry/derivative thermogravimetry (TG/DTG) and DSC techniques are used to evaluate the compatibility between ketoprofen and several excipients including corn starch, microcrystalline cellulose, colloidal silicon dioxide, lactose, PVP K30, magnesium stearate and talcum. The results of the study demonstrated that DSC helps us to ascertain any incompatibilities in the formulation components. These may include the changes in appearance, in endothermic or exothermic peaks, or in enthalpy curves. In a similar study, it has been evaluated the compatibility of the acetylsalicylic acid, a non-steroidal anti-inflammatory drug, with pharmaceutical excipients of common use such as diluents, binders, disintegrants, lubricants and solubilising agents. The results confirmed the utility of DSC as a sensitive and a specific technique in assessing the drug-excipient compatibility. Although DSC is frequently used due to its inexpensive and eco-friendly nature, it is important to understand that it may not provide accurate results in every situation. For example, amorphous API are known to reduce the enthalpy of fusion of the API. DSC often involves exposing the formulations to temperatures that may degrade excipients (as high as 300°C) and are physiologically unrealistic. As a result, DSC may sometimes be misleading and is often used in combinations with other techniques to ensure accuracy. This technique, however, can be used in combination with SEM to search for physical incompatibilities within a formulation.

Thermogravimetric analysis

Thermal testing improves the thermogravimetric analysis (TGA). This test, and the DSC, examines the mass of formulation lost as a percentage with increasing temperature. Additionally, thermogravimetry and derivative thermogravimetry can determine the reactivity of each excipient with the API or with each other. The TGA is used, in addition to the DSC to check the compatibility of acetylsalicylic acid with 11 other excipients. The thermogravimetric analysis, derivative of thermogravimetric analysis, and DSC revealed that all excipients, aside from polyvinyl pyrrolidone (PVP) and magnesium stearate, have been compatible with acetylsalicylic acid. In another study, the compatibility of ketoprofen with similar, commonly used excipients using DSC, TGA, DTGA, PXRD and FTIR is assessed. The TGA results along with other techniques revealed a possible interaction between the ketoprofen and PVP K30, and between ketoprofen and magnesium stearate. In a study on the compatibilities between excipients and sildenafil citrate has been conducted, the DSC and TG curves showed that after heating to a range of 190 - 229.5°C, 28.8% of citric acid was evaporated. What remained was the sildenafil base that later decomposed at higher temperatures. The TG curves in this analysis helped to understand each temperature range at which excipients would be lost.

Isothermal microcalorimetry

Isothermal microcalorimetry (IMC), or isothermal stress testing, is another method that helps the determination of the integrity of the pharmaceutical formulations. The test involves storing the excipients for three to four weeks, with or without moisture, at temperatures above 50°C. This process simulates drug ageing and stimulates excipient interactions. The test has the capacity to determine compatibilities but is limited by its time-consuming and arduous nature. After a predetermined storage period, the contents of the formulation are analysed using methods such as HPLC and DSC. IMC is used in combination with DSC to understand the compatibilities between promethazine HCl and lactose monohydrate, and zinc stearate. It has been found that after three months of storage of IMC, at accelerated stability conditions, the tablet formulation had an acceptable level of reactivity and was thermally stable. This test not only helped with determining incompatibilities, but also offset the misleading results commonly associated with DSC.

Hot stage microscopy

Methods involving microscopy are used to study the drug formulation morphology and to identify any physical incompatibilities associated with the excipients. A study has been conducted to evaluate the compatibility of ibuproxam and excipients using DSC. Hot-stage microscopy (HSM) has been used as an adjunct to DSC. The process required only a small amount of sample, and the microscopy results confirmed that the incompatibilities found in the DSC analysis was due in part by the dissolution of excipient at an elevated temperature. In a different study, conducted by Aigner et al, HSM has been used to find the thermal behaviour of aceclofenac[56]. DSC revealed one sharp endothermic peak at 153.1°C. Magnesium Stearate, an excipient used in this formulation, showed three endothermic peaks on the DSC analysis at 89.2°C, 104.5°C, and 203.5°C. The HSM analysis showed that the magnesium stearate melted first and subsequently dissolved the aceclofenac. HSM thus essentially explained the disappearance of aceclofenac and the peak associated with magnesium stearate on the DSC. It is thus advisable that when developing formulations, both DSC and HSM be used in conjunction to ensure accuracy and compatibility of drug excipients.

Non-thermal Techniques

Infrared, near Infrared and Raman Spectroscopy

Infrared (IR), near-infrared (NIR) and Raman spectroscopy are the most commonly used non-thermal techniques for the screening of drug-excipient compatibility. These techniques provide a unique fingerprint to the API and the excipients based on their physical and chemical properties. Due to the highly sensitive nature of these techniques, any little deviations in the physico-chemical properties of the API as a result of the interactions with the excipients are readily detected. Commonly observed physico-chemical changes due to drug-excipient interactions include polymorph transitions, dehydration, formation of hydrates/solvates, changes in the deformation behaviour of powders etc. Some of the common advantages of these techniques include rapid analysis, quick and easy detection of incompatibilities due to spectral shifts and the detection of interaction by-products. The compatibility of aceclofenac with various tableting excipients such as Carbopol 940, hydroxypropyl methylcellulose, microcrystalline cellulose, Aerosil 200 and magnesium stearate were investigated by Aigner et al. using DSC and FT-IR. The study results showed the occurrence of interaction between aceclofenac and magnesium stearate resulting in the formation of magnesium salt of aceclofenac. The other excipients were found to be compatible with the drug i.e. no significant interaction was observed between aceclofenac and other excipients studied. Similarly, Pani et al. assessed the compatibility of nateglinide with various excipients in the development of immediate release tablets of nateglinide using DSC, IR and IST. The IR results revealed the absence of any significant incompatibilities between the API and the tested excipients. Blanco et al. evaluated the polymorphic transition in Dexketoprofen Trometamol (DKP) production samples obtained by direct compression and wet granulation using Multivariate Curve Resolution - Alternating Least Squares (MCR–ALS) methodology to obtain the NIR spectra for samples without pretreatment. The results showed that significant polymorphic transition occurred in DKP during wet granulation; whereas no changes were observed with samples processed via direct compression. Dave et al. investigated the influence of plasticiser (triethyl citrate, TEC) level on the breaking force of extended-release matrix tablets prepared by roller-compaction. The multivariate analysis of the results demonstrated the feasibility of NIR spectroscopy in evaluating the influence of TEC levels on the breaking force of prepared tablets. Kogermann et al. explored the dehydration of piroxicam monohydrate in compacts using terahertz pulsed spectroscopy (TPS), Raman spectroscopy, and reflectance near-infrared (NIR) spectroscopy[57]. The study results concluded that the Raman and NIR spectroscopy were suitable for monitoring the loss of moisture along with the structural changes that occurred during the dehydration of samples.

Powder X-ray Diffraction

In the preformulation stage of the drug development process, powder x-ray diffraction (PXRD) is used to characterise the crystalline nature of materials. PXRD is a widely used polymorph screening technique for the API. Each crystalline material exhibits a unique x-ray diffraction pattern, as displayed by the peak intensities against a range of diffraction angles (2θ). Any interactions between the API and excipients that results in a change in the crystalline form of the API is generally exhibited as a shift, appearance or disappearance of these peak intensities. Thus, PXRD analysis can provide useful information regarding the influence of drug-excipient interactions on the polymorphic changes in the API. PXRD analysis may also be useful in the evaluation of API polymorphic transitions occurring as under the influence of moisture and temperature changes during processing, albeit only in the absence of interference from any excipient peaks. Tita et al. assessed the compatibility between ketoprofen and several excipients such as corn starch, microcrystalline cellulose, colloidal silicon dioxide, lactose, polyvinyl pyrrolidone K30, magnesium stearate and talc using DSC, TGA, FTIR and

PXRD. The PXRD data confirmed the DSC and TGA results indicating a possible interaction between the KT with polyvinyl pyrrolidone K30 and magnesium stearate, as demonstrated by the changes in the intensity of peaks as well as disappearance of certain peaks observed in the spectra of individual components. In a similar study, Tita et al. evaluated the compatibility of the acetylsalicylic acid (ASA) with pharmaceutical excipients including diluents, binders, disintegrants, lubricants and solubilising agents using DSC, TGA, FTIR and PXRD. The x-ray analysis results confirmed a possible chemical interaction between the ASA with polyvinyl pyrrolidone K30 and magnesium stearate, and a possible physical interaction with colloidal silicon dioxide and stearic acid. In another study, Roumelli et al. demonstrated the compatibility of trandalopril with α-lactose monohydrate, microcrystalline cellulose, and pre-gelatinised starch using PXRD analysis of the physical mixtures of the drug with the selected excipients.

Solid-state Nuclear Magnetic Resonance Spectroscopy

Solid-state nuclear magnetic resonance (ssNMR) spectroscopy has emerged as a common analytical tool for the analysis of drug-excipient interactions in recent years. This technique identifies the interactions between the API and the excipients through variations in the chemical shift occurring as a result of change in the electron density around the interaction sites. Some of the known advantages of this technique include higher selectivity, limited interference from excipients and the ability to detect polymorphic transitions in the API. In addition, the presence and influence of water on the drug-excipient interactions are easily detected by this method. The main drawback of this technique is the duration of analysis, which often can be lengthy and complex. Chen et al. investigated the acid–base reactions of solid materials, a common type of drug–excipient interaction using binary mixtures (1:1) of pure α-form indomethacin and sodium bicarbonate as model drug and excipient respectively. The ssNMR results, along with those obtained from PXRD analysis confirmed the transformation of the mixtures into the micro-crystals of sodium indomethacin trihydrate, indicating the presence of drug-excipient interaction. In another study, Skotnicki et al. evaluated the compatibility of bisoprolol fumarate with amorphous valsartan using DSC, TMDSC, ssNMR and PXRD. The study results indicated a strong interaction between bisoprolol fumarate and valsartan above 60°C[58]. The ssNMR data provided the information on the incompatibility at a molecular level. Schachter et al. characterised the nature of interaction between ketoprofen and polyethylene oxide (PEO) in a solid dispersion formulation using ssNMR along with other analytical techniques. The 13C single pulse/magic angle spinning NMR indicated the presence of hydrogen bonds between the carboxylic group of ketoprofen and the ether oxygen of PEO, indicating a drug-excipient interaction.

Microscopic Techniques

Scanning Electron Microscopy

The interactions between the API and the excipients often result in polymorphic transitions and changes in crystal habits of the API. Scanning electron microscopy (SEM) provides useful information on such changes by characterizing the surface morphology of pharmaceutical APIs. Although SEM may not independently provide information on the nature of drug-excipient interaction at a molecular level for example, chemical and thermal transitions; combining SEM with other analytical techniques such as DSC/TGA, HSM, and other thermal techniques can significantly benefit to the overall characterisation of the incompatibilities. Mura et al. assessed the compatibility of ibuproxam with commonly used excipients such as corn starch, Avicel, sodium carboxymethyl cellulose, polyethylene glycol 4000 (PEG-4000), palmitic acid, stearic acid, Ca- and Mg-stearate, polyvinyl polypyrrolidone (PVPP) and polyvinyl pyrrolidone K30 (PVP K30). The results obtained from the SEM analysis were in general, in agreement with and confirmatory to those obtained from DSC and HSM.

Chromatographic Techniques

High Performance Liquid Chromatography

High performance liquid chromatography (HPLC) is the most widely used analytical technique for determining the API content in a formulation. This technique can be very useful in situations where the drug-excipient interaction may lead to a quantitative change in the API. In drug-excipient compatibility studies, the formulations or the drug-excipient mixtures are subjected to high temperatures for a predetermined period of time i.e. isothermal stress testing (IST) to accelerate any chemical incompatibilities. This is followed by determination of drug content using HPLC analysis, thus identifying any quantitative loss of drug as a result of interactions with the excipients. Gu et al. screened the compatibility of moexipril HCl, an angiotensin-converting enzyme (ACE) inhibitor, with commonly used filters, disintegrants, lubricants, glidants, and coating agents using IST along with HPLC. The HPLC results confirmed the presence of interactions between the drug and the excipient. The results also indicated that neutralization of the acidic drug by the basic excipients suppressed drug degradation. In another study, Julio et al. evaluated the compatibility of sildenafil citrate with colloidal silicon dioxide, cross-carmellose sodium, lactose, mannitol and sucrose using DSC, HSM and HPLC. The accelerated stability studies results showed the presence of incompatibilities between the drug and the selected excipients. However, it was also observed that some incompatibilities detected by HPLC, were not detected by DSC and vice-versa. The study demonstrated the benefits of complementing the thermal techniques with HPLC in detecting incompatibilities and providing more robust and accurate approaches for preformulation studies. Along with the commonly recognised advantages of HPLC such as accuracy and robustness, the main drawback of the technique is that this technique is time consuming and complex. To evaluate the drug-excipient compatibility, this is a very useful supportive tool in preformulation studies.

Liquid State Incompatibility Reaction

The reactions occur in the liquid state are easier to detect as compared to solid state reactions. For detection of unknown reactions responsible for incompatibility of two liquids, the program set up is similar to as in case of solid dosage forms. According to the stability guidelines decided by FDA, following conditions are to be evaluated in solution/ suspension preparations of the bulk drug substances:

Acidic or alkaline pH

Presence of added substances, such as, chelating agents, stabilisers, etc.

Effect of stress testing conditions............

High Oxygen and Nitrogen atmospheres.

Procedures to be followed are:

Place the drug in solution of additives,

Both flint and amber vials are used,

In many cases, autoclaved samples are examined. This will provide following information:

Susceptibility to oxygen,

Susceptibility to light (exposed),

Susceptibility to heavy metals

In case of oral liquids, compatibility with ethanol, glycerin, sucrose, preservatives, buffering agents, colouring agents, flavouring agents etc. are carried out.

Exercise

Multiple Choice Questions

1. The physical or chemical stability and the morphology of the drug product depend mainly on ....
   a) The selection of an appropriate polymorph,
   b) Appropriate granulation method
   c) The selection of an appropriate cocrystal of excipient
   d) None of the above

2. The pharmaceutical industry is developing new molecules with different modalities, such as, ...
   a) Macrocycles, b) Peptides,
   c) All of the above d) None of the above

3. Co-processed API can be defined as *a* drug substance, manufactured in a drug manufacturing facility, that contains the API in addition to one or more covalently bonded...........
   a) Active component
   b) Non-active component,
   c) Binder
   d) Disintegrant

4. When equilibrium attains between a crystalline phase and its surroundings, the statistical amount of growth units exchanged between the two phases is ....
   a) Sometimes not same
   b) Sometimes same
   c) Not same and change with time
   d) The same and does not change with time.

5. When equilibrium attains between a crystalline phase and its surroundings, the statistical amount of growth units exchanged between the two phases remains ....
   a) Same and does not change with time.
   b) Different and that changes with time.
   c) Same but changes with time.
   d) None of the above

6. Which of the following statement is correct?
   a) The crystal structure, on which the surface structures (i.e., the profiles) of the faces depend, these crystal defects are caused by external factors.
   b) The supersaturation, nature of solvent, solution composition, impurities, physical conditions (temperature, solution flow, electric and magnetic field, microgravity, ultrasound, etc.) are the internal factors.
   c) The supersaturation, nature of solvent, solution composition, impurities, physical conditions (temperature, solution flow, electric and magnetic field, microgravity, ultrasound, etc.) are the external factors.
   d) The supersaturation, nature of solvent, solution composition, impurities, physical conditions (temperature, solution flow, electric and magnetic field, microgravity, ultrasound, etc.) are the mixed factors.
7. Kinetic roughening of the crystals occurs...........
   a) Above the roughening temperature when supersaturation exceeds the d critical value.
   b) Below the roughening temperature when supersaturation does not exceed the critical value
   c) Above the roughening temperature when supersaturation does not exceed the critical value.
   d) Below the roughening temperature when supersaturation exceeds the critical value
8. The flow properties of solid depend on several parameters, such as........
   a) Particle size distribution,
   b) Moisture
   c) All of the above
   d) None of the above
9. For shear to failure the normal stress acting on the specimen is decreased to a value σ_{sh}, which is ....
   a) More than the normal stress at pre-shear, σ_{pre}.
   b) Less than the normal stress at pre-shear, σ_{pre}.
   c) Less than the shear stress, τ,
   d) Less than the normal principal stress σ_1

10. If several yield loci are measured at different stress levels, that is, with different normal stresses at pre-shear, σ_{pre}, ...
    a) Each yield locus represents another state of consolidation and another bulk density.
    b) Each yield locus represents same state of consolidation and same bulk density.
    c) Each yield locus represents same state of consolidation and another bulk density.
    d) Each yield locus represents another state of consolidation and same bulk density.

11. When an aircraft is modified by attaching external payload to it,.....................
    a) The dynamic behaviour of the aircraft does not change.
    b) The behaviour of the aircraft changes.
    c) The behaviour of the aircraft does not change.
    d) The dynamic behaviour of the aircraft changes.

12. In a structural modification problem the additional dynamic stiffness matrix due to structural modification is given by..........
    a) $[\Delta A] = [D] - [D_0]$
    b) $[D] = [\Delta A] + [D_0]$
    c) $[\Delta A] = [K_0] - [D_0]$
    d) $[\Delta A] = [D] - [H_0]$

    where, $[D]$ and $[D_0]$ are the dynamic stiffness matrices of the modified and original structures, respectively, $[\Delta D]$ is the dynamic stiffness matrix of the modifying structure, $[K_0]$ is the stiffness mass of the original structure, and $[H_0]$ is the structural damping matrices of the original structure.

13. Making logical and systematic changes to NPs is ....
    a) An effective way to decrease their potency and activity spectrum and therefore counter resistance mechanisms.
    b) An effective way to increase their potency and activity spectrum and therefore counter resistance mechanisms.
    c) An ineffective way to decrease their potency and activity spectrum and therefore counter resistance mechanisms.
    d) An ineffective way to increase their potency and activity spectrum and therefore counter resistance mechanisms.

14. Drug-excipient incompatibility can affect ....
    a) The safety, and therapeutic effect.

b) The safety, and appearance.
c) The therapeutic efficacy, appearance, or elegance
d) The safety, therapeutic efficacy, appearance, or elegance

15. The techniques for evaluation of drug-excipient compatibility are diverse with respect to their…
a) The type of stress,
b) Duration of analysis,
c) All of the above
d) None of the above

16. The commonly reported methods include thermo-analytical techniques such as……….
a) Differential scanning calorimetry, isothermal microcalorimetry,
b) Thermogravimetric analysis, differential thermal analysis, hot stage microscopy
c) All the above
d) None of the above

17. Which of the following states DSC?
a) Differential scanning calorimetry
b) Differential scanning colorimetry
c) Diffusional scanning calorimetry
d) Diffusional scanning colorimetry

18. IMC stands for…………..
a) Internal Microcalorimetry
b) Isothermal Microcalorimetry
c) Isothermal Micro colorimetry
d) Industrial Microcalorimetry

19. Mark the following statement true or false
a) Methods involving microscopy are used to study the drug formulation morphology and to identify any physical incompatibilities associated with the excipients.
b) True
c) False

20. Mark the following statement true or false
a) The drug-excipient compatibility studies are carried out for the purpose of identifying, quantifying and prediction of potential interactions (physical or chemical).
b) False
c) True

Short Questions

1. What is molecular optimization? Write down the commercial applications of co-processing of APIs.
2. What is crystal habit? What are the factors that can influence the crystal habit?
3. Write down the procedures used to study the change in crystal habit.
4. Explain the uniaxial compression test.
5. What is meant by Time consolidation (caking)?
6. What is the importance of drug-excipient compatibility study?
7. Name the methods used for study of drug-excipient incompatibility study.
8. Discuss the thermogravimetric analysis.
9. Discuss the isothermal microcalorimetry.
10. Write a note on hot state microscopy.

Long Questions

1. What is meant by the term molecular optimization, write in brief.
2. Write down in short, the various aspects of crystal morphology.
3. What do you know about polar crystals and kinetic roughening?
4. Describe the flow properties of a powder or a bulk solid.
5. How does introduction of water-soluble groups would help to improve the water solubility of NPs.?
6. Explain the term, 'solid state reaction'.
7. Describe the methods of isothermal calorimetry and hot stage microscopy.
8. What are the non-thermal methods used for drug-excipient incompatibility test. Discuss the method of scanning electron microscopy.
9. What is chromagraphic method such as High performance liquid chromatography?
10. What do you know about Solid-state nuclear magnetic resonance spectroscopy? What for this method is used?

Answers

1	2	3	4	5	6	7	8	9	10	11	12	13	14	15	16	17	18	19	20
a	c	b	d	a	c	d	c	b	a	d	a	b	d	c	d	a	b	b	c

References

1. Lee, S. L.; O'Connor, T. F.; Yang, X.; Cruz, C. N.; Chatterjee, S.; Madurawe, R. D.; Moore, C. M. V.; Xu, L. X.; Woodcock, J. Modernizing Pharmaceutical Manufacturing: from Batch to Continuous Production. Journal of Pharmaceutical Innovation 2015, 10, (3), 191-199.
2. Final Business Plan ICH Q13: Continuous Manufacturing for Drug Substances and Drug Products International Council for Harmonisation of Technical Requirements for Pharmaceuticals for Human Use Geneva, Switzerland 2018.
3. Matsuda, Y. Global Regulatory Landscape. Aaps Pharmscitech 2019, 20, (1).
4. Wang, Y.; O'Connor, T.; Li, T.; Ashraf, M.; Cruz, C. N. Development and applications of a material library for pharmaceutical continuous manufacturing of solid dosage forms. International Journal of Pharmaceutics 2019, 569.
5. Kawashima, Y., Imai, M., Takeuchi, H., Yamamoto H., Kamiya, K., Hino, T. Improved flowability and compactibility of spherically agglomerated crystals of ascorbic acid for direct tableting designed by spherical crystallization process. Powder Technology 2003, 130, 283-289.
6. Maghsoodi, M.; Hassan-Zadeh, D.; Barzegar-Jalali, M.; Nokhodchi, A.; Martin, G. Improved Compaction and Packing Properties of Naproxen Agglomerated Crystals Obtained by Spherical Crystallization Technique. Drug Development and Industrial Pharmacy 2008, 33, (11), 1216-1224.
7. Pena, R.; Nagy, Z. K. Process Intensification through Continuous Spherical Crystallization Using a two-Stage Mixed Suspension Mixed Product Removal (MSMPR) System. Crystal Growth & Design 2015, 15, 4225-4236.
8. Chen, H. B.; Guo, Y. W.; Wang, C. G.; Dun, J. N.; Sun, C. C. Spherical Co-crystallization-An Enabling Technology for the Development of High Dose Direct Compression Tablets of Poorly Soluble Drugs. Cryst Growth Des 2019, 19, (4), 2503-2510.
9. Chen, H. B.; Wang, C. G.; Sun, C. C. Profoundly Improved Plasticity and Tabletability of Griseofulvin by in Situ Solvation and Desolvation during Spherical Crystallization. Cryst Growth Des 2019, 19, (4), 2350-2357.
10. Sheikh, A. Y.; Pal, A.; Viswanath, S.; Tolle, J. C. Agglomerative crystallization of ABT-510 in a partially miscible solvent system. Journal of Pharmaceutical Sciences 2008, 97, (3), 1202-1212.

11. Orlewski, P. M.; Ahn, B.; Mazzotti, M. Tuning the Particle Sizes in Spherical Agglomeration. Crystal Growth & Design 2018, 18, (10), 6257-6265.
12. Chen, H. B.; Aburub, A.; Sun, C. C. Direct Compression Tablet Containing 99% Active Ingredient-A Tale of Spherical Crystallization. Journal of Pharmaceutical Sciences 2019, 108, (4), 1396- 1400.
13. Chen, H.; Chenguang, C.; Kang, H.; Haynes, C. L.; Aburub, A.; Sun, C. C. Microstructures and pharmaceutical properties of ferulic acid agglomerates prepared by different spherical crystallization methods. International Journal of Pharmaceutics 2020, 574, 73-79.
14. Valeur, E.; Gueret, S. M.; Adihou, H.; Gopalakrishnan, R.; Lemurell, M.; Waldmann, H.; Grossmann, T. N.; Plowright, A. T. New Modalities for Challenging Targets in Drug Discovery. Angewandte Chemie-International Edition 2017, 56, (35), 10294-10323.
15. Benet, L. Z.; Hosey, C. M.; Ursu, O.; Oprea, T. I. BDDCS, the Rule of 5 and drugability. Advanced Drug Delivery Reviews 2016, 101, 89-98.
16. Wu, C. Y.; Benet, L. Z. Predicting drug disposition via application of BCS: Transport/absorption/elimination interplay and development of a biopharmaceutics drug disposition classification system. Pharmaceutical Research 2005, 22, (1), 11-23.
17. New Drugs at FDA: CDER's New Molecular Entities and New Therapeutic Biological Products. (08 Nov 2019),
18. Ghosh, A.; Louis, L.; Arora, K. K.; Hancock, B. C.; Krzyzaniak, J. F.; Meenan, P.; Nakhmanson, S.; Wood, G. P. F. Assessment of machine learning approaches for predicting the crystallization propensity of active pharmaceutical ingredients. Crystengcomm 2019, 21, (8), 1215-1223.
19. Wicker, J. G. P.; Cooper, R. I. Beyond Rotatable Bond Counts: Capturing 3D Conformational Flexibility in a Single Descriptor. Journal of Chemical Information and Modeling 2016, 56, (12), 2347-2352.
20. Li, Z.; Lin, X.; Shen, L.; Hong, Y. L.; Feng, Y. Composite particles based on particle engineering for direct compaction. International Journal of Pharmaceutics 2017, 519, (1-2), 272-286.
21. Good Manufacturing Practice Guide for Active Pharmacutical Ingredients Q7 GUIDELINE, I. H. T., Ed. 2000.
22. Q7 Implementation Working Group ICH Q7 Guideline: Good Manufacturing Practice Guide for Active Pharmaceutical Ingredients Questions and Answers GUIDELINE, I. H. T., Ed. 2015.

23. Choi, H.; Lee, H.; Lee, M. K.; Lee, J. Polymer-Directed Crystallization of Atorvastatin. Journal of Pharmaceutical Sciences 2012, 101, (8), 2941-2951.
24. Kaialy, W.; Larhrib, H.; Chikwanha, B.; Shojaee, S.; Nokhodchi, A. An approach to engineer paracetamol crystals by antisolvent crystallization technique in presence of various additives for direct compression. International Journal of Pharmaceutics 2014, 464, (1-2), 53-64.
25. Tian, F.; Saville, D. J.; Gordon, K. C.; Strachan, C. J.; Zeitler, J. A.; Sandler, N.; Rades, T. The influence of various excipients on the conversion kinetics of carbamazepine polymorphs in aqueous suspension. Journal of Pharmacy and Pharmacology 2007, 59, (2), 193-201.
26. CHMP Assessment Report: Zelboraf. EMA/CHMP, Ed. London, UK, 2012.
27. CHMP Assessment Report: Tybost. EMA/CHMP, Ed. London, UK, 2013.
28. Quality Working Party questions and answers on API mix EMA/CHMP/CVMP/QWP, Ed. 2016.
29. Madurawe, R. D., An FDA Perspective on Expanding Continuous Manufacturing to the Drug Substance -Drug Product Interface. In ISPE Annual Meeting, Las Vegas, 2019.
30. Regulatory Classification of Pharmaceutical Co-Crystals Guidance for Industry. (CDER), U. S. D. o. H. a. H. S. F. a. D. A. C. f. D. E. a. R., Ed. 10001 New Hampshire Ave., Hillandale Bldg., 4th Floor Silver Spring, MD 20993-0002, 2018.
31. H.J. Scheel: Historical Introduction. In: Handbook of Crystal Growth. 1a. Fundamentals, ed. by D.T.J. Hurle (North-Holland Elsevier, Amsterdam 1993) pp. 3-42
32. I.N. Stranski: a) Zur Theorie des Kristallwachstums, Ann. Univ. Sofia 24 (1927) 297; b) Z. phys. Chem. 136 (1928) 259-278
33. A.A. Chernov: Morphology and kinetics of crystal growth from aqueous solutions. In: Morphology and Growth Unit of Crystals, ed. by I. Sunagawa (Terra Scientific Pu.Co., Tokyo 1989) pp 391-417
34. Sunagawa: Surface Microtopography of Crystal Faces. In: Morphology of Crystals (Terra Scientific Pu. Co., Tokyo 1987) pp 321-365; Sunagawa: Crystals, Growth, Morphology and Perfection (Cambridge University Press, Cambridge 2005)
35. W.A. Tiller: The science of crystallization: microscopic interfacial phenomena (Cambridge University Press, Cambridge 1991)
36. K. Sangwal, R. Rodriguez-Clemente: Surface Morphology of Crystalline Solids (Trans. Tech. Pu, Zurich 1991)

37. B. Simon, R. Boistelle: Crystal growth from low temperature solutions, J. of Crystal Growth 52 (1981) 779-788.
38. Z. Berkovitch–Yellin: Towards the ab initio determination of crystal morphology, J. Am. Chem. Soc. 107 (1985) 8239-8253
39. P. Bennema: Growth and Morphology of Crystals: Integration of Theories of Roughening and Hartman-Perdok Theory. In: Handbook of Crystal Growth. 1a. Fundamentals, ed. by D.T.J. Hurle (North-Holland Elsevier, Amsterdam 1993) pp 477-581.
40. E. van Veenendaal, P.J.C.M. van Hoof, J. van Suchtelen, W.J.P. van Enckevort, P. Bennema: Kinetic roughening of the Kossel (100) surface, J. of Crystal Growth 198 (1999) 22-26
41. T.N. Thomas, T.A. Land, T. Martin, W.H. Casey, J.J. DeYoreo: AFM investigation of the step kinetics and hillock morphology of the {100} face of KDP, J. of Crystal Growth 260 (2004) 566-579.
42. R. Rodriguez-Clemente, S. Veintemillas-Verdaguer, F. Rull-Perez: Mechanism of crystal growth from boiling water solutions of soluble inorganic salts, mainly KDP. In: *Morphology and Growth Unit of Crystals*, ed. I. Sunagawa (Terra Scientific Pu. Co., Tokyo 1989) pp 479- 512
43. Jenike, A.W.: Storage and flow of solids, Bull. No. 123, Engng. Exp. Station, Univ. Utah, Salt Lake City (1964)
44. Schulze, D.: Powders and Bulk Solids – Behavior, Characterization, Storage and Flow, Springer Berlin – Heidelberg – New York – Tokyo (2008)
45. Carr, J.F., Walker, D.M.: An annular shear cell for granular materials, Powder Technology 1 (1967/68), pp. 369–373
46. Schwedes, J., Schulze, D.: Measurement of flow properties of bulk solids, Powder Technology 61 (1990), pp. 59–68
47. Schulze, D.: Powders and Bulk Solids – Behavior, Characterization, Storage and Flow, Springer Berlin – Heidelberg – New York – Tokyo (2008)
48. Molerus, O.: Schüttgutmechanik, Springer Verlag, Berlin – Heidelberg – New York – Tokyo (1985)
49. The Institution of Chemical Engineers (Eds.): Standard shear testing technique for particulate solids using the Jenike shear cell (1989)
50. Schulze, D.: Development and application of a novel ring shear tester, Aufbereitungstechnik 35 (1994) 10, pp. 524–535
51. Schulze, D.: Flowability and time consolidation measurements using a ring shear tester, Powder Handling & Processing 8 (1996) 3, pp. 221–226.

52. Schulze, D.: The measurement of the flowability of bulk solids. In: Brown CJ, Nielsen J (Eds.) Silos – Fundamentals of theory, behaviour and design. E & FN Spon, London und New York (1998), pp. 18–52

53. Cragg GM, Newman DJ. Natural products: a continuing source of novel drug leads. Biochim Biophys Acta. 2013;1830(6):3670–3695.

54. Lipinski CA, Lombardo F, Dominy BW, et al. Experimental and computational approaches to estimate solubility and permeability in drug discovery and development settings. Adv Drug Deliv Rev. 2012;64:4–17

55. Harding, L., S. Qi., Hill, G., Reading, M., Craig, D.Q.M.; The development of microthermal analysis and photothermal microspectroscopy as novel approaches to drug-excipient compatibility studies. Int. J. Pharm., 2008. 354(1-2): p. 149-157.

56. Aigner, Z., Heinrich, R., Sipos, E., Farkas, G., Ciurba, A., Berkesi, O., Szabo´-Re´ve´sz, P.; Compatibility studies of aceclofenac with retard tablet excipients by means of thermal and FT-IR spectroscopic methods. J. Therm. Anal. Calorim., 2011. 104(1): p. 265-271.

57. Kogermann, K., Zeitler, J.A., Rantanen, J., Rades, T., Taday, P.F., Pepper, M., Heinamaki, J., Strachan, C.J.; Investigating dehydration from compacts using terahertz pulsed, Raman, and near-infrared spectroscopy. Appl. Spectrosc., 2007. **61**(12): p. 1265-1274.

58. Skotnicki, M., Aguiler, J.A., Pyda, M., Hodgkinson, P.; Bisoprolol and Bisoprolol-Valsartan Compatibility Studied by Differential Scanning Calorimetry, Nuclear Magnetic Resonance and X-Ray Powder Diffractometry. Pharm. Res., 2014.

CHAPTER - 2

Formulation Additives

Introduction, Study of Different Formulation Additives, Factors Influencing their Incorporation, Role of Formulation Development, Role of Processing, New Developments in Excipient Science, Design of Experiments Factorial Design for Product, Design of Experiments – Process Development

INTRODUCTION

Drugs are always administered in the form of a dosage form containing two basic parts: the active pharmaceutical ingredient (API) and some additives. Additives are therapeutically inactive substances. These additives are obtained from different sources based on biological, minerals, chemical, or synthesis. Most pharmaceutical dosage forms could not be produced without the use of additives. The quantity of additives used in the formulation should be generally optimum. Depending on whether they are organic or inorganic substance. They may be of different character, up to highly complex materials. Initially, the safety of additives was ignored, and no distinct safety evaluation was usually performed because they were therapeutically inactive. But they are not dormant; they have considerable impact on the drug substance. Hence, their safety and effectiveness in terms of bioavailability and stability in a dosage form should be quantified. Several examples have demonstrated that partial understanding of additive's functionality can directly affect process control and the final product. Some additives are inert in nature, but some can form toxic reactions in the concentrations used in a dosage form. The Federal Food, Drug, and Cosmetic Act of 1938 has sanctioned after the disaster of sulphanilamide in 1937 in which an additive which was not tested for effectiveness found accountable for the casualty of several children who took the formulation as reported by the U.S. Department of Health and Human Services, Administration, 2005. Earlier it was considered that additives, or their impurities, can be linked with unfavorable events, either by direct action or by creation of undesirable products. However, this fact has been distorted over times and at present, it is accepted that the added substances 'lethality should not be disregarded, because it can directly interact with the active pharmaceutical ingredient (API), with the body or with other additives, which may result in a potential change in the connection between toxicity and effectiveness[1]. The hazards and advantages of using additives should always be assessed on the basis of not merely their manufacturing and quality but also of their safety and toxicity. Good Manufacturing Practices (GMPs), Toxicology Assessment, Good Laboratory Practices, and Good Distribution Practices requirements are also required for additives like API. Otherwise, the dosage forms would face the exceptional challenges in terms of attaining pharmaceutical grade material and in regulatory control. Since, the added substances are an indispensable content of every single pharmaceutical dosage form, it is significant for the pharmaceutical researcher to perceive the distinctive sorts or evaluations of added substances. It is further essential to understand whether newly added substances will be necessary considering the cost, accessibility, and biopharmaceuticals properties inside the definition. It is necessary to note that how these new added substances can get administrative approval. The manufacturers of the added substances generally, supply their material to various end clients; that is, pharmaceutical industries, food industries, and others. Hence, the suppliers of added substances remained unaware of the last utilisation of their items. It became a problem for the suppliers to help their end clients with respect to their actual requirements. However, the added substances for pharmaceutical use might require additional quality, usefulness, and safety requirements. For this reason, the Good Manufacturing Practices (GMP) has included the requirement of interaction between the user and manufacturer of a particular substance[1].

STUDY OF DIFFERENT FORMULATION ADDITIVES

Kinetic principles is involved in additive interactions that occurs frequently. These interactions may be either drug- additive, additive-additive types. These interactions are either due to physical interaction such as modification of the speed of dissolution or uniformity of the dosage, or chemical interaction such as degradation of drug and/or the formation of degraded products[2]. Although additives are thought of inert substance, they have the tendency to react with drug substance, also with other excipients and primary packaging components. In fact, impurities present in additives can also deteriorate the active pharmaceutical ingredients. The different types of interactions have been shown in Fig 2.1.

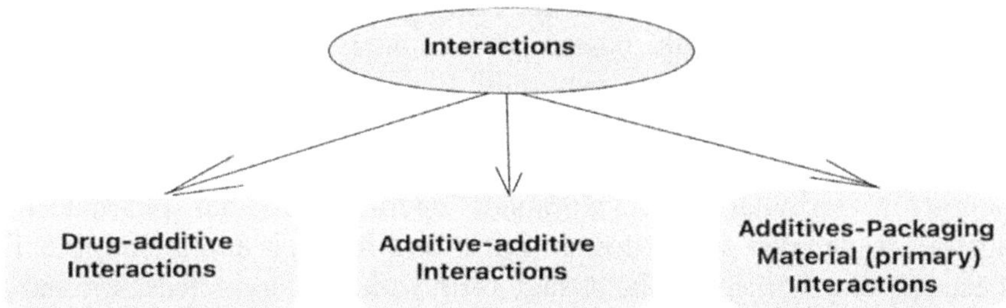

Fig.2.1 Types of interactions.

Drug-Additive interactions: The API remains in close contact with additives in pharmaceutical formulations. Generally, the additives are present in larger quantities than the drug. Incompatibilities between them may result in drug-additive interactions. This type of interactions may be classified into three categories:

(1) physical,

(2) chemical, and

(3) physiological/biopharmaceutical.

Physical interactions are different from chemical interactions. The reactants retain their molecular entity.

Chemical interactions involve chemical reactions that result in the formation of different molecule(s). The important variations between physical and chemical interactions are that in physical interactions the molecules are not chemically changed or modified by any means, for example, esters are susceptible to change in pH, and also the presence of alkaline earth metal and salts. The Millard reaction occurs in primary amines due to reducing sugar.

Physiological interactions involve interactions between the additive(s) and the body fluids after administration, for example, change in dissolution time, pH, disintegration time, etc. This interaction is advantageous in control release formulations.

Additive-additive interactions:

Although the additive- additive interactions occur very rarely, but it is very important to establish the stability of additives present/used in a formulation before the operation starts. Sometimes, additive-additive interactions can be undesirable, or they are desired to contribute to the formulations to get the required product attributes, for example, use of co-processed additives[3].

Pharmaceutical additives are secondary constituents present in both pharmaceutical formulation and over the counter (OTC) drug formulations. Additives are classified on the bases of their function and interactions affecting drug administration due to their chemical and physicochemical properties. The major classes are the coating additives, emulgents, taste and smell-improvers, ointment bases, antioxidants, consistency or viscosity enhancers, and disintegrating materials. Few additives have more than one function, such as, methylcellulose functions as both coating material, viscosity enhancer, disintegrating agent, or binder in tablets[3]. Additives perform the key function in formulation development operation in the pharmaceutical industries to develop stable dosage forms and for their administration. They are used to take delivery of the dosage form with ease, to increase the stability of active ingredients, to be used as filler so that it can properly obtain a dosage form, or to serve as preservatives for enhancing the shelf life of the product or

API. A selection of additive can result in harsh intoxications, as experienced by epileptic patients in Australia in the late 1960s who were using phenytoin capsules. The calcium sulphate that was used as a diluent in the capsule had been substituted with lactose and this substitution was believed to be harmless. However, lactose aggravated an abrupt and massive release of phenytoin higher than the toxic threshold[4]. The functional roles of an additive in the dosage form and on the drug, substance consist of:

- Influence on solubility and bioavailability of the active ingredient(s).
- Improving stability of the API in finished products and also inside the subject after administration.
- Preserve physiochemical property of drug substance.
- Work as preservatives, lubricant, adhesives, propellants, glidants, flavours, colours, disintegrant, diluents and bulking agents, fragrances, coating agents, sweetening agents, polishing agents etc.
- Protecting physical and chemical entity of dosage form.
- Amending predetermined physiological or immunogenic response toward API.
- Maintenance of the formulation for long period: Additives are incorporated in formulations to improve stability or enhance the time of the product in its original form for its shelf-life period.
- To form bulk of content if API does not have required concentration for making a dosage.
- Get better patient acceptance.
- Helps to improve the bioavailability of active constituents: In most of the cases, an API, for example, aspirin is poorly absorbed or soluble in body fluid easily. In these instances, additives are incorporated which support the absorption of the drug from the external environment to inside the body.
- Increase the safety and stability throughout the product shelf life.

Therefore, the additives are substances that aid, improve, and maintain the health of the patients. It can be direct or indirect. Mucilage and gums are naturally obtained for both new and old dosage forms. Natural substances have the advantages over synthesis because of their chemically stability, non-toxicity, low price, and biodegradability. The additives are used in different types of dosage forms based on the functions of the additives.

1. Additives used for solid dosage forms are disintegrating agent, binders, plasticisers, etc., for example, 5% starch paste acts as a binder in solid formulations, while in dry form it works as disintegrant.

2. Additives used for liquid dosage forms are solvents, antimicrobial agents, emulsifying agents, co-solvents, flavour, buffers, sweetening agents etc.
3. Additives used for making the semisolid dosage form are gelling agent, preservative, emollients, suppository bases, solubilising agents, etc.

Additives used in Solid Dosage Forms

Solid dosage forms contribute a lot for the treatment of patients and a large population depends upon the solid dosage forms for their wellness. Broadly, solid dosage forms include but are not limited to tablets, capsules, freeze-dried (lyophilised) powders, powder aerosol formulations, spray-dried powders, etc. Solid dosage forms, such as tablets, granules, and powders, have lots of advantages for both patients and medical practitioners. All the solid dosage forms utilise a number of additives which may include diluents, binders, lubricants, etc. Depending on their use in solid dosage forms additives are classified as follows:

- **Diluents/fillers:**

  These additives increase the bulk content of the dosage form whenever the active constituent in the formulation is of less quantity. Example: lactose, lactose anhydrous, lactose spray dried, directly compressible starch, hydrolysed starch, MCC, other cellulose derivatives, dibasic calcium phosphate dihydrate, mannitol, sorbitol, sucrose, etc.

- **Binders:**

  These may be dry powders or liquid; they are added at a specific stage in wet granulation to promote formation of granules or to provide cohesive force between particles during direct compression for mechanical strength. Example: cellulose, methyl cellulose, polyvinyl pyrrolidine, polyethylene glycol (PEG), gelatine, polyvinylpyrrolidone, hydroxypropyl methyl cellulose, sucrose, starch, etc.

- **Disintegrants:**

  Disintegrants are added to the formulation to facilitate the fragmentation of the tablet and capsule into smaller particles that will provide increased surface area and thus aid a quick release of the API from formulation. Example: starch, starch derivatives, clay, cellulose, alginates, Polyvinylpyrrolidone, cross-linked sodium carboxymethyl cellulose (NaCMC), etc.

- **Wetting Agents:**

  In solid dosage form wetting agents aid water uptake by reducing surface tension and thereby enhancing disintegration and dissolution. Example: Sodium lauryl sulphate.

- **Chelating Agents:**

  Chelating agents tend to respond with overwhelming metal particles inactivating their synergist action in the oxidation of medicaments by forming soluble complexes. Example: ethylene diaminetetraacetic acid, glycine, citric acid, or tartaric acid, etc.

- **Lubricants:**

  Lubricants are intended to decrease the friction between surfaces in mutual contact like tablets and die cavity. It works to make efficient ejection of tablet from die cavity. Example: stearic acid salt, surfactants, waxes, etc.

- **Glidants:**

  Glidants are used to improve the flowability of granular mixture by reducing inter-particle friction and that is used in the pharmaceutical production of tablets and capsules. Actually, glidants, lubricant, and anti-adherent have a close relationship because in different concentration glidants work as lubricants and anti-adherents. Example: talc, corn starch, etc.

- **Film Former:**

  Coating is a process in which coating material is spread over a surface of a dosage form like tablet and capsule in order to remove disadvantages of uncoated tablet like taste and odour. Example: ethyl cellulose, PG, cellulose acetate phthalate, HPMCP, etc.

- **Plasticiser:**

  Glycerine and Sorbitol are the two most common plasticisers. Glycerine is in general used with oil-based fills. Sorbitol is not soluble in PEG and therefore will not leach out of the shell int Titanium dioxide is used as opacifier to produce an opaque shell to avoid photodegradation of light sensitive components and also to hide the content colour or appearance.

- **Stabiliser:**

  It is a chemical that is used to prevent degradation by environmental stresses, and physical and chemical stress during manufacturing. These may contribute to changes that affect quality of product. These additives play a vital role in turning an unstable drug or formulation into unacceptable one. Example: saccharides work to stabilise lyophilised protein formulation[5].

- **Adsorbent:**

  In solid dosage form if there is a requirement to add a liquid or semisolid material in the formulation; adsorbents absorb or adsorb the liquid part on to the dry powder. Example: magnesium oxide, bentonite, etc.

- **Flavours:**

  Used to improve the flavour to mask the taste and can give a pleasant and acceptable taste to the colorants used in the formulation to increase the patient compliance like formulation for paediatric patient. Example: food-drug and cosmetics and drug and cosmetics approved dyes and lakes.

- **Sweeteners:**

  Lactose, sugars, and artificial sweetener, etc. are used to give sweet taste of the dosage forms/ formulations.

- **Preservatives:**

  Preservatives are an important part of formulation, they prevent the development of microorganisms. For example, benzoate derivatives like methyl and propyl are used as preservatives.

Additives used as Spray-Dried Powders

Spray drying is a process where a drug solution is sprayed through a nozzle into a chamber that simultaneously has hot air blown into it for evaporating the moisture content of formulation to convert a mixture from its liquid form to a powder. Trehalose is used to prevent denaturation of protein in dry powder formulation; polysorbate 20 to stabilise aggregation of proteins; silica to increase the flow of powder; polyvinylpyrrolidone prevented the sublimation of salicylic acid during spray-drying; dibutyl phthalate were used. as plasticisers for controlled-release microspheres of theophylline and sulfamethazine pre-pared by spray drying.

Additives used in Controlled Release Solid Dosage Forms

Controlled release dosage is formed by using polymeric additives which coat around a drug core by micro-encapsulation or as a matrix in which the drug is embedded. It includes water-soluble resins (gelatine, starch, polyvinyl-pyrrolidone, and water-soluble celluloses), water-insoluble resins (polymethacrylate, silicones, and water-insoluble celluloses), waxes and lipids (paraffin, beeswax, stearic acid), enteric resins (shellac cellulose acetate phthalate). Surfactant like tween 20 and PEG additives have been used in micro-encapsulation of macromolecules for various effects.

Formulation Additives used for Designing of Semisolid Dosage Form

It contains a major portion of pharmaceutical formulations. It is used to deliver a drug by way of skin, cornea, rectal tissue, nasal mucosa, vagina, buccal tissue, urethral membrane, and external ear lining. But topically applied drugs have some problems in their permeation, but to minimize this issue additives play a vital role in delivering the drug in an efficient manner. Additives work on the physical properties of the vehicle, which make them capable to change the stratum corneum property, e.g., alcohol, or the mucosa to deliver the drug effectively. Semisolid dosage forms usually are intended for localized drug delivery. Semisolids have rheological properties in which they impart solid-like properties until they are disturbed; disturbance easily breaks down particle forces. Semisolids includes creams, ointments, pastes, and gels.

Bases: The base is the central ingredient used in semisolid dosage formulation. Base of ointment does not merely act as the transporter of the drug but influences the absorption of drug. Bases are categorized as follows:

Water-soluble base: They are mixtures of high and low MW PEG which have the general formula $CHCH_2$ CH_2OCH_2 CH_2OH CH_2OH. The characteristics of these bases are:

- Low molecular weight as liquids; those with moderately higher molecular weight are unctuous and the high molecular weight are solids.
- No water is required for their preparation.
- Suitable combination of high and low molecular weight PEG yield material having ointment-like consistency. It melts when applied to the skin.
- Presence of many polar groups make it water soluble.
- Also called greaseless ointment bases.

The macrogols or carbowax are polycondensate mix materials of ethylene oxide and water and they are denoted by their average molecular weights, e.g., microgel 1500 (semi-solid), 200, 300 (viscous), 3000, 4000 (waxy), etc.

PEG: Like paraffine, their consistency differs from viscous liquids to waxy solids; for example, PEG 200, PEG 400, PEG 1000, PEG 1540, and PEG 6000. Different grade of PEGs are mixed together to get desired consistency of formulation.

Water-miscible bases: Excess of water is used to make them soluble, that is why formulation using these bases can be removed after use or application, e.g., cetrimide, cetomacrogol. For o/w type, e.g., antifungal benzoic acid ointment.

Importance of water-miscible bases:

- Promptly miscible with the exudates.
- Reduced impedance with ordinary skin functioning.
- Effective in touch with the skin, in view of their surfactant content.
- Elevated corrective agreeableness, and it makes less probability of the patients discontinuing treatment.
- Easy expulsion from the hair.

Absorption base: The absorption bases have absorbing or emulsifying property. The name does not express their action on the skin. These bases absorb considerable amounts of water, but their consistency will not change (sometimes called emulsifiable ointment bases) Preparations of these bases not contain any water but if water may be used then it converts to w/o type emulsion.

Some commonly used bases are discussed below:

- **Wool Fat (Anhydrous Lanolin):**

  Fat obtained from the wool of sheep. Water solubility is very poor but can absorb water of about 50%. Hence, preparation using wool fat can hold the water in a large amount. It is used with other bases for better consistency.

- **Hydrous Wool Fat (Lanolin):**

  It is a mix of wool fat and water (70:30%). It is a w/o emulsion. It can be incorporated as an emollient.

- **Wool Alcohol:**

  It is emulsified part wool fat. Wool fat is alkaline treated from which cholesterol and alcohol is separated. It has around 30% cholesterol. It absorbs water to maximum extent in w/o formulation (emulsifying agent).

- **Beeswax:**

  It is purified wax obtained from honeycomb of honeybees, contains very low quantity of cholesterols and acts as a stiffening agent in preparation. It is available in two types yellow and white.

- **Cholesterol:**

  Widely available from animal sources. Source of cholesterol is wool fat. It helps in absorbing water in preparation.

- **Oleaginous Base:**

  These are mixture of oils and fats. Important one is hydrocarbons, i.e., petrolatum, paraffin, and mineral oils.

- **Petrolatum (Yellow Soft paraffin) MP 3856°C:**

  It is a mixture of hydrocarbons obtained from heavy lubricating oil. Antioxidants, e.g., butylated hydroxytoluene (BHT), etc. may also be used with this base to make the formulation stable.

- **White Soft Paraffin (White Petroleum Jelly, White Petrolatum):**

  It is a mix of semisolid hydrocarbons, also known as white petroleum jelly. It is decolorized by percolating yellow paraffin. When you apply it to the skin it leaves a layer of oil on the surface of the skin that prevents water evaporating from the skin surface.

- **Hard Paraffin (Paraffin)**

  It colourless, odourless wax type mix of solid hydrocarbons obtained from petroleum. Above 50°C it solidifies. It is used as a stiffening agent.

- **Liquid Paraffin (Liquid Petrolatum/White Mineral Oil):**

  It is transparent, colourless refined mineral oil which is a mix of liquid hydrocarbons obtained from petroleum used in cosmetics. On long storage, it may oxidize, therefore antioxidant like tocopherol or BHT incorporated in preparation. It may combine with other bases for desired consistency.

Additives used for Designing Liquid Dosage Form

Compared to solid dosage form, liquids are processed and formulated as solutions, suspensions, and emulsions according to the dosage form required or API solubility and stability. Powder may also be delivered as syrups, solutions, suspensions, and emulsions by reconstitution in which powder and vehicle are combined prior to delivery. Liquid formulation (LDF) requires various additives which are elaborated as follow:

- **Vehicles:**

  Complex formation, or the use of surfactants. Example of solubilizers in LDF are ethanol, PET that carry drug APIs and other additives in dissolved or dispersed state. Aqueous Vehicles: water (SWFI, WFI, USP purified water), propylene glycol, ethyl alcohol, glycerine.

- **Oily Vehicle:**

  Vegetable oils, mineral oils, organic oily bases or emulsified bases.

- **Solubilisers:**

  Breaking the hydrogen bond between the particles so they get soluble in water. Solubility can be modified by use of cosolvent, pH change, coGs such as PEG-400, etc.

- **Sweeteners:**

  Generally, sweeteners are used in between 30% and 50% of the total formulation concentration except for cold syrups that contain 80% of sweetener.

- Natural Sweeteners: Sucrose, lactose, mannitol, etc.
- Artificial Sweetener: Aspartame, saccharin, etc.
- **pH Modifiers and Buffering Agents:** Buffers used to control or prevent changes in the formulation pH which could prevent and increase the stability.
- **Antimicrobial Preservatives:**

  Preservative used in preparation to prevent the growth of microbes so it should be of wide spectrum. It should be nontoxic, no sensitizing, compatible with other additives, and have no taste and odour, e.g., parabens (0.015%0.2% w/v.), Phenol, benzyl alcohol (2%), chlorocresol, etc. (AULTON pharmaceutics).

- **Surfactant:**

  Anionic Sodium lauryl sulphate (SLS), 2-naphthalene sulfonate sodium, docusate sodium.

- **Cationic:**

  Cetylpyridinium chloride.

- **Non-ionic:**

  Poloxamer, polysorbate.
- **Suspending Agent and Viscosity Modifying Agent:** Cellulose derivatives:

  MCC (and derivatives such as carboxymethylcellulose (CMC));
- **Clays:** magnesium aluminium silicate; sodium alginate, xanthan gum, carbomer povidone, tragacanth, guar gum; colloidal silicon dioxide; BHA, BHT, EDTA; fumaric acid tartaric acid, ascorbic acid, alpha tocopherol, citric acid[5].
- **Colour:**

  Different colorants are frequently used in the liquid dosage forms and most of the time the purpose is to enhance the elegance of the formulation and thereby the acceptability of the dosage forms, e.g., food, drug, and cosmetic colours.

Classification of Additives

The substances which are used to aid, improve, and maintain the health of patients. It can be direct or indirect. Mucilage and gums commonly are obtained for both new and old dosage forms. Substances available naturally are chemically stable, nontoxic, and economical, biodegradable. For this reason, these are advantageous and easily obtainable[6]. Additives can be classified on the basis of:

1) On the basis of the source
   - Animal source, such as, Stearic acid, Honey, Lactose, Gelatine, Musk, Lanolin, etc.
   - Vegetable sources, such as, Turmeric, Guar gum, Acacia, Starch, Peppermint, etc.
   - Mineral source, such as, Talcum, Asbestos, Kaolin, Calcium phosphate, Silica, Paraffin, etc.
   - Synthetic source, such as, Polyethylene glycols, Boric acid, Polysorbates, Boric acid, etc.
2) On the basis of their therapeutic value
   - Anaesthetics, such as, chloroform, etc.
   - Laxative, such as bentonite, psyllium, xanthan gum, guar-gum, etc.
   - Astringent, such as, cinnamon, alum, citric acid.
   - Carminative, such as, cinnamon water, dill water, anise water.
   - pH modifier, such as citric acid.
   - Nutrient sources, such as, agar, lactose, etc.

3) On the basis of their functions
   1) Disintegrating agent, binders, plasticisers, etc., such as, 5% starch paste acts as a binder in solid formulations, in dry form it works as disintegrant are used as additives in solid dosage forms.
   2) Solvents, antimicrobial agents, emulsifying agents, cosolvents, flavour, buffers, sweetening agents, etc. are used as additives in liquid dosage forms.
   3) For semisolid dosage form: gelling agent, preservative, emollients, suppository bases, solubilising agents, etc. are used as additive.
   4) On the basis of their therapeutic value
      - Anaesthetics,
      - Laxative,
      - Astringent,
      - pH modifier, and
      - Nutrient sources.

FACTORS INFLUENCING THEIR INCORPORATION

Physicochemical Properties

- **Molecular Size and Diffusivity**

A drug must diffuse through a variety of biological membranes during a course of time in the body. In addition to diffusion through these biological membranes, drugs present in many extended-release formulations must diffuse through a rate-controlling polymeric membrane or matrix. The ability of a drug to diffuse in polymers, called diffusivity or diffusion coefficient D, is a function of its molecular size or molecular weight. For most of the polymers, it is possible to relate log D empirically to some function of molecular size as

$$\log D = -s_v \log u + k_v = -s_M \log M + k_m$$

Where, v is molecular volume, M is molecular weight, s_v, s_M, k_v and k_m are the constants. The value of D, is related to the size and shape of the cavities as well as size and shape of drugs. In general, the values of diffusion coefficient for drugs of intermediate molecular-weight, such as 150 to 400 Da through flexible polymers range from 10^{-6} to 10^{-9} cm^2/sec, with values in the order of 10^{-8} being most common[7]. A value of approximately 10^{-6} is typical for these drugs through water as the medium. For drugs with a molecular weight larger than 500 Da, the diffusion coefficients in many polymers are frequently so small (less than 10^{-12} cm^2/sec) that they are difficult to be quantified. Thus, high-molecular-weight drugs are expected to display very slow-release kinetics in extended release devices using diffusion through polymeric membranes or matrices as the releasing mechanism.

- **Aqueous Solubility**

Solubility is defined as *the amount of material that remains in solution in a given volume of solvent containing undissolved material at a given temperature*. It is the thermodynamic property of a compound. The fraction of drug absorbed into the portal blood is a function of the amount of drug in the solution in the GI tract, which is alternatively called the intrinsic permeability of the drug Before absorption of a drug, the drug must go into solution in the aqueous phase surrounding the site of administration and then partitioned into the absorbing membrane[6]. The aqueous solubility of a drug influences its dissolution rate, establishes its concentration in solution and the driving force for diffusion across the membranes. Thus, dissolution rate depends on the aqueous solubility, as shown by the Nomes-Whitney equation that, under sink conditions,

$$\frac{dC}{dt} = k_D \, A.C_s \qquad .....(2.1)$$

Where, $\frac{dC}{dt}$ is the dissolution rate,

k_D is the dissolution rate constant,

A is the total surface area of the drug particles, and

C_s is the aqueous saturation solubility of the drug.

The dissolution rate is constant and remains constant, but the important point to note is that the initial rate is directly proportional to Cs. Therefore, the aqueous solubility of a drug can be used as a first approximation of its dissolution rate. Drugs with low aqueous solubility have low dissolution rate and usually suffer from oral bioavailability problems. The aqueous solubility of weak acids or bases is governed by the pKa value of the compound and the pH of the medium. For a weak acid

$$S_t = S_0\left(1+\frac{K_a}{[H^+]}\right) = S_0(1+10^{pH - pKa}) \qquad .....(2.2)$$

Where, S_t is the total solubility (both the ionised and unionised forms) of the weak acid,

S_0 is the solubility of the unionised form.

K_a is the acid dissociation constant, and

$[H^+]$ is the hydrogen ion concentration in the medium.

Similarly, for a weak base

$$S_t = S_0\left(1+\frac{[H^+]}{K_a}\right) = S_0\,(1+10^{pKa - pH}) \qquad (2.3)$$

Where, S_t is the total solubility (both the conjugate acid and freebase forms) of the weak base,

S_0 is the solubility of the free-base form, and

K_a is the acid dissociation constant of the conjugate acid.

Equations 2 and 3 predict that the total solubility of a weak acid or base with a given pKa can be affected by the pH of the medium.

Considering the pH partition hypothesis, the importance of Equations 2 and 3 relative to drug absorption is evident. The pH – partition hypothesis simply states that the unionised form in the stomach (pH = 1 to 2), their absorption will be excellent in such an acidic environment. On the other hand, weakly basic drugs exist primarily in the ionised form (conjugate acid) at the same site, and their absorption will be poor. In the upper portion of the small intestine, the pH is more basic (pH = 5 to 7), and the reverse will be expected for weak acids and bases. The ratio of Equation 2 or 3 written for either the pH of the gastric or intestinal fluid and the pH of blood is indicative of the driving force for absorption based on pH gradient. For example, consider the ratio of the total solubility of aspirin in the blood and gastric fluid.

$$R = (1 + 10pHb - pK_a)/(1+10pHg - pK_a) \qquad .....(2.4)$$

Where, pHb is the pH of blood (pH 7.4), pHg is the pH of the gastric fluid (pH 2), and pKa of aspirin is about 3.4.

Substituting these values into Equation 4 gives a value for R of 103.8, indicating that aspirin is readily absorbed within the stomach. The same calculation for intestinal pH (about 7) yields a ratio close to 1, indicating less driving force for aspirin absorption within the small intestine. Ideally, the release of an ionizable drug from an extended-release system should be programmed in accordance with the variation in pH of the different segments of the gastrointestinal tract so that the amount of preferentially absorbed forms, and thus the plasma level of the drug, will be approximately constant throughout the time course of drug action. The Bio-pharmaceutical Classification System (BCS) allows estimation of likely contribution of three major factors solubility, dissolution and intestinal permeability which affect the oral drug absorption[7].

Classification of drugs according to BCS

- Class I: High solubility-High permeability
- Class II: Low solubility-High permeability
- Class III: High solubility-Low permeability
- Class IV: Low solubility-Low permeability
- **High solubility**

  When the largest dose of a drug dissolves in 250 ml of water over a pH range 1- 8, this solubility is called high solubility.

- **High permeability**:

  When the extent of absorption is > 90%, the Class III and Class IV drugs become poor candidates for S.R/C.R dosage forms. Compound with solubility less than 0.1mg/ml prevent the significant solubilisation, and the compounds with solubility are below 10 mg/ml, this presents difficulties related to solubilisation during formulation[8]. In general, the extremes in aqueous solubility of a drug are undesirable for formulation into an extended-release product. A drug with very low solubility, a slow dissolution rate will be achieved and thus, dissolution rate-limited absorption will be observed. This will yield an inherently sustained blood level. In most cases, formulation of such a drug into an extended-release system may not provide considerable advantages over conventional dosage forms. If a poorly soluble drug is formulated into an extended-release system, a constraint would be placed on the type of delivery system. For example, in any system if the drug is diffused through a polymer as the rate-limiting step, the drug release would be unsuitable for a poorly soluble drug, since the driving force for diffusion is drug concentration in the polymer or in the solution, and this concentration would be low. On the other hand, for a drug with very high solubility and a rapid dissolution rate, it is often quite difficult to decrease its dissolution rate and slow its absorption[9]. A drug of high-water solubility can dissolve in water or gastrointestinal milieu readily and tends to release the huge quantity of drug from its dosage form and thus, will be absorbed quickly, leading to a sharp increase in the drug concentration in the blood. Compared to less soluble drugs, it is often difficult to keep it separately of a highly water-soluble drug in the dosage form (such as tablet) and retard the drug release, particularly when the dose of the drug is high. Preparing a slightly soluble form of a drug with normally high solubility is possible for producing extended–release dosage forms[8,9]. The pH dependent solubility, particularly in the physiological pH range would be another problem for S.R/C.R formulation because of the variation in the pH throughout the gastro intestinal tract and hence, a variation in dissolution rate is observed, for example, Phenytoin. The drugs which are poor candidates for S.R/C.R release systems:

- Drugs, limited in the absorption by their dissolution rates are: Digoxin, Warfarin, Griseofulvin, and Salicylamide.

- Drugs poorly soluble in the intestine (acid soluble basic drugs) are: Diazepam, Diltiazem, Cinnarizine, Chlordiazepoxide, and Chlorpheniramine.

- **Drugs having lower solubility in stomach:**

- **pKa - Ionisation Constant**

The pKa is a measure of the strength of an acid or a base. The pKa allows us to determine the charge on a drug molecule at any given pH. Drug molecules which are active in the undissociated state and the unionised molecules can cross these lipoidal membranes more rapidly than the ionised species.

The amount of drug that exists in unionised form is a function of dissociation constant of the drug and at the pH of fluid at the site of absorption. For a drug to be absorbed, it must be in unionised form at the absorption site. Drugs which exist in ionised form at the absorption site are poor candidates for sustained/controlled dosage forms[10].

- **Partition Coefficient**

Partition coefficient influences not only the permeation of drug molecules across the biological membranes, but also diffusion across the rate controlling membrane or matrix. Between the time when a drug is administered and when it is eliminated from the body, it must diffuse through a variety of biological membranes that act primarily as lipid-like barriers. A major criterion in evaluation of the ability of a drug to penetrate these lipid membranes (membrane permeability) in its apparent oil/water partition coefficient, is defined as

$$K = \frac{C_O}{C_W} \qquad .....(2.5)$$

Where, C_O is the equilibrium concentration of all forms of the drug in an organic phase at equilibrium, and C_W is the equilibrium concentration of all forms in an aqueous phase In general, drugs with extremely large values of K are very oil-soluble and will partition into membranes quite readily. The relationship between tissue permeation and partition coefficient for the drug generally is defined by the Hansch correlation, which describes a parabolic relationship between the logarithm of the activity of a drug or its ability to be absorbed and the logarithm of its partition coefficient. The explanation for this relationship is that the activity of a drug is a function of its ability to cross membranes and interact with the receptor. As a first approximation, the more effectively a drug crosses the membranes, the greater its activity. There is also an optimum partition coefficient of a drug. Below this optimum partition coefficient there is decreased lipid solubility, and the drug will remain localized in the first aqueous phase it contacts. At values larger than the optimum partition coefficient the drug shows poorer aqueous solubility but increased lipid solubility. The drug will not partition out of the lipid membrane once it gets in. The value of K at which optimum activity is observed is approximately 1000/1t in n-octanol/water. Drugs with a partition coefficient, higher or lower than the optimum are, in general, poorer candidates for formulation into extended–release dosage forms, for example, the third generation dihydro-pyridines have an added additional property to this class of drugs - high lipophilicity. Currently one of these drugs commercially available is Lercanidipine. As a result of the lipophilic character, this compound is relatively quickly cleared from the plasma building up within phospholipid bilayer of cell membranes. The dihydropyridine [DHP] thus accumulated can interact with its target, the DHP site of target, the L– type calcium channel lying within the double layer of the cell membrane. This phenomenon explains the slow onset and long duration of action. The sustained release of drugs which exhibit this type of property will offer no special advantages over conventional dosage forms[11].

- **Stability**

  One important factor for the loss of drug is through acid hydrolysis and/or metabolism in the GIT when the dosage form is administered orally. It is possible to significantly improve the relative bioavailability of a drug, that is, unstable in G.I.T when placed in a slowly available controlled release form. Thus, the drugs unstable in the stomach, for them the most appropriate controlling unit would be one that release its contents only in the intestine. In case of the drugs, unstable in the intestinal environment, are the most appropriate for controlled/extended release provided that the dosage form releases its contents, only in the stomach. Hence, the drugs with significant stability problems in any particular area of the G.I. tract are less suitable for formulation into controlled release systems that deliver the contents uniformly over the length of GIT[12].

  The drugs which are unstable in the stomach (acid) are rabeprazole, pantoprazole, omeprazole, iansoprazole, esomeprazole, rifampicin, mesalazine, erythromycin, riboflavin.

  The drugs which are unstable in the intestine and colon (Alkaline) are captopril, ranitidine, etc.

Pharmacokinetic and Pharmacodynamic Considerations

- **Release Rate and Dose**

  Conventional dosage forms include solutions, suspensions, capsules, tablets, emulsions, aerosols, foams, ointments, and suppositories. These dosage forms can release the active ingredients into an absorption pool immediately. This is illustrated by the following simple kinetic scheme.

$$\text{Dosage Form} \xrightarrow[\text{Drug Release}]{k_r} \text{Asorption Pool} \xrightarrow[\text{Asorption}]{ka} \text{Target Area} \xrightarrow[\text{Elimination}]{ke}$$

The absorption pool means a solution of the drug at the site of absorption, and the terms kr, ka and ke are first order rate constants for drug release, conventional dosage form means that kr >>> ka, alternatively, the absorption of drug across a biological membrane, the intestinal epithelium, is the rate-limiting step in delivery of the drug to its target area. For non-immediate-release dosage forms, kr $<<<$ $k_{e,}$ that is, the release of drug from the dosage form is the rate-limiting step. This causes the above kinetic scheme to reduce to

$$\text{Dosage Form} \xrightarrow[\text{Drug Release}]{k_r} \text{Target Area} \xrightarrow[\text{Elimination}]{k_e}$$

In fact, the absorptive phase of the kinetic scheme is insignificant compared with the drug release phase. Thus, a non-immediate-release delivery system must be developed primarily to alter the release rate by affecting the value of k_r.

Although it is not necessary or desirable to maintain a constant level of drug in the blood or target tissue for all therapeutic cases, this is the ideal starting goal of an extended-release delivery system. In some cases, the optimum therapy is achieved by providing oscillating, rather than constant drug levels. An example of this is antibiotic therapy, where the activity of the drug is required only during the growth phase of the microorganism.

The ideal goal in designing an extended-release system is to deliver drug to the desired site at a rate according to the needs of the body (a self-regulated system based on feedback control). However, this is a difficult assignment. Although some attempts have been made to achieve this goal, such as with the self-regulating insulin pump. There is no commercial product available in the market that can represent this type of system. In the absence of feedback control, we are left with a simple extending effect. The primary question is, at what rate should a drug be delivered to maintain a constant blood drug level. The rate of release of the drug should be the same by continuous intravenous infusion of the drug which is given to the patient at a constant rate just equal to its rate of elimination. This implies that the rate of delivery must be independent of the amount of drug remaining in the dosage form and constant over time. That is, release from the dosage form should follow zero-order kinetics, as shown by

$$K_r^o = \text{Rate In - Rate Out} - k_e.C_d.V_d$$

Where, K_r^o is the zero-order rate constant for drug release (amount/time),

k_e is the first-order rate constant for overall drug elimination (time^{-1}),

C_d is the desired drug level in the body (amount/volume), and

V_d is the volume of the space in which the drug is distributed. T

The values of k_e, C_d, and V_d are required to be calculated to calculate k_r^o. These values can be obtained from appropriately designed single-dose pharmacokinetic studies. The above equation indicates the method to calculate the zero-order release rate constant necessary to maintain a constant drug concentration in blood or tissue. For the simplest case, the drug is eliminated by first order kinetics. However, for many drugs, more complex elimination kinetics and other factors affecting their disposition are involved. This affects the nature of the release kinetics necessary to maintain a constant drug level in blood. It is important to recognize that while zero-order release may be desirable theoretically, non-zero-order release may be equivalent clinically to constant release in many cases. The extent of intra and inter subject variation is observed for many drugs, the modest changes in drug tissue levels do not result in an improvement in clinical performance. Thus clinically, a non-constant drug level may be indistinguishable from a constant drug level. To achieve a therapeutic level promptly and sustain the level for a given period of time, the dosage form generally consists of two parts: (1) an initial/priming dose, D_i, that releases the drug immediately, and (2) a maintenance /sustaining /booster dose, Dm.

The total dose, W, thus required for the system is

$$W = D_i + D_m$$

For a system in which the maintenance dose releases the drug by a zero-order process for a specified period of time, the total dose would be

$$W = D_i + k_r^o T_d - k_r^o T_p$$

Where, T_d is the total time required for extended release from one dose. If the maintenance dose begins release of drug at the time of dosing (t = 0), it will add to that which is provided by the initial dose, thus increasing the initial drug level. In this case a correction factor is needed to account for the added drug from the maintenance dose

$$W = D_i + k_r^o T_d - K_r^o T_p$$

The correction factor k_r^o Tp is the amount of drug, r that has been provided during the period from t = 0 to the time of the peak drug level, T_p. No correction factor is required if the dosage form is constructed in such a way that the maintenance dose does not begin to release the drug until time T_p.

It already has been mentioned that a perfectly invariant drug blood or tissue level versus time profile is the ideal starting goal of an extended-release system. The way to achieve this, in the simplest case, is use of a maintenance dose that releases its drug by zero-order kinetics. However, satisfactory approximations of a constant drug level can be obtained by suitable combinations of the initial dose and a maintenance dose that releases its drug by a first–order process. The total dose for such a system is

$$W = D_i + (k_e C_d / k_r V_d)$$

Where, k_r is the first-order rate constant for drug release (time' and k_e, C_d, and V_d have been defined previously. If the maintenance dose begins releasing the drug at t = 0, a correction factor is required just for the zero-order case. The correct expression in this case is

$$W = D_i + (k_e C_d / k_r) V_d - D_m k_e T_p$$

To maintain the drug levels in blood within the therapeutic range over the entire time course of therapy, most extended-release drug delivery systems are, like conventional dosage forms, administered as multiple rather than single doses. For an ideal extended-release system that releases drug by zero-order kinetics, the multiple dosing regimen is analogous to that used for a constant intravenous infusion.

Since, an extended-release system is designed to reduce repetitive dosing, it naturally will contain a greater amount of drug than a corresponding conventional form. The typical administered dose of a drug in a conventional dosage form will give some indication of the total amount of drug required in an extended-release preparation. For the drugs requiring large conventional doses, the volume of the sustained dose may be too large to be practical or acceptable, depending on the route of administration. The same may be true for drugs that have a large release rate from the extended-release system (drugs with short half-lives).

If the dose of a drug is high (a daily dose exceeding 500 mg), it becomes more challenging to develop a sustained release oral dosage form. For short half-life drugs, to provide once a day tablet, it requires not only that a large amount of drug to be incorporated in a dosage unit to provide the daily dose, but the dosage units would be small in size to allow for ease of swallowing by the human. The requirement for small sizes would leave little space in the dosage unit for other ingredients required to control the drug release. The size of the dosage unit becomes even more critical with highly water-soluble drugs, even a larger amount of inactive ingredients (more than 50% of the total weight) is usually required to provide the sustained release property, according to the conventional SR methods[13].

Biological Factors

- **Absorption**

  The rate, extent, and uniformity of absorption of a drug are important factors when considering its formulation into an extended-release system. The most critical case of oral administration is when

K_r <<< K_a. Let us assume that the transit time of drug through the absorptive area of the gastrointestinal tract is between 9 – 12 hours, then the maximum absorption half-life should be 3 – 4 hours. This requires a minimum absorption rate constant Ka is about 0.17– 0.23/hr for about 80 – 95% absorption over a 9 – 12 hr transit time.

- For a drug with a very slow rate of absorption (K_a<< 0.17/hr), the first order release rate constant K_r less than 0.17/hr results in poor bioavailability in many patients. Therefore, slowly absorbed drug would be difficult to be formulated into extended-release systems where the criterion Kr<<<Ka must be maintained. If the drug is erratically absorbed due to variable absorptive surface of gastrointestinal tract, design of the sustained/controlled release product would be more difficult, for example, the oral anticoagulant– dicoumarol, Iron, etc.
- Drugs absorbed by active transport system are unsuitable for sustained/controlled drug delivery system, such as methotrexate, enalapril, riboflavin, pyridoxine, 5-fluorouracil, 5-bromo uracil, nicotinamide, fexofenadine, methyldopa.
- Drugs absorbed through amino acid transporters in the intestine, such as, cephalosporines, gabapentin, baclofen, methyldopa, levodopa.
- Drugs transported through oligo-peptide transporters, such as captopril, lisinopril, cephalexin, cefadroxil, cefixime.
- Drugs required to exert a local therapeutic action in the stomach are unsuitable for sustained /controlled drug delivery, such, misoprostol, 5-fluorouracil, antacids, anti-helicobacter pylori agents.
- **Absorption Window**

  Some drugs show region specific absorption which is related to differential drug solubility and stability in different regions of G.I.T, as a result of changes in environmental pH, degradation by enzymes, etc. These drugs show absorption window, signifying the region of G.I tract where primarily absorption occurs. Drugs released from sustained/controlled release systems, after crossing the absorption window goes waste with little/no negligible absorption. Hence, absorption window can limit the bioavailability of orally administered compounds and can be a major obstacle to the development of sustained/controlled release drugs[14]. Drugs exhibiting the site specific absorption in stomach or upper parts of small intestine (absorption window) are acyclovir, captopril, metformin, gabapentin, atenolol, furosemide, ranitidine, levodopa, sotalol, salbutamol, riboflavin, sulphonamides, loratadine, cephalosporines, tetracyclines verapamil, thiamine, sulpiride, quinolines, baclofen, nimesulide, cyclosporine, etc.

- **Distribution**

In the overall elimination kinetics, the distribution of a drug into vascular and extra vascular spaces in the body is an important factor. Apparent volume of distribution and ratio of drug in tissue to plasma (T/P) concentration are used to describe the distribution characteristics of a drug.

For drugs which have apparent volume of distribution higher than real volume of distribution i.e., drugs which are extensively bound to extra vascular tissues eg: chloroquine, the elimination half-life is decreased i.e., the drug leaves the body gradually provided drug elimination rate is limited by the release of drug from tissue binding sites and that drug is released from the tissues to give concentrations exceeding the threshold level or within the therapeutic range, one can assume that such drugs are inherently sustained. The larger the volume of distribution, the more the drug is concentrated in the tissues compared with the blood. It is the drug in the blood that is exposed to hepatic or renal clearance, so that when the distribution volume is large these mechanisms have fewer drugs to work on. By contrast, if the volume of distribution is small, most of the drug in the body is in the blood and is accessible to the elimination process. To avoid the ambiguity inherent in apparent volume of distribution as estimation of amount of drug in body, the T/P ratio is used. If the amount of drug in central compartment 'P' is known, the amount of drug in peripheral compartment 'T' and hence the total amount of drug in the body can be calculated by

$$\frac{T}{P} = k_{12}(k_{21} - \beta)$$

Where, β = slow disposition rate constant.

Table 2.1 Drugs with apparent volume of distribution higher than total volume of distribution.

Drug	App. Vol. Distribution (lts)
Chloroquine	12950
Haloperidol	1400
Digoxin	500
Doxepin	1400
Flurazepam	1540
Azithromycin	2170
Amiodarone	4620

Table 2.2 Relationship between $\frac{T}{P}$ ratio and V_{dss}.

Drug	$\frac{T}{P}$ ratio	V_{dss}	Drug	$\frac{T}{P}$ ratio	V_{dss}
Diazepam	2.85	130	Theophylline	0.9	40
Digoxin	4.3	500	Furosemide	0.96	5
Procainamide	14.35	62	Meperidine	2	3000

Table 2.3 Use of T/P ratio in conjunction with total body clearance at steady state to gain further view into drug disposition.

T/P ratio	Total body clearance	Disposition characteristics
High	High	Weak tissue binding
High	Low	Strong tissue/protein binding
Low	Low	Strong protein binding
Low	High	Weak plasma protein binding

- **Metabolism**

  The metabolism of a drug can either inactivate an active drug or convert an inactive drug to active metabolite. Complex metabolic patterns would make the S.R/C.R design much more difficult particularly when biological activity is wholly or partly due to a metabolite as in case isosorbide 2, 5-dinitrate.

There are two areas of concern related to metabolism that significantly restrict SR product design. First, if a drug upon chronic administration is capable of either inducing or inhibiting enzyme synthesis, it will be a poor candidate for a S/R/C.R product because of the difficulty of maintaining uniform blood levels of a drug.

Second, if there is a variable blood level of a drug through either intestinal (or tissue) metabolism or through first pass effect, this also will make formulation of SR dosage form difficult, since most of the process are saturable, the fraction of the drug loss would be dose dependent and that would result in significant reduction in bioavailability if the drug is slowly released over a extended period of time[15].

Fluctuation of drug-concentration in blood (serum) due to intestinal metabolism after oral dosing have been observed, for example, salicylamide, isoproterenol, chlorpromazine, clonazepam hydralazine and levodopa.

Fluctuation of drug-concentration in blood (serum) due to first pass hepatic metabolism after oral dosing, for example, nortriptyline, phenacetin, morphine, propranolol.

Fluctuation of concentration of drug in blood (serum) due to enzyme induction are poor candidates for Sustained/controlled release dosage forms, for example, griseofulvin, phenytoin, primidone, barbiturates, rifampicin, meprobamate, cyclophosphamide.

Fluctuation of concentration of drug in blood (serum) due to enzyme inhibition are poor candidates for Sustained/Controlled release dosage forms, isoniazid, cimetidine, amiodarone, erythromycin, fuconazole, ketoconazole, MAO –inhibitors, para - aminosalicyclic acid, allopurinol, coumarins.

- **Dose Dependent Bioavailability**

  In case of propoxyphene, the bioavailability of the drug depends on its dose. Only 18% of 65 mg dose, 28% of 130 mg dose, 33% of 195 mg dose can reach the systemic circulation due to first pass effect. As a result, making of the S.R/C.R dosage form of this drug is less desirable.

- **Elimination Half Life**

  Half-life is the time taken for the amount of drug in the body (plasma concentration) to fall by half and is determined by both clearance (C_l) and volume of distribution (V_d)

$$t_{1/2} = 0.693.\frac{V_d}{C_l}$$

Half-life is increased by increasing in volume of distribution or a decrease in clearance, and vice-versa. The larger the volume of distribution the more the drug is concentrated in the tissues compared with the blood. If the volume of distribution is small, most of the drug in the body is in the blood which is then moved for the elimination process.

For drugs that follow linear kinetics, the elimination half-life is found constant and does not change with dose or concentration of the drug. For drugs that follow non-linear kinetics, the elimination half-life and drug clearance both change with dose or concentration of the drug. Drugs with short half-lives (< 2 hrs) and high dose are not suitable for formulation into sustained/controlled release systems. Because the necessary dose size and drugs with long half-lives (> 8 hr) are inherently sustained. Sustained release products for drugs having intrinsically long biologic half-lives are available. As expected, little or no therapeutic advantages have been shown in these products over conventional dosage forms, for examples, of meprobamate (11.3 hr), amytriptyline (21 hr). Sustained release corticosteroids are not necessary for the therapy, undesirable for the side effects, and un-physiological for the diurnal variations in cortisol secretions. In fact, SR formulations of prednisolone sodium phosphate and methyl prednisolone have been shown to be equally effective as conventional oral tablets offering no advantages over the latter.

- **Drug -Protein Binding**

  The drug can bind to components such as blood cells and plasma proteins and also to tissue proteins and macromolecules. Drug-protein binding is a reversible process. As the concentration of free-drug in the blood decreases, the drug-protein complex dissociates to liberate the free drug and maintain equilibrium. Due to this reversible binding of a drug, the free-drug concentration is maintained for long time in the blood resulting to a long biological half-life. Due to the high molecular size a protein bound drug is unable to enter into hepatocytes, resulting in reduced metabolism. The bound drug is not available as a substrate for liver enzymes there by further reducing the rate of metabolism.

  The glomerular capillaries do not permit the passage of plasma-protein and drug-protein complexes. Hence, only unbound drug is eliminated. The elimination half-life of drugs generally increases when the percent of drug bound to plasma increases. Such drugs need not be formulated into sustained/controlled release formulations. Since blood proteins are mostly re-circulated, not eliminated, high drug-protein binding can serve as a depot for drug producing a prolonged drug action.

  The role of protein binding as a factor in formulation of S.R/C.R dosage forms can be explained by considering angiotensin-II antagonist class of drugs. The drugs of this class are highly protein bound (> 99%). Tasosartan is a long-acting AT-II receptor blocker shows protein binding of 99.8%, while it's long acting active metabolite enoltasosartan has a protein binding of 99.9%. In a study AT-II receptor blockade effect of single doses of tasosartan (100 mg oral and 25mg IV) and enoltasosartan (25 mg IV) have been compared. It has been found that tasosartan induced rapid and sustained blockade of AT-II receptors. Tasosartan blocked 80% of AT-II receptors within 1–2 hrs of drug administration and still had 40% effect for 32 hrs. On the other hand, the blockade induced by the enoltasosartan was markedly delayed and hardly reached 60 -70% despite IV administration and high plasma levels. This delayed *in vivo* blockade effect for enoltasosartan appears to be due to high and tight protein binding, leading to decrease in affinity for receptors and slower receptor association rate[16].

- **Duration of action**

  Duration of action is the time period for which the blood levels remain above the MEC of the drug and below the MSC levels or more specifically within the therapeutic window. Drugs acting for long duration are unsuitable candidates for formulation of S.R/C.R dosage forms.

The long duration of action of ACE inhibitors is determined by plasma half-life and the affinity of binding to tissue ACE. Drugs with short plasma half- life and high tissue binding such as quinapril remains active for 24 hrs. Other drugs such as lisinopril have weaker tissue ACE binding but much long plasma half-life is also long acting. In contrast captopril which has relatively short duration of action has weaker tissue ACE binding and short plasma half-life. Proton pump inhibitors forms covalent bond with parietal cells and is irreversible and inhibits acid secretion for life period of bonded parietal cell (18-24 hrs).

Receptor occupation, Tissue binding, Half-life, Metabolism, Partition coefficient Irreversible binding to cells are some parameters which are responsible for long duration of action of drugs[17]. Since inhibition lasts for 24 hrs or more, these proton pump inhibitors are dosed once daily and offer no significant advantage if formulated in sustained release dosage form.

- **Therapeutic Index**

It is most widely used to measure the margin of safety of a drug.

$$TI = TD_{50} / ED_{50}$$

The longer the value of TI, the safer the drug. Drugs with very small value of therapeutic index are poor candidates for formulation into sustained release products. A drug is considered to be safe if its T.I value is greater than 10.

ROLE OF FORMULATION DEVELOPMENT

The reason why do some companies consistently perform better than other companies in the industry is the research. Research has shown that even though the tends to be a gradual long-term convergence of above-average and below-average profit rates towards the mean, persistent differences in companies' profits remain into the indefinite future. These companies do have the competitive advantages that enable them to earn above average profits over a long period of time.

Today the modernization in the strategy is used to answer these questions; that is, the "positioning" school[18.] Porter claimed that a sustainable competitive advantage could be achieved by creating a defendable position within the industry against its competitive forces. An alternative approach to this strategic management is the resource-based that the company can create a competitive advantage from the use of their distinctive resources and internal capabilities. The importance of analysing distinctive competencies has already been described[19,20]. However, little research was done in this area until a recent group of scholars refined and extended the work and developed the resource-based view of the company[21-24]. The term "dynamic capabilities" is used to stress the importance of history (path dependency) of current capabilities and the importance of a firm to renew, augment, and adapt its capabilities in the future to sustain a competitive advantage[25].

- **Technological learning**

  A dynamic capabilities framework of strategy focuses on how a firm will build their core competencies over time and develop sustainable competitive advantages. Emphasis is given to the need for firms for continuous improvement by upgrading their products and improving the productivity. Continuous improvement is only accomplished if the firm is successful at shining, which can be described as the act of bringing in or creating new knowledge[26]. Thus, organizational learning can be considered the preeminent capability in the dynamic capabilities framework. Many researchers only attempt to analyse a specific type of organizational learning, such as, adaptive, vicarious, experiential learning or a specific part of the process. There are very few rigorous empirical studies based on computer simulation[27,28].

Explicit, or codifiable, knowledge is that which can be transferred from one individual to another using some type of formal communication system, whereas tacit knowledge is that which cannot be formally communicated, but instead is deeply rooted in one's experience and own "mental model." Thus knowledge is not just the flow of information, but is viewed as the stock of a company's expertise and the understanding of information. The knowledge may be embedded in individual people, physical capital, organizational routines, or the organization's culture[29]. All organizational learning occurs through individuals but it is more than the cumulative result of organizational members 'learning[30].

Pharmaceutical formulation development is related to *the discovery of a new drug substance to the successful development of a commercial drug product*. Formulation development scientists must determine the most appropriate route to achieve effective drug delivery based on the need of patient, then optimize the characteristics of the formulation on the basis of a knowledge of the drug product's bioavailability and processing requirements. Drug development is a high trend in the pharmaceutical industries. With growing responsibilities to study the drug candidates from discovery to human clinical trials as soon as possible. Most of the pharmaceutical industries have provided a portion of the development of their potential new drugs. Outsourcing decreases the timeline of product development and a cost-effective alternative. The needs of the people can be considered and fast solution can be provided to the company and people necessary for outsourcing give a multiple cost structure, increasing resources and spending and decreasing when the demand decreases. Formulation can determine patentability, lifecycle of a pharmaceutical product. Companies use this formulation development rules and regulations and personnel into their product development to grow better. In large pharmaceutical companies, specific departments may exist as the physical Characterisation of drug substances and formulation issues. In many cases, various department are work at deferent places so there handling is very much important by single authority so that the development get speed up and the formulation development timeline decreases. the concept of preformulation was known to us around 1950 as result of focus industrial pharmaceutical product development. it is stage of the pharmaceutical product development during which the physicochemical properties of the drug of drug substance are characterised and established the psychochemical and biopharmaceutical properties gives appropriate formulation and delivery methods. The steps involved in pharmaceutical formulation development are shown in Fig 2.2.

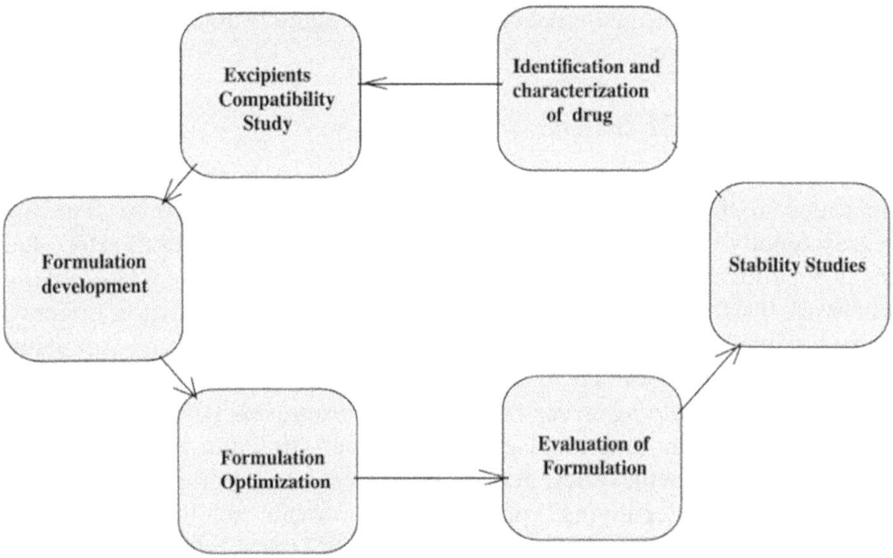

Fig.2.2 Steps involved in formulation development activities.

- **Step I:** Identification and Characterisation of drug

  The identification and characterisation of drug is very important because it can affect the final product. The effect of various characters that can make drug more potent or toxic

- **Step II:** Excipients Compatibility Study

  If the excipient used are more compatible with the drug, there would be more chances of drug formulation towards success and effect of drug also increase.

- **Step III:** Formulation development

  The next stage deals with the formulation development using the different chemicals as excipients that are suitable for drugs.

- **Step IV:** Formulation Optimization

  In this stage formulation like vaccine are produced in such a way that this type of formulation has as minimum as possible excipients. In this step lots of studies than normal formulation are conducted and large amount of the knowledge is required.

- **Step V:** Formulation Evaluation

  The evaluation studies help to improve the already, made formulation by changing the part of formulation like the vehicle types. The evaluation process should be such that the formulation has been prepared in correct way using the optimized excipient.

- **Step VI:** Stability Studies

  It deals with the stability of the formulation by doing various tests so that the stability of formulation can increase, it also helps to improves the shelf life of formulation[31].

ROLE OF PROCESSING

Many active pharmaceutical ingredients (API), such as medicinal herbs, prebiotics in their solid form are highly hygroscopic in nature. The high hygroscopicity causes many issues such as alterations to their physicochemical properties, cause difficulties in subsequent formulation processes, instability during their shelf life, and eventually, adverse effects on their bioavailability. Hygroscopicity, commonly known as 'moisture-sensitivity', can be defined as the *susceptibility of a solid to absorbing or adsorbing and retaining water from their environment.* Highly hygroscopic solids possess polar functional groups or water-attracting binding sites for hydrogen bonding with water, making them relatively hydrophilic or capable of exhibiting 'water-loving' properties. By virtue of their hydrophilic properties, water uptake or moisture absorption by the solids can occur.

Moisture absorption is governed by five factors:

1) Difference between the partial vapour pressure of water in the environment and the equilibrium moisture concentration of the solid;
2) Surrounding temperature;
3) Exposed surface area of the solid;
4) Velocity of the moist air; and
5) Reactivity of the solid to water, which is a characteristic of the solid itself.

All these factors can contribute to the solids' water-binding tendencies by moisture gradient and the availability and accessibility of its polar chemical groups such as hydrogen bonding sites to water, which changes depending on the surface area, chemical composition, crystal structure orientation and presence of any disorganized structure of the solid.

The adverse effects of moisture on pharmaceutical solid dosage forms are of three types:

1) It may cause drug degradation through unwanted chemical reactions such as hydrolysis, which forms impurities and reduces the amount of actives in the formulation. Some crystalline bioactive, regardless of whether they are API or nutraceuticals, may transform into hydrates when water is integrated into their lattice in stoichiometric or non-stoichiometric ratios through hydrogen and/or covalent bonding with the anhydrous actives, changing their physicochemical properties, and affecting their solubility, stability, and bioavailability[32]. It is found that the bioavailability of anhydrous ampicillin is higher than that of trihydrate due to differences in aqueous solubility. It has been discovered that the dissolution rate and bioavailability of nitrofurantoin tablets is reduced after two months under several storage conditions.
2) Moisture may bring on phase transitions by lowering glass transition temperatures and acting as a plasticizer in amorphous solids. It may induce recrystallization of intended amorphous forms, which were formed for their enhanced solubility, back into stable crystalline forms with decreased solubility and bioavailability. Other than plasticization of amorphous bioactive, it may also cause deliquescence of crystalline bioactive, which is the liquefaction and dissolution of water-soluble solids in the absorbed water.
3) Moisture uptake can bring about the wetting of solids, impacting not only their stability but also the flow property, compactibility, dosing accuracy, and hardness of the powders. In tablet compression, hygroscopic solids may adhere to the punches and cause caking and clumping. Measures such as controlling relative humidity (RH), and the use of adsorbents, lubricants and glidants may be taken in these formulation steps.

In case of hygroscopic drug forms, packaging is critical for its protection against moisture in the air, from the time of production to use. Two main points must be regarded in the packaging of hygroscopic drug forms: (1) It must be conducted under controlled humidity conditions to minimize the amount of water vapour occupying the headspace of the package, and (2) Careful consideration must be taken for the choice of the packaging material, to not only ensure that it is inert but that it provides ample moisture protection based on their water vapour permeation rate. Some common packaging materials are polyvinyl chloride (PVC), and polychlorotrifluoroethylene.

The aforementioned formulation strategies, such as, coating, encapsulation have been widely used in solid dosage form for various objectives, such as, taste masking, controlled release, and improved pharmacokinetics.

It is worth mentioning that the issue of hygroscopicity in pharmaceutical solid dosage form formulation is expected to become bigger in the future because problems with low solubility, poor bioavailability, and polymorphic conversion have continuously plagued the quality of pharmaceutical solid dosage forms. Alternative forms of APIs, such as ionic liquids (IL) and therapeutic deep eutectic solvents (THEDES) have emerged as viable solutions. API-ILs and THEDES have shown great scope in solving the issues of conventional solid dosage forms by providing physicochemical properties such as higher solubility, enhanced thermal stability, faster dissolution rate, and absence of polymorphism.

Formulation Strategies to Reduce or Control Hygroscopicity

Widely practiced formulation strategies to reduce hygroscopicity of pharmaceuticals can be categorised into four groups,

(1) Film coating—to form a thin film acting as moisture-barrier around the solid core containing the active ingredients;

(2) Encapsulation—to envelop the active ingredients with polymers via spray-drying/freeze drying or complex coacervation;

(3) Co-processing with excipients—to formulate the active ingredients with hydrophobic excipients to divert water away from the actives; and

(4) Crystal engineering—to transform the crystalline form of the active ingredient to less- process to evaporate the solvents and allow the polymers to fuse into a hygroscopic crystal forms.

- ***Film Coating***

  Film coating may be defined as *forming a moisture-resistant film around the solid dosage core to protect hygroscopic cores from contact with water vapour in the surroundings*[33]. It has many advantages, such as fast processing, small space utilisation, automation potential, better mechanical film properties, limited increase to tablet size, and ease of customisation for specific formulation needs. In general, there are three types of film coatings: (1) aqueous solvent coating, (2) organic solvent coating, and (3) dry powder coating.

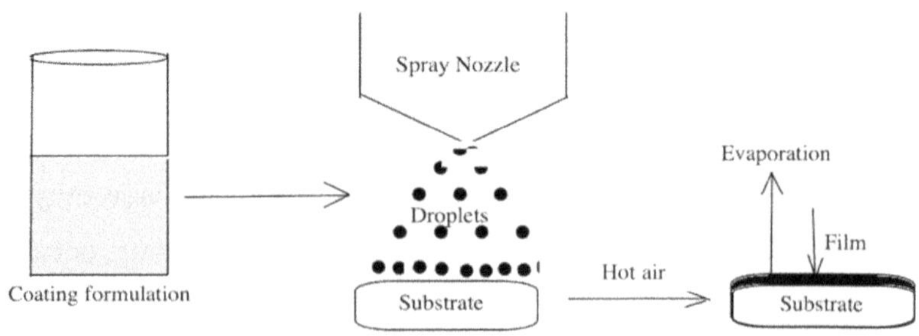

Fig.2.3 Schematic diagram of Film coating.

For aqueous solvent coating, water-soluble polymers are dissolved to form aqueous coating solution; while the micronised powders of water-insoluble polymer are dispersed in water to prepare aqueous coating suspension. The organic coating solution is prepared by dissolving the suitable polymer. The coating solution is then sprayed appropriately over the solid dosage form, so that on heating there remains a coating film over the dosage form. Alternatively, dry powder has been used to coat to eliminate or minimise the use of solvents and water together. It works by applying fine polymer particles and additional excipients onto the solid surfaces, after curing at elevated temperature so that film coating is formed. This technology is still in the developmental stage. In the formulation of film coatings, polymers, plasticisers, and pigments play important role. Plasticisers are used to reduce the T_g of films to impart polymer chains with extra flexibility. These allow the coalescence of molecules so that firmer bonds with appropriate tensile strengths. Thus, they strengthen the adhesion of the film to the surface of the tablets. Pigments are insoluble in water used to cover intermolecular gaps that have formed during film formation.

- ***Encapsulation***

  Encapsulation is *the process of coating the drug powders with a material to shelter the powders from adverse environmental conditions*. To protect their therapeutic functionalities, control release, mask unpleasant taste, increase solubility, and incorporate them into dry systems. Encapsulation may also help with hygroscopicity reduction for shelf-life extensions and ease of preparation. The encapsulated drug in the particle structure is the core, and it is dispersed in a matrix of wall material. Some common encapsulation techniques are spray-drying, freeze-drying, and coacervation[34,35].

The most popular wall materials used for encapsulation include polysaccharides such as maltodextrin (MD), chitosan (CS), gum Arabic (GA), and alginate (ALG). Polysaccharides are generally recognised as safe (GRAS) by the Food and Drug Administration (FDA). They have structures that confer stability during controlled release, are cheap, have low viscosities at high ratios, high solubilities in aqueous solutions, good emulsification ability, and are edible and biodegradable. These properties make them fitting for encapsulation techniques. However, their moisture-resistant properties may be limited by their hydrophilicity. Proteins are less popular but used as well, and some common ones are gelatine (GE), whey protein isolate (WPI) and soy protein isolate (SPI). Proteins present advantages such as nutritional benefits, good solubility, emulsification, and gelation abilities, making them suitable for encapsulation techniques too.

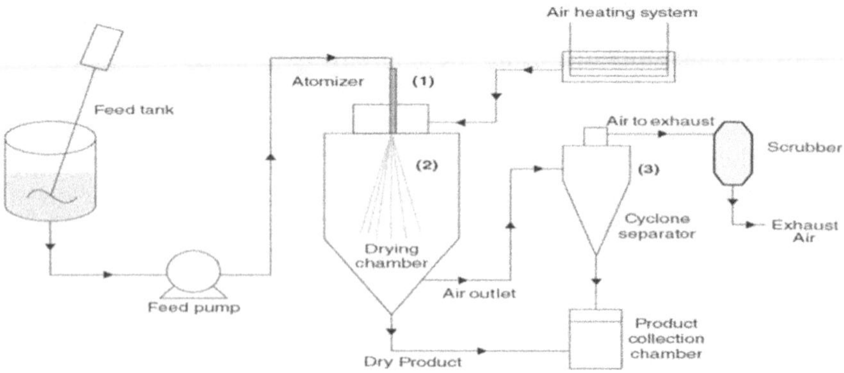

Fig.2.4 Schematic diagram of spray-drying mechanism (1) atomizer, (2) sprayed droplets, (3) product collector.

- ***Encapsulation by Spray Drying***

  Spray-drying is the conversion of a liquid solution, emulsion or suspension into dry material through a single step. Briefly speaking, the dry materials are produced by atomisation of the liquid under hot air flow which immediately removes moisture, creating a solid particulate material that is separated through cyclone and received in a container.

- ***Encapsulation by Coacervation***

  Micro-encapsulation by coacervation is achieved by phase separation of one or more macromolecules from the initial solution followed by environment of this phase uniformly around the suspended or emulsified drug in the same media[36]. There are two types of coacervation processes, simple and complex coacervation.

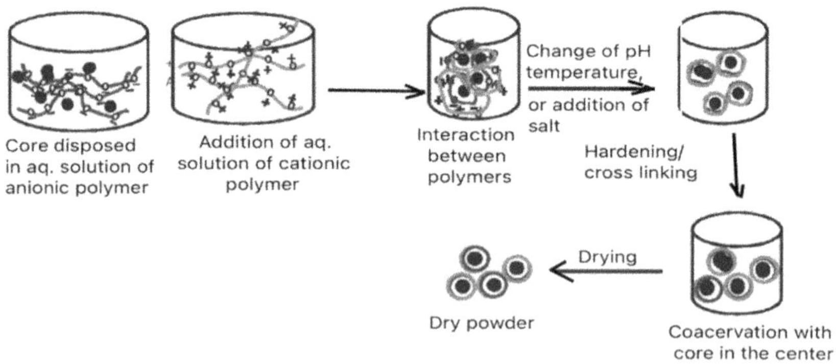

Fig.2.5 Schematic diagram of complex coacervation technique.

When a single polymer is used for coacervation process, and coacervations are formed through dehydration mechanism by addition of crosslinker salts or by desolvation liquid, it is called simple coacervation. While in the complex coacervation process, two or more oppositely charged polymers form ionic or electrostatic interactions which causes phase separation and polymers form ionic or electrostatic interactions leading to phase separation and formation of coacervates are formed.

The complex coacervation is commonly used due to simple processing, lower expense, scalability, and reproducibility, higher encapsulation and loading efficiency[37].

- ***Double-Emulsion Complex Coacervation for Hydrophilic drugs***

  Although the complex coacervation method is promising one, it is suitable for hydrophobic drugs because of the necessity of phase separation between the core and hydrophilic aqueous biopolymer solution. For hydrophilic drugs, a two-step adaption process is required. For hydrophobic drugs, a two-step adaption process is typically required, where they are first emulsified in a primary water/oil (W/O) emulsion, followed by double water/oil/water (W/O/W) emulsion in the biopolymer solution, before encapsulation by coacervation is feasible[38].

Reduction in hygroscopicity can be obtained by this method. The biopolymers used for encapsulation of hygroscopic cores should be less hygroscopic than the cores for reduction of hygroscopicity. Besides hygroscopicity of biopolymers, the drying step after coacervation can also affect the hygroscopicity of the products. The spray-dried extracts have been found to have lower hygroscopicity than the freeze-dried extracts because there is more driving force and surface area for moisture evaporation in spray drying. Moreover, the freeze-dried samples possess highly porous surfaces, increasing their susceptibility to water absorption.

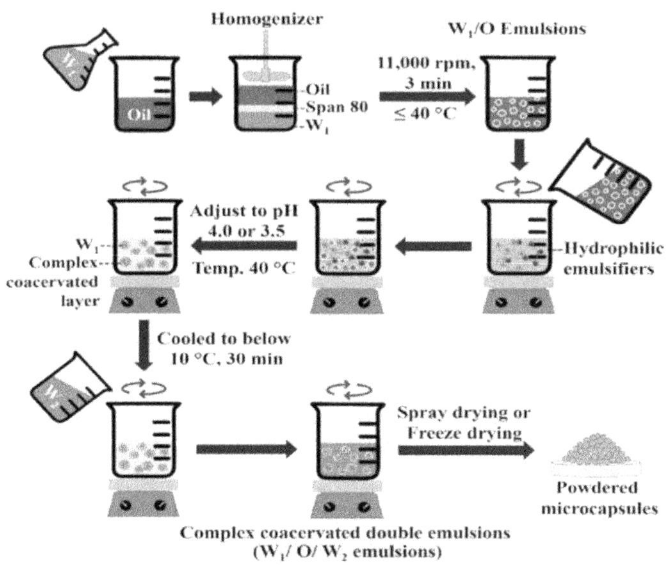

Fig.2.6 Schematic diagram of double emulsion complex coacervation process.

- ***Coacervation by Gelation***

  Gelation is a simple coacervation. It needs a single polymer and a cross-linker to make coacervation with itself. Although less popular than complex coacervation method such as gelation can still be effective to encapsulate hygroscopic drugs. Film containing LAC demonstrated that reductions in hygroscopicity can be possible due to its hydrophobicity and good moisture-protective properties[39].

- ***Co-Processing with Excipients***

  Usually, solid dosage forms comprise the active ingredient coupled with different excipients to aid in its preparation and therapeutic functions. The excipients added should mostly be inert in terms of therapeutic effects and should not produce undesired alterations such as phase or stability changes in the drugs during manufacturing and storage[40]. Excipients may be added to improve the hygroscopicity and stability of solid dosage forms through their interactions with ambient moisture. Excipients can be added to formulations through mixing with or without the help of water, binder, or dissolution solution, followed by melting or solvent evaporation. Common co-processing techniques are wet granulation, dissolution, physical mixing, followed by freeze drying, oven drying, or fluid bed drying, or ambient drying.

- ***Hydrophilic Excipients***

  Similar to amorphous excipients, hydrophilic excipients can bring stability to the drugs due to their ability to absorb substantial amounts of water and bind to them tightly, restricting the availability and mobility of water to reach the hygroscopic activities. For porous excipients such as calcium silicate (FLR) have been added to the formulation containing TCM. The addition of FLR allowed the formulation of granules due to the high water-sorption ability of FLR, where it can carry. up to 4 to 5 times its own weight of water due to its abundance of pores, transferring water very slowly to the extract, successfully yielding granules.

NEW DEVELOPMENTS IN EXCIPIENT SCIENCE

A presentation was given at Rutgers University in March 1995 on possible future developments in the field of excipients. This presentation was subsequently developed into a review paper. It is worth reviewing what has happened in the field of pharmaceutical excipients since 1995. Report on other developments that have impacted excipients, and also take a look into the future to try to anticipate possible changes that will impact excipients, from the perspectives of both excipient manufacturers and excipient users. In addition, other desirable developments will also be discussed.

The original report[41] looked at possible future developments related to excipients in three categories:

- New excipients
- Particle engineering
- Other factors influencing excipients

New excipients

There would be introduction of few new chemical excipients. This has largely been borne out in practice. Five new chemical excipients have been introduced into the US market that have been used in commercial pharmaceutical finished products. It should be noted that, in the case of sulfobutyl ether betadex sodium and fumaryl diketopiperazine, and possibly for the other new excipients. The new excipient was an unmet technical requirement that could not be solved using existing means. Recently, a new surfactant excipient based on novel chemistry has been announced (FM1000 from The Dow Chemical Company) for use in protein drug products[42].

Particle Engineering

This has been suggested that new grades of existing excipients would continue to be introduced to meet the requirements of user and the needs of new enabling technologies, such as, hot-melt extrusion, spray dried amorphous dispersions, etc. There are only so many variations which can be made to an excipient to achieve a new grade for it to continue to meet, such as, compendial specifications. If it no longer complies with the monograph specification, it becomes more difficult to cause potential users to use the excipient. There is an expectation on the part of regulatory authorities that, if a pharmacopeia monograph exists for the excipient, the excipient used in human medicines, both for investigational use or for commercial use/sale, must comply with that monograph. It may be possible to modify the monograph, but this takes time. The revision of the monograph to extend the definition of the excipient may have to wait for the excipient to be included in a marketed product. There is the issue of potential excipient safety questions during product marketing authorisation review, and there is also the need to develop a suitable specification which can be accepted by the regulatory agencies. With the current move to Quality by Design (QbD) the question of suitability of specification is a potential issue for all excipients. The regulatory agencies require that the suitability of the excipient for use in a drug product should be justified and acceptance of the compendia specification will likely not be sufficient. It has also been suggested that the co-processed excipients would be more likely to be introduced. Their safety can be bridged to that of the individual components provided there. This has largely been the case with several co-processed combinations of excipients having been launched. New co-processed excipients continue to be announced. It seems likely that this trend will continue for the foreseeable future. The current options for particle engineering do not overcome the issue of excipient chemical incompatibility. These 'new 'excipients, whether co-processed or new grades of existing materials, will have the same reactive groups. These will have the same potential to react with and degrade a susceptible active pharmaceutical ingredient (API). Such chemical reactivity can only be overcome by using different excipients not containing the reactive group(s). This is not always easily achieved.

Other factors influencing excipients are:

- Just-in-Time (delivery of excipients to the user's site)
- Automation (of pharmaceutical product manufacturing)
- Materials science approach to excipient characterisation
- Validation
- Developments in (pharmaceutical product) manufacturing technology
- The interface between (pharmaceutical product) development and production
- Globalisation
- Harmonisation

Just in time

This is a logistic strategy whereby materials (API and excipients) are delivered to the manufacturing site just in time to be tested, released, and used. There are savings related to reduced quantities in inventory and storage. It also works so well for pharmaceutical materials such as APIs and excipients because the ability to control their manufacture to achieve the necessary consistency in physical characteristics.

Automation of Pharmaceutical Manufacturing

The discussion focused on three aspects of automation: (1) computer-integrated manufacture (CIM), (2) lights out manufacture and (3) robot workstations. It can be agreed that the first two aspects have been achieved, at least for tablet manufacture, with the approval of marketing authorisations for products produced by continuous manufacturing in both the US and Europe. The robot workstation concept is related to the concept of form, fill and seal. In this case, the concept is to compress and immediately pack the individual unit doses using workstations that could be installed in, such as, isolation cabinets to reduce operator exposure to hazardous drugs and/or assure product stability by excluding, such as, moisture or oxygen. As far as is known to the author, this concept has not been commercialised; the technology exists in other industries. The nearest approach to the concept in pharmaceutical product manufacture would be the packaging of effervescent tablets coming directly off the tablet press to reduce the issues with the storage of the unpacked tablets in bulk.

The materials science approach to the characterisation of Pharmaceutical Materials

Progress has been made in this area. The Quality by Design (QbD) concepts have been used in pharmaceutical development projects. In QbD there is a requirement of the regulatory authorities that the marketing authorisation applicant demonstrate enhanced understanding of their excipients (and API) and how they can affect the pharmaceutical finished product, critical quality attributes (CQAs). The applicant is required to justify the use of each excipient, the specifications, and demonstrate that any critical material attributes (CMAs) are properly controlled. This requires that the applicant characterise their excipients beyond those tests listed in the pharmacopeial monograph. These aspects, and others, form the Control Strategy for the release of batches of finished product. Moreover, in the EU the applicant is expected to justify and assess that the excipient has been manufactured to an acceptable level of cGMP and is fit for its intended purpose. This has not happened, and probably will never happen, because excipient functionality (performance) is very much linked to its use, i.e. the particular product formulation in which it is being used. Each formulation and its processing are different, as are the likely CMAs and functionality tests. In addition, there can be many ways to assess a particular performance characteristic, for example, the Handbook of Pharmaceutical Excipients, 2nd Ed.[43] lists seven different test conditions for the determination of compression characteristics with several different types of equipment being used in the different test procedures. There may be a correlation between the different procedures with some materials, that may not be the case for all materials.

Validation

The pharmaceutical industry has been operating according to the three-batch validation procedure whereby three batches are manufactured at commercial scale and if all three batches meet the specifications, the product and process are considered validated. However, it has been recognised that this does not always ensure that subsequent routine product manufacture meets specification. The United States Food and Drug Administration (FDA) has stated publicly that there are products on the market that had been validated according the three-batch validation process, but in general, one in two batches fails. The FDA now encourages continuous verification of product manufacture to demonstrate that each batch manufactured is fit for the purpose and that the Control Strategy is still satisfactory to assure the suitability of the released finished pharmaceutical product. Second sourcing of excipients is a part of a risk mitigation strategy. However, if this is contemplated from the outset, it should be included in the QbD Design of Experiments (DoE).

Developments in (Pharmaceutical Product) Manufacturing Technology

The increase in manufacturing output may be contemplated, such as increased speed of compression on a rotary tablet machine, and make the point that there is a limit, beyond which even the most compactible material will fail to compact properly. The reality is that the improvements in equipment design have focused on adding better sensors to allow more and better data capture linked to better control of manufacturing output. While the manufacturing equipment is more sophisticated today, the manufacturing or filling speeds have not dramatically increased for either oral solid dosage forms or liquid dosage forms. There have been other developments in pharmaceutical manufacturing technology. The first 3D-printed tablet product has been approved in the US. In addition, hot-melt extrusion (HME) has emerged as an alternative to spray drying for the manufacture, such as, amorphous polymer dispersions of poorly water-soluble drugs. There are now drugs approved for sale in the US market that are manufactured using HME. Another major development in pharmaceutical manufacturing technology has been the adoption of continuous manufacturing for pharmaceutical products. These newer manufacturing technologies will place extra demands on the excipients in terms of designed functionality and consistency of performance.

The interface between (Pharmaceutical Product) Development and Production

As a consequence of the introduction of the FDA's SUPAC (Scale-Up and Post-Approval Changes) Guidance documents and the introduction of QbD, there has been considerable progress in smoothing the transition from pharmaceutical product development to routine commercial manufacture. Although the SUPAC documents strictly relate to the products which have been launched and are thus, in commercial production, these documents indicate the thought of FDA on scale up and equipment changes in general. The transition to the use of QbD concepts in the development of pharmaceutical products and the introduction of the concepts of risk assessment and risk mitigation have put us to understand better the pharmaceutical formulations, their manufacturing processes, and the effects of scale changes.

Globalization

The pharmaceutical industry and the excipient manufacturers have continued to witness the process of globalisation. For example, Pfizer has taken over Warner Lambert-Parke Davis, Pharmacia and Wyeth, Novartis and the merger of Ciba-Geigy and Sandoz, Roche took over Genentech, Sanofi acquired Genzyme, and there have been others. Among the excipient companies

Rettenmaier took over the Mendell division of Penwest Pharmaceuticals to form JRS Pharma and Dow Chemicals and Dupont are in the process of merging and splitting. At the same time, Dow Dupont took over FMC Biopolymer. Many companies in both the pharmaceutical products and excipients areas have expanded into India and China. Both the pharmaceutical and excipient sectors are global and will continue to be so.

Harmonization

There has been considerable progress in the area of pharmacopeial harmonization of excipient monographs and general chapters. It must also be stated that progress has not always been smooth. Of the approximately 60 excipients on the harmonization list, out of which approximately 40 have been harmonized, but none have been harmonized completely. There has been little to no progress took place during the first10 years of the harmonization effort under the Pharmacopeial Discussion Group (PDG). It has been found that there was typically one test, sometimes two, that the pharmacopoeias could not agree on. The PDG then introduced the concept of 'harmonization by attribute 'to overcome this. In fact, the pharmacopoeias indicate in the monograph, what they have agreed on and what they could not agree on. It may not be perfect, but it is much better than nothing. There has been better progress in the area of general chapter harmonization with some general chapters being completely harmonized. Pharmaceutical excipients for use in medicines for human or veterinary use are required to be manufactured to an acceptable standard of current Good Manufacturing Practice (cGMP). There were no universally accepted GMP rules for excipients, and this is still the case today. The International Pharmaceutical Excipients Council (IPEC), in particular IPEC-Americas and IPEC Europe, issued the first version of their Good Manufacturing Guide for Bulk Pharmaceutical Excipients in 1996. Subsequently, the IPEC worked with the Product Quality Group (PQG) on revisions to the guide. The layout of the Guide is based on the structure of ISO 9001. The ISO 9001 Standard was revised and reissued in 2017. The IPEC-PQG Guide has been revised in 2017 but is currently being further updated. Third-party certification of excipient manufacturers is a current topic of discussion and has been for some years. Quite simply, with the number of customers for a particular excipient manufacturing site, about hundreds. There is simply not enough time available to accommodate all the site audit requests. Even if one company is the largest pharmaceutical company in the world, its business may only be a small fraction of output of the manufacturing plant since many pharmaceutical excipients are used in far greater quantities in other industries such as food, construction and oil and gas. Third-party certification has been proposed as a possible means to overcome this 'audit crunch'. Currently, there are two very similar schemes available, both based on ISO 9001; The EXCiPACT scheme and the ANSI/NSF/IPEC 363 standard[44]. The EXCiPACT scheme is an add-on to ISO 9001 and requires that the manufacturing site be certified to ISO 9001. The ANSI standard is stand-alone and does not require ISO certification. Both schemes are intended to be identical to all intents and purposes. The Rx-360 consortium has a joint audit scheme whereby one audit is performed on behalf of a group of companies. This is not a certification scheme of EXCiPACT or ANSI type.

Developments which have Impacted Excipients

- **Risk Mitigation Strategies**

  In the mid- to late- 1990s, the risk mitigation on the part of excipient users in the supply of their excipients was a hot topic. One aspect which was investigated was the option for alternate sourcing. There may have been some successes; however, there were also some failures. The failures highlighted the fact that, in many cases, it is not known enough about the APIs, excipients and their variability to be able to predict, with certainty. The same grade of an excipient from a different manufacturer, or different manufacturing site from the same manufacturer, can be successfully substituted in a particular formulation. It must also be remembered that inclusion in the DoE, in and of itself, is not sufficient to allow a change to the alternate source to be made at some later date, such as, due to interruption of supply of the excipient due to a manufacturing plant shutdown. In order to be able to switch in a timely manner to the alternate sourced excipient, regulatory authorities expect the alternate source to be used on a regular basis during routine commercial manufacture, such as, 10 – 20% of batches be made on a continuing basis using the alternative source excipient. This acknowledges that excipients have some inherent variability and that their manufacturing processes can drift in ways that may not be obvious to the excipient manufacturer or user. Continued use of the alternate source excipient during routine manufacture will allow the excipient user to have an understanding of any changes in the variability of the alternate source excipient over time.

DESIGN OF EXPERIMENTS – FACTORIAL DESIGN FOR PRODUCT

Since introduction of the Quality-by-Design (QbD) concepts, it has been accepted that quality of pharmaceutical products should be designed and built during the manufacturing process. According to Juran[45], most of the quality problems are associated with the way in which a pharmaceutical product has been designed. A poor-designed pharmaceutical product will not provide adequate safety and efficacy, whether the product has been tested for many times and analysed to verify its quality[46]. Thus, QbD starts with the recognition that the quality will not be improved by merely increasing analyses of pharmaceutical products. In other words, quality must be built into the product. QbD is 'a systematic approach' to pharmaceutical development that begins with predefined objectives and emphasizes product and process understanding and process control, based on sound science and quality risk management. Application of QbD will provide the knowledge and scientific understanding to support pharmaceutical development[46]. Pharmaceutical QbD goals may include to:

a) Achieve meaningful product quality specifications;

b) Increase process capability and reduce product variability;

c) Increase pharmaceutical development and manufacturing efficiencies; and

d) Increase cause-effect analysis and regulatory flexibility.

Throughout the world use of risk-based approaches and pharmaceutical QbD have been encouraged by most of regulatory agencies[47]. The concept of Pharmaceutical QbD has been used to improve the manufacturing of the pharmaceutical products in terms of 'Six-sigma' approach. 'Six-sigma' is a system of practices to achieve the process improvement. This results in a significant reduction of products which are chance of out-of-specification (OOS). The significant number of out-of-specification (OOS) results indicates that this is an issue to pharmaceutical industries[48].

In these days quality and quantity has equal significance when comes to the production. Accordingly, the standard operation procedures (SOP), in process quality control (IPQC) and Total quality management (TQM) came into existence. The reasons behind all these developments are to reduce or eliminate the errors and save time, energy, cost and to achieve consistent quality. Reliable predictions based on scientific speculations achieve greater credibility and robustness of a product as well as process. In conventional experimental approach, QA is assured by physical testing and inspection, specifications are based on history of batch, focus only on reproducibility, discourages changes thus freezing the process, specifications depend on batch history. QbD thus, can be used preferentially in the reliability of data and is more flexible. The design of experiments (DOE) became a useful tool for determining specific factors affecting defect-levels in a product. The historical background of DOE goes back to 1920s, when Prof. Ronald Fisher,[49] a British statistician developed groundbreaking applications in discoveries. This method now became universal software tool for engineers and researchers.

Types of statistical designing are factorial designs, sequential simplex techniques, response surface methodology, D- optimal techniques and I-optimal techniques. Out of these, the factorial designs is the most applicable in pharmacy.

But before discussing the concept of factorial design, we need to personalise, some common terminologies which is stated and elaborated as below.

Optimization

Optimization means a perfect, effective or functional of a method/ process/ product. Thus, it is the determination of the experimental conditions resulting in its optimal performance. That is, optimization is to achieve the best possible results out of a given circumstances.

Objective

The objective of optimization program is to indicate either the property of interest (criteria) or the goal of an optimization experiment.

Variables

During development of a product or process several factors are found to affect the process or product, at various % of influence. Variations may be independent, dependent, quantitative and qualitative. These factors are called variables. Independent variable are under direct control of the investigator are concentration of drug, polymer composition etc.

Dependent variable are the response of the finished product such as tablet/ microsphere based on the influence of dependent variables, such as, drug release profile etc.

Quantitative variables are those which can be measured and can be expressed in terms of numerical values, such as, temperature, pressure, concentration.

Qualitative variables include type of carrier/ polymer etc. The dependence can be linear or non-linear.

Response

The variable that is calculated and that measures the relationship between the change in level of each of the factors and the change in response.

Factor

A factor is an assigned variable. Quantitative factor has a numerical value (1%, 2%), qualitative factors include batch of materials, excipients, treatment, diet, labs, analysts etc. Single factor design fits into one way ANOVA.

Levels

Levels of a factor are the values or designations assigned to the factor. Some of the factors and levels are shown in table no.2.4.

Effect

It is the change in response by a varying level of a particular factor.

Table 2.4 Description of factor and level.

Factor	Level
Concentration	mg, µg
Temperature	25°,70°
Drug treatment	Drug, placebo

Design Space

Design space refers to the establishment of range of process parameters that has been demonstrated to provide QA. Within the design space, if some work is done, generally it is not considered as a change of the approved ranges for process parameters and formulation attributes. If any movement out of space is done, it may be considered as a change and would normally require a regulatory post approval change process[50,51].

Factorial experimental design:

To achieve reliable and consistent information with minimum number of experiments implementation of QbD utilizing the design space would be necessary.

Advantages of Factorial Designing

1. Quality can be incorporated into product as well as process, based on scientific understanding.
2. Specifications will be fixed on the basis of performance of the product.
3. Focus is given on understanding and controlling of robustness.
4. Within the design space, process becomes flexible.
5. Submission of the report can be explained by the product and process knowledge.

There are number of variables that can influence[52,53] the results of a research on product and process development. These variables are called as "factors" in factorial design. However, there are some factors which have never been considered or these might have been discovered during the process. Byrne and Taguchi classified the factors that can be important for the outcome of an experiment into *controllable* (noise) and *non-controllable* (non-noise) categories. Noise factors are further described as *difficult, impossible* and *expensive for controlling*. Generally, the researchers use controllable factors. Thus, the random factors and co-variants are rarely used. ANOVA and multiple regression analysis are based on factorial approaches. Software are available to support the calculations.

For the first-degree models, the factorial design (FD) is also called as experimental designs, this is the most common technique. The simplest method of setting up of a design of experiments (DoE) is to take 2 or more variables (n) and conduct the test at different levels. In a full factorial design method, all the factors are combined with each other on all levels and the number of experiments becomes f^{n} where f is the number of factor and n is considered as the level. Therefore, 3^2 full factorial design requires nine experiments, 4^2 requires 16 and 5^2 requires 25 number of experiments to be conducted. If the level becomes 3, then the number of experiments to be conducted would be 3^3, 4^3 and 5^3. Thus, when the number of experiments becomes more, it really becomes unmanageable levels. Therefore usually 2 levels considered are to minimize the number of experiments. If each factor has the same number of levels are considered and the design is said to be symmetric, such as 2^2, 3^3 etc. If the number of levels differ from the factor the design is called asymmetric, such as, 2^3, 3^2 etc. But if it becomes necessary to conduct the design for all required experiments, the fractional factorial design (FFD) should be considered. Here, the number of experiments have been cut short systematically.

The fractional factorial design is a fraction ($1/x^{p}$) of the complete FD.

Where p is degree of fractionation. The total number of experiments for FFD can be given by f^{n-p}. Each experimentation is called as "trial" or "run". Standard symbols, data interpretation, experimental design representation and interaction have been mentioned in table no. 2.5, 2.6.

Table 2.5 Standard symbols for particular ratio of drug: excipients.

Formulation	Standard symbols	Effect (%drug release)
Low drug- low excipient	1	10 %
Low drug- high excipient	a	10%
High drug- low excipients	b	20%
High drug- high excipient	ab	30%

Note: low and high value refers to low and high concentration presented for the drug and excipients.

Interaction = [ab-b]- [a-(1)] / 2 = 5%

Table 2.6

Experiment	f1	f2	f3	Interpretation
1	-1	-1	-1	Zero level interaction
2	-1	+1	-1	Main factor effect f2
3	+1	-1	-1	Main factor effect f1
4	-1	-1	+1	Main factor effect f3
5	+1	+1	+1	Interaction between f1, f2, f3.

Central Composite Design (CCD)

Central composite design (CCD) is a special and advanced form of full factorial design first described by Box et al. Instead of square and cube, 2^2 and 2^3 are represented by circular or spherical respectively. In addition to 2^n full factorial design, a centroid experiment (axial points) and a set of experiments (star points) are also involved. To get circular or spherical domains, the star points situated in a definite distance from the centroid along the axis from the centre point are required.

Fractional factorial design is opposite to Taguchi model. To avoid the above problems, the fractional factorial designs have been introduced. In this case, the large multi fractional studies should be divided into blocks. Within each block experiments have been conducted randomly. Blocks must be performed one at a time. Correction in the factorial design can be made between the blocks. Advantage of such study is that first block may reveal all information required. Some free software downloads are also available regarding factorial designing[54].

Demonstration of Factorial Designing:

Adetogun GE et al. in his experiment has demonstrated the implementation of factorial designing. To study the type of gum as a binding agent (B), its concentration (C) and relative density (D) of the tablet on tensile strength (TS), brittle fracture index (BFI), disintegration time (DT) and crushing strength-friability/ disintegration time ratio (CSFR/ DT) of paracetamol tablets, have been performed as experiments in a factorial design, formulations statistics. Here each of high variables have been utilized as "high level" (subscript H) and "low level" (subscript L). Number of experiments were 2^3, that is, 8. Thus the combinations were:

$B_LC_LD_L$, $B_LC_LD_H$, $B_LC_HD_L$, $B_LC_HD_H$

$B_HC_HD_H$, $B_HC_HD_L$, $B_HC_LD_H$, $B_HC_LD_L$

Where, B_L represents formulation with binding agents Delonix regiaseed gum + tragacanth or acacia gum + tragacanth.

B_H represents formulation with binding agents tragacanth + acacia gum or delonix regia seed gum + acacia gum.

C_H and C_L represent high (5% w/w) and low concentration (2% w/w) of gum binding agent respectively.

D_L and D_H represents tablet relative density of 0.80 and 0.90 respectively.

By grouping the results from the combinations into a number of sets, it became possible to assess the effects that each of the three variables (B, C, D) had on the mechanical/ disintegration properties of the tablets and determine whether the variables have been interacting independently of each other.

The effects of increasing B, from its low to high level, on the mechanical/ disintegration parameters have been found by summing up all "high" levels of B and subtracting the sum of "low" levels of B.

$\frac{1}{4}$ $[(B_HC_HD_H + B_HC_HD_L + B_HC_LD_H + B_HC_LD_L) - (B_LC_LD_L + B_LC_LD_H + B_LD_HD_L + B_LC_HD_H)]$

The same procedure has been adopted for C and D. Then, the results of combinations, n, which appear "high" and "low" levels have been summed up and the sum of the combinations was subtracted to obtain the interaction coefficient. For example, for B and C:

$\frac{1}{4}$ $[(B_LC_LD_L + B_LC_LD_H + B_LC_HD_L + B_LC_HD_H) - (B_HC_HD_H + B_HC_HD_L + B_HD_LD_H + B_HC_LD_L)]$

When a zero result is obtained, it indicates no interaction; but if the interaction coefficient is found different from zero, then the two variables concerned would be interacting with each other. If the difference between the coefficients is found more than zero, the interaction would also be higher. The results were subjected to the analysis of variations (ANOVA) at a 5 % probability level[55].

Disadvantages of Factorial Designing

1. Insignificant variables may not be able to be detected on time.
2. To separate the aliased effects from each other is not possible.
3. If the result indicates undesired effects and all the experiments undertaken at that level are of no use.
4. The entire experimental plan has to be redesigned and repeated at worse condition.
5. The process may not be economic and consumes more time.

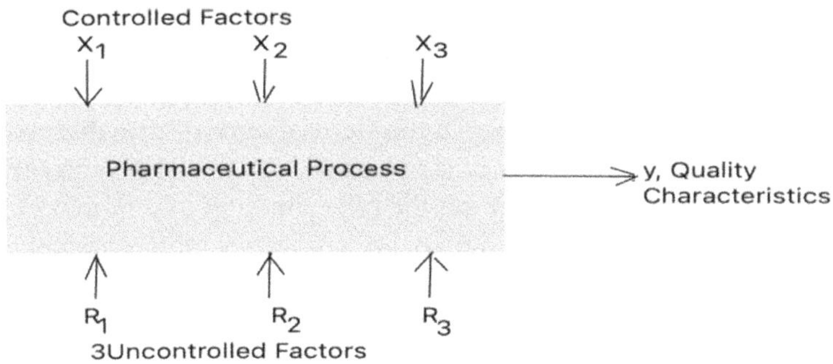

Fig.2.7 Schematic presentation of a process.

DESIGN OF EXPERIMENTS – PROCESS DEVELOPMENT

During the planning stages of research rather than at the final phases of experimentation, Fisher practically highlighted the need to consider statistical analysis. He emphasized that a statistician should be consulted when an experiment is finished. It is often merely to ask him to conduct a postmortem examination. The statistician can perhaps say why the experiment died of. Obviously, the pioneer scientist has strongly supported a proactive approach in his research, which includes the essence of the current regulatory framework that can govern the development of pharmaceutical products[56]. Thereafter, this work has been expanded and disseminated by Quality gurus such as Walter A. Shewhart, William E. Deming, and Joseph M. Juran. They promoted the requirement for a process centered culture to build the quality into the products. Juran used the term "Quality by Design"[57] to emphasize the importance of planning quality into goods and services. Juran made a roadmap comprising of five steps: (1) identifying the customer, (2) determining his needs, (3) translating the needs into product features, (4) developing the process, and (5) transferring it to operations. Almost half a century before Juran, W.E. Deming proposed his profound knowledge, comprising four major points, (1) based on system thinking, (2) understanding variation, (3) theory of knowledge, and (4) psychology[58]. He also underlined the importance of process focus versus product testing in assuring quality, quoting that "If you can't describe what you are doing as a process, you don't know what you're doing" and "You cannot inspect quality into the product; it is already there". Deming actually promoted Shewhart's work[59] on continuous quality improvement through Plan-Do-Study-Act (PDSA) cycles and statistical process control using control charts. The pharmaceutical sector is process-based and quality oriented, thus it would be expected to adopt the aforementioned paradigms early after their introduction. However, Quality by Design was actually suggested by the regulatory authorities (FDA, EMA) at the beginning of the new millennium, recognizing that "quality cannot be tested into products, i.e. quality should be built in by design". Design of Experiments (DoE) is the main component of the statistical toolbox to deploy Quality by Design in both research and industrial settings. While the first DoEs have been applied by Fisher in the field of agriculture, their use entered the chemical process industries during the 1950s, as these were affected by the key paper of Box and Wilson on the experimental attainment of optimum conditions. It should be noted that there are numerous mathematical modelling techniques, for addressing pharmaceutical development and more specifically within the QbD and Process Analytical Technology (PAT) concept, for example, multivariate data analysis (MVDA) methods which focus on historical data, can comprise a point of departure for DoE. Therefore, MVDA in conjunction with DoE can be used for analysing non-designed and designed factors. However, considering the proactive culture of QbD, DoE is considered as the main systematic approach. This requires the implementation of statistical thinking at the starting point of pharmaceutical development, which is the central point of Fisher's legacy. The first reference of DoE application to pharmaceutical dosage form design is considered the paper by Marlow and Shangraw[60],

The introduction of the ICH Q8 guideline has created a favourable environment for the use of DoE, a dramatic increase of relevant scientific work and industrial application has been noticed, further supported by the introduction of user friendly soft wares facilitating construction and analysis of the designs.

Advantages of DoE

DoE shows several advantages over OFAT[61–63]. In particular, experimental design strategies:

1) Maximising the process knowledge, with the minimum use of resources.
2) Provide accurate information, in the most efficient way possible.
3) Identify factor interactions.
4) Characterise the relative significance of each factor.
5) Allow for the prediction of the process behaviour within the design space.
6) Establish a solid cause and effect relationship between CPPs and CQAs.
7) Enable the optimization of CQAs through appropriate selection of CPP settings, thus establishing a Proven Acceptable Range (PAR), i.e. a characterised range of a process parameter for which operation within this range, while keeping other parameters constant, will result in a product meeting the relevant quality criteria.
8) Allow for multiple response optimization. As pharmaceutical products exhibit several CQAs, the latter require simultaneous optimization.

9) Make the product or process more robust, in other words relatively insensitive against external and non-controllable influences.
10) Assure protection from outliers through their effective identification within the structured experimental matrices.

In contrast, OFAT approaches target on the identification of local sub-optimum regions based on changing one factor at a time. This obsolete, time-consuming technique is incapable of supporting the simultaneous study of several factor changes or identifying causal relationships including interactions. Such deficiencies make OFAT inappropriate for QbD applications.

Therefore, the design of experiment (DoE) can be defined as a structured and organised method which is used to determine the relationships between the factors that can. affect a process and output of that process. Alternatively, the design of experiment is a way to achieve the knowledge of a process, through the establishment of mathematical relationships between process inputs and its outputs.

Thus, a process would be a value-added activity by transforming a numbers of process inputs into the outputs. This would be done under the influence of various factors, categorised as controllable and uncontrollable, the latter is described as noise. They occur randomly and have an overall minimal effect compared to the controlled ones[64]. However, within the concept of experimental design, Montgomery differentiates the process variables into potential design and nuisance factors. These are subsequently classified as controllable, uncontrollable or noise. The latter correspond to uncontrolled and unavoidable variation, which is expressed through the experimental error.

The effect of the controlled factors on the quality characteristics of the final product varies according to a general pattern which is known as the Pareto principle, indicating that a relatively small number of factors are responsible for the substantial percentage of the effect. This is also called as the 20:80 rule, stating that 20% of the causes (factors) are responsible for 80% of the results (responses).

The most influential factors have been defined in ICH Q8 as Critical Process Parameters (CPPs). The process parameters whose variability has an effect on a critical quality attribute of the product. Therefore, these should be monitored and controlled to ensure that the process produces the desired quality. The latter is the sum of the product's characteristics, which should consistently comply with predefined ranges, widely known as specifications.

The ICH Q8 defines Critical Quality Attributes (CQAs) as physical, chemical, biological, or microbiological properties or characteristics that should be within an appropriate limit, i.e. range or distribution to ensure the desired product quality. DoE is an approach where the controlled input factors of the process are systematically and purposefully varied in order to determine their effects on the responses. The overall scope is the connection of the CPPs (x_1, x_2,.x_i) with the CQAs (y_i) through mathematical functions y¼ f(x), as described in Figure 2.8.

Factorial (Process) Designs

In factorial designs, intentionally and simultaneously the process parameters are varied according to a predetermined matrix of factor levels combinations. Their main difference from mixture designs is that each factor can be adjusted independently of the others. Factors are usually represented by capital letters (A, B, C ...), while their lower and higher levels are designated with (-) or -1 and (+) or +1, respectively. In case a middle level exists, this is described as (0).

This is obviously a coded representation of the levels, which, however, corresponds to actual values of the parameters, according to the following equation:

$$X_{coded} = (X_{actual} - X_{mean}) / [(X_{high} - X_{low}) /2] \quad .....(2.1)$$

Full factorials include all possible combinations of factor levels. The number of experiments required is provided by the following equation:

$$\text{Number of experiments} = \text{Levels}^{\text{Factors}} \quad .....(2.2)$$

For example, a full two-level factorial for three factors requires 2^3 =8 experiments.

Fig 2.8 shows simple two-level factorial designs for two and three factors.

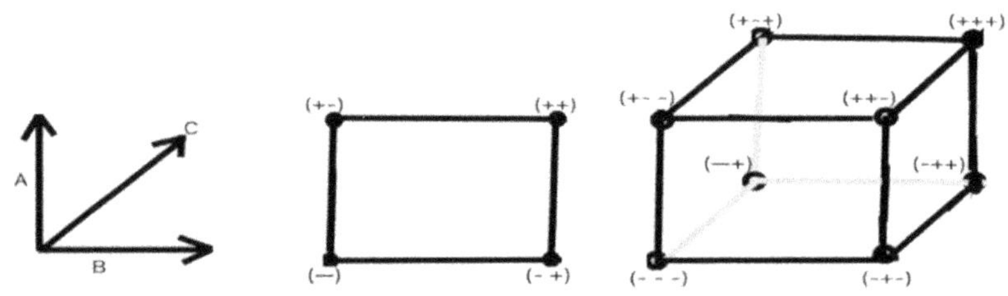

Fig.2.8 Schematic diagram of two level full factorial designs for two (A and B, center) and three (A, B, and C, right) factors.

The fractional factorial designs show a part of the relevant full design, typically $\frac{1}{2}$ or $\frac{1}{4}$....... of the full factorial design. They are typically used when the number of factors is more than 4 –5, for screening purposes. The term "resolution" means the ability of a design to estimate the effects and interactions without confounding. The most common resolution ranks are as follows.

- Resolution III designs indicate that main effects are not named as other main effects but may be named as two factor interactions, while some of the latter may be named to each other. These can be misleading when two-factor interactions significantly affect the response.

- Resolution IV designs indicate that the main effects are not named as other main effects or two factor interactions but could be named with three factor interactions. Moreover, two-factor interactions are named with each other. These form an appropriate choice for screening purposes, as the main effects will be clear of any two-factor interactions.
- Resolution V (or higher) designs have practically the same performance as full factorials. These can effectively reduce the required number of experiments. These indicate that no main effect or two-factor interaction has the name as with other main effects or two-factor interactions. The latter could be named as three-factor interactions. Assuming that three-factor (and higher) interactions are not significant or likely to occur. All the main effects and two-factor interactions can be measured.

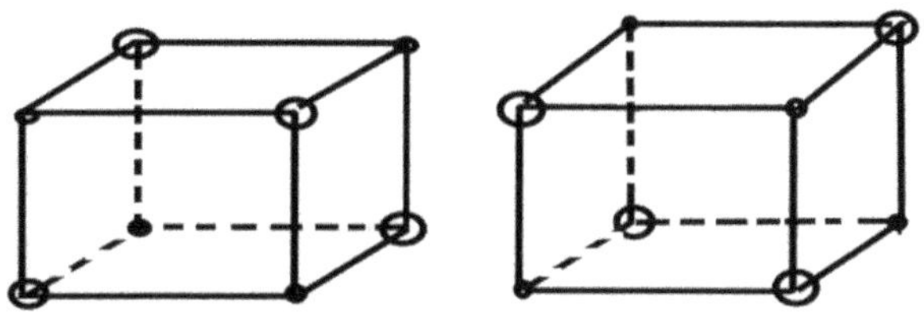

Fig.2.9 Graphical representation of a half fractional factorial at two levels for four factors.

When the resolution of design is lower, the ambiguity during the interpretation of the results is increased. A half fractional two-level factorial for four factors is presented in Figure 2.10. Each cube represents the levels of the three first factors, A, B, C, at the two different levels of the fourth factor D. It is quite known that in this case only half of the design (circled points) is executed, that is, eight out of the total 16 points of the relevant full factorial design. The scope of a DoE is the development of mathematical equations that can relate the factors to the responses. The latter can depend on either to the factors themselves (main effects) or their interactions. Main effect of a factor is the average change observed in the response, while this specific factor changes from its low to high level. It is measured as the difference between the average response at the high factor level minus the average response at the same factors at low level. In several cases, apart from the main effects, interactions between the factors are observed and should be carefully addressed. An interaction between two factors A and B is presented as AB, and means that the effect of factor A on the response is different at the various levels of factor B. In this case the interaction is calculated as the half of the difference of the response of factor A at the low level and high levels of factor B or Interaction AB $= \frac{1}{2}$ [Effect of A at (B^+) - Effect of A at (B^-)]

Exercise

Multiple Choice Questions

1. Whether the statement below stated is true or false?
   a) The additives have considerable impact on the drug substance.
   b) True
   c) False
2. Which type of interactions are commonly found to take place between drug substance and additive present in the formulation?
   a) Additive- additive interactions
   b) Additive-packaging packaging material
   c) Oxidative interaction.
   d) None of the above
3. According to the Bio-pharmaceutical Classification System, a dug substance can be said to be Class III when.............
   a) Its solubility is high, and its permeability is low.
   b) Its solubility is low, and its permeability is high.
   c) Its solubility low, and its permeability is low.
   d) Its solubility high, and its permeability is high.
4. The solubility of the drug is called high, when ....
   a) The largest dose of a drug dissolves in 250 ml of water over a pH range 7- 10
   b) The largest dose of a drug dissolves in 250 ml of water over a pH range 1- 6
   c) The largest dose of a drug dissolves in 250 ml of water over a pH range 1- 3,
   d) The largest dose of a drug dissolves in 250 ml of water over a pH range 1- 8,
5. The permeability of a drug substance would be called high, when................
   a) When the extent of absorption is > 90%,
   b) When the extent of absorption is > 50%,
   c) When the extent of absorption is > 30%,
   d) When the extent of absorption is > 10%,

6. Which of the following drugs is limited by the absorption by their dissolution rates?
   a) Diazepam,
   b) Digoxin,
   c) Chlorpheniramine,
   d) Furosemide.
7. Which of the following is a water-soluble base?
   a) Cholesterol
   b) Wool-fat
   c) Mixture of high molecular weight PEG and low molecular weight PEG
   d) Wool-alcohol
8. Sodium lauryl sulphate is an..............
   a) Non-anionic
   b) Cationic
   c) Non-ionic
   d) Anionic
9. Which of the following is a natural sweetener?
   a) Mannitol
   b) Saccharine
   c) Aspartame
   d) All of the above
10. Which of the following is physicochemical property?
    a) Release rate and dose
    b) pH-ionisation constant
    c) Absorption
    d) Therapeutic index
11. In the pharmaceutical industries, drug development is a ....
    a) Low trend
    b) Medium trend
    c) High trend
    d) None of the above
12. Moisture absorption is governed by.................
    a) The partial vapour pressure of water in the environment
    b) Source of heat
    c) Surface area of the solid
    d) Velocity of the moist air

13. Dry powders can be used for film coating to minimize or eliminate the use of.....
    a) Solvent
    b) Water
    c) Both
    d) None

14. Which of the following material is not popularly used as wall material in microencapulasion?
    a) Dextran
    b) Maltodextrin
    c) Gum Arabic
    d) Chitosan

15. Fill in the blank correctly using any one of following phrase words.

    The new grades of existing excipients would not continue to be introduced to meet the requirements of user and the needs of new enabling technologies, such as, ...'
    a) Hot-melt extrusion,
    b) Spray dried amorphous dispersions,
    c) Spay dried crystalline dispersion,
    d) None of the above

16. Which of the following is correct?
    a) Calcium silicate (FLR) is a porous compound.
    b) True
    c) False

17. Fill in the blank correctly with the words given in (b), (c) and (d)
    a) ....needs a single polymer and a cross-linker to make coacervation with itself.
    b) Complex compound
    c) Complex coacervation
    d) Gelation

18. Which of the following statements is correct one?
    a) For preparation of W/O/W emulsion of hydrophobic drugs, a two-step adaption process is typically required,
    b) For preparation of O/W/O emulsion of hydrophobic drugs, a two-step adaption process is typically required,
    c) For preparation of W/O/W emulsion of hydrophilic drugs, a two-step adaption process is typically required,
    d) For preparation of W/O/W emulsion of hydrophobic drugs, a two-step absorption process is typically required,

19. Fill in the blank correctly using any one of following phrase words.

    'The excipients added should mostly be inert in terms of t............. effects, and should not produce undesired alterations such as phase or stability changes in the drugs during manufacturing and storage.

    a) prophylactic
    b) chemical
    c) therapeutic
    d) physical

20. Which of the following statements is correct one?

    a) The FDA now encourages 3-bach verification of product manufacture to demonstrate that each batch manufactured is fit for the purpose.
    b) The FDA now encourages continuous verification of product manufacture to demonstrate that each batch manufactured is fit for the purpose.
    c) The FDA now encourages 5-batches verification of product manufacture to demonstrate that each batch manufactured is fit for the purpose.
    d) The FDA now encourages 10-batches verification of product manufacture to demonstrate that each batch manufactured is fit for the purpose.

Short Questions

1. What are the functional roles of an additive in the dosage form and on the drug substance?
2. What are commonly bases used in different types of formulation. Write down one or two lines of each of them.
3. Explain elimination half-life of drug.
4. Classify the additives used in pharmaceutical formulations.
5. Explain the relation between 'therapeutic window 'and 'therapeutic efficacy 'of a drug substance.
6. What are the different steps involved in formulation development?
7. Write down formulation strategies to reduce or control hygroscopicity.
8. What in meant by 'particle engineering'?
9. What is 'Central composite design (CCD)'?
10. What are the advantages of factorial design?

Long Questions

1. What are the additives used in solid dosage form? Are the same additives used in semi-solid and solid dosage forms – justify your answer.
2. Explain the additives used to design a liquid dosage form.
3. Explain high permeability of drug substances.
4. How can the partition coefficient of a drug can influence a formulation? Is there any link between partition coefficient and ionization constant-explain.
5. Explain the effect of protein-drug binding on the therapeutic efficacy of a drug substance.
6. What are the adverse effects of moisture on pharmaceutical solid dosage forms? Write down the five factors that govern the moisture absorption.
7. How are the film coating and coacervation related to each other? Write down the process of Double-Emulsion Complex Coacervation for Hydrophilic drugs.
8. What are various techniques of encapsulation? What is meant by co-processing with excipients?
9. What do you about new development in excipient science?
10. How can you develop a process with design of experiments?

Answers

1	2	3	4	5	6	7	8	9	10	11	12	13	14	15	16	17	18	19	20
b	c	a	d	a	b	c	d	a	b	c	d	c	a	c	b	d	a	c	b

References

1. Tekade, R.K., Maheshwari, R., Jain, N.K.; Toxicity of nanostructured biomaterials A2 Narayan, Roger. Nanobiomaterials. Woodhead Publishing; 2018. 9.
2. Katdare, A.; Excipient Development for Pharmaceutical, Biotechnology, and Drug Delivery Systems. Informa Healthcare USA, Inc., New York, NY.; 2006.
3. Katdare, A.; Excipient Development for Pharmaceutical, Biotechnology, and Drug Delivery Systems.; Informa Healthcare USA, Inc., New York, NY.; 2006.
4. Kalazs, H., Antal, I.; Drug Excipients; Current Medicinal Chemistry; 13, 2535 – 2563, 2006.

5. Weber, R., Ruppik, M., Rickenbach, M., Spoerrii, A., Furrer, H., Battegay, M., Cavassini, M., Calmy, A., Bernasconi, E., Schmid, P., Flepp, M., Kowalska, J., Ledgerber, B.; Decreasing mortality and changing patterns of causes of death in the Swiss HIV Cohort Study; Swiss HIV Cohort Study (SHCS); 24 September 2012.

6. Ramesh Kumar, S., Mohan, S.D.; Pharmaceutical excipient development from natural source, compressed.; Asian J. Pharm. Heal. Sci.; 2, 620626, 2014.

7. Alfonso.R. Remington's "The science and practice of pharmacy", 20th edition,. pp. 903-929. 2002.

8. Bechgaard. H and G.H. Nelson. Controlled release multiple units and single unit doses.; Drug Dev. Ind. Pharm; 4, 1978.

9. Madhukat, Mansukal Doshi, Milind, Dattatraya Joshi, Bharat Pravinchandra Mehta. Pharmaceutical composition for controlled drug delivery system, patent No: US 7,157,100 B2, Jan. 2, 2007.

10. James Swarbrick, James C. Boylan. Encyclopedia of Pharmaceutical Technology. pp. 369-394, 2007.

11. Gasser R, Klein W, Koppel H, Lercanidipine, a new third generation Ca-antagonist in the treatment of hypertension, Journal of clinical and basic cardiology :169-174, 1999.

12. Venkataraman Daar.S N, Chester.A, Kliener.L. An overview of Controlled-release systems, Handbook of Pharmaceutical Controlled release technology, Marcel dekker Inc: 1-30, 2000.

13. Brahma Singh. N, Kwon Kim. H. Drug delivery Oral route, Encyclopedia of pharmaceutical technology, vol no 1. pp. 1242-1261, 2007.

14. Staney Davis S. Formulation strategies for absorption windows. Drug Discovery Today. Vol 10, No 4, 2005.

15. Joseph Robinson. R, Vincent H. L. Lee, Controlled drug delivery fundamentals and applications, Marcel Dekker Inc, New York:3-61, 2002.

16. Marc Maillard. P, Julie Hans-R. Brunner, and Michel Burnier. "Tasosartan, Enoltasosartan, and Angiotensin 2 Receptor Blockade: The Confounding Role of Protein Binding",The journal of pharmacology and experimental therapeutics. pp. 649-653, 2005.

17. Del cavillo, J Mullol, J Barta, Davila, Jauregui, J Montoro, J sastre, AL Valero, Comparative pharmacology of the H1 anti histamines, J Investig Allergol Clin Immunol, 16:3-12, 2006.

18. Porter, M.; *Competitive Strategy.* New Yoi-k: Free Press, 1980.

19. Penrose, E. T.; The Theory of the Growth of the Firm.; Ncw York: Wiley. 1959.
20. Andrews, K. R.; The Concept of Corporate Strategy. Jones-Irwin, 197I.
21. Grant, R. M.; "The resource-based theory of competitive advantage," Calif: Manage. Rev., vol. 33, no. 3, pp. 114-135, 1991.
22. Mahoney, J. T. and Pandian, J. R.; "The resource-based view within the conversation of strategic management," Strategic Manage. .I.; 13, *5* , pp. 363-380, 1992.
23. Reed, R. and DeFillipi, R. J.; "Causal ambiguity, barriers to imitation, and sustainable competitive advantage;" Acad, Manage. Rev.; 15, 1, pp. 88-102, 1990.
24. Werimfelt, B.; "A resource-based view of the firm," Strategic Manage J.; 5, pp 171-181, 1984
25. Teece, D J., Pismo, G and., Shuen, G.; "Dynamic capabilities and strategic management," working paper; Univ Calif Berkeley; 1992
26. Kogut, B. and, Zander, U.; "Knowledge of the firm, combinative capabilities, and the replication of' technology," Orgonic. Sci.; 3, 3, pp. 383-397, 1992.
27. Duncan, R. and Weiss, A.; "Organizational learning: Implications for organizational design," in Research in Organi7ationnl Behavior. vol. I , B. Staw, Ed. Greenwich, CT: JAl, 1979.
28. Fiol , C. M.and Lylcs, M. A.; "Organizational Iearning," Arad. Mannge. Rev.. vol. 10, pp. 803-813, 1985.
29. Starbuck, W. H.; "Learning by knowledge-intensive firms," J Manage Studies,; 29, pp 713-740, 1992
30. Hedberg, B.; "How Organizations learn and unlearn," in Handbook of Organizational Design,; 1, P. C. Nystrom and W. H. Starbuck, Eds. Ncw York: Oxford, 1981
31. Shaikh, A.C., Shaikh, S. S., Shaikh, A.M., Gaikwad, M. S., Shinde, P.B.; Review- Formulation Development Studies; IJCRT; 10, 3 2022.
32. Khankaria, R.K., Grant, D.J.W.; Pharmaceutical hydrates.; Thermochim. Acta; 1995, *248*, 61–79.
33. Yang, Q., Yuan, F., Xu, L., Yan, Q., Yang, Y., Wu, D., Guo, F., Yang, G.; An Update of Moisture Barrier Coating for Drug Delivery.; Pharmaceutics,; *11*, 436, 2019.
34. Aguilar-Toala, J.E., Quintanar-Guerrero, D., Liceaga, A.M., Zambrano-Zaragoza, M.L.; Encapsulation of bioactive peptides: A strategy to

improve the stability, protect the nutraceutical bioactivity and support their food applications.; RSC Adv;. 12, 6449–6458., 2022,

35. Giroldi, M., Grambusch, I.M., Neutzling Lehn, D., Volken de Souza, C.F.; Encapsulation of dairy protein hydrolysates: Recent trends and future prospects.; Dry. Technol.; 39, 1513–1528, 2021.

36. Mendanha, D.V., Molina Ortiz, S.E., Favaro-Trindade, C.S., Mauri, A.; Monterrey-Quintero, E.S.; Thomazini, M. Microencapsulation of casein hydrolysate by complex coacervation with SPI/pectin.; Food Res. Int.; 42, 1099–1104, 2009.

37. Timilsena, Y.P.; Akanbi, T.O.; Khalid, N.; Adhikari, B.; Barrow, C.J. Complex coacervation: Principles, mechanisms and applications in microencapsulation.; Int. J. Biol. Macromol.; 121, 1276–1286, 2019.

38. Kanha, N., Regenstein, J.M., Surawang, S., Pitchakarn, P., Laokuldilok, T.; Properties and kinetics of the in vitro release of anthocyanin-rich microcapsules produced through spray and freeze-drying complex coacervated double emulsions.; Food Chem.; 340, 127950, 2021.

39. Huang, X., Ganzle, M., Zhang, H., Zhao, M., Fang, Y., Nishinari, K.; Microencapsulation of probiotic lactobacilli with shellac as moisture barrier and to allow controlled release.; J. Sci. Food Agric.; 101, 726–734, 2021.

40. Yang, Y., Cheow, W.S.; Hadinoto, K.; Dry powder inhaler formulation of lipid-polymer hybrid nanoparticles via electrostatically-driven nanoparticle assembly onto microscale carrier particles.; Int. J. Pharm.; 434, 49–58, 2012.

41. Moreton, R.C.; Tablet excipients to the year 2001: A look into the crystal ball; Drug Dev. Ind. Pharm.; 22, (1), 11 – 23, 1996.

42. Katz, J.S., Nolin, A., Yezer, B.A., and Jordan, S.; Dynamic properties of novel excipient suggest mechanism for improved performance in liquid stabilization of protein biologics; Mol. Pharm.; 16, 282 -291, 2019.

43. Appendix II: HPE Laboratory Methods, in Handbook of Pharmaceutical Excipients, 2nd Ed., Wade A and Weller PJ (eds.), American Pharmaceutical Society, Washington, DC and The Pharmaceutical Press, London, UK,, pp 625 – 632, 1994.

44. NSF/IPEC/ANSI 363 – 2014 Good Manufacturing Practices (GMP) for Pharmaceutical Excipients, Joint Committee on Pharmaceutical Excipients, Ann Arbor, MI.

45. Yu LX, Amidon G, Khan MA, Hoag SW, Polli J, Raju GK, Woodcock J. Understanding pharmaceutical quality by design. AAPS J. 2014;16(4):771-783.

46. Sangshetti JN, Deshpande M, Zaherr Z, Shinde DB, Arote R. Quality by design approach: regulatory need. Arab J Chem. 2017;10 (Suppl 2):S3412-S3425.

47. Bhutani H, Kurmi M, Singh S, Beg S, Singh B. Quality by design (QbD) in analytical sciences: an overview. Pharma Times. 2014;46(8):71-75.

48. Peraman R, Bhadraya K, Reddy YP. Analytical quality by design: a tool for regulatory flexibility and robust analytics. Int J Anal Chem. 2015;2015:1-9.

49. Hald AA. History of mathematical statistics. New York: Wiley; 1998.

50. Fridrun Podczeck, Aims and objectives of experimental design and optimization in formulation and process development, in: Larry Augsburger L, Stephen Hoag W. Pharmaceutical dosage forms: tablets 3rd ed. (2), Informa Health Care, New york, 2008.

51. Sanford Bolton, Charles Bon. Pharmaceutical Statistices. Practical and Clinical applications, 4th ed. (135), Mark Dekker, NY, 2005.

52. Singh B, Ahuja N. Book review on Pharmaceutical experimental design, Int J Pharm., 248, 195- 247, 200

53. Design Space and PAT- Q8ICH. Draft guidance on pharmaceutical development by Kovalycsik, Wyeth research vaccines Rand D. Quality operations.

54. Krupakar BR. Design of experiments for pharmaceutical formulation development; Pharmainfo.net.; 6 (4), 2008.

55. Adetogun, GE., Alebiowu, G.; Evaluation of the qualitative effects of variables on a paracetamol tablet formulation prepared with gum as binding agent,; J pharm. Res.; 8 (4), 176-180, 2009.

56. ICH Q8(R2), Pharmaceutical Development, Guideline, Available from: http://www.ich.org/fileadmin/Public_Web_Site/ICH_Products/Guidelines/Quality/Q8_R1/Step4/Q8_R2_ Guideline.

57. Juran JM. Quality by design, the new steps for planning quality into goods and services. US: The Free Press; 1992.

58. Deming WE Institute, Available from: http:// demining.org/therman/theories/profound knowledge, last accessed 4 Nov 2016.

59. Shewhart WE. Economic control of quality of manufactured product. New York: D. Van Nostrand Company; 1931.

60. Marlow E, Shangraw RF. Dissolution of sodium salicylate from tablet matrices prepared by wet granulation and direct compression. J Pharm Sci 1967;56:498–504.

61. Montgomery DC. Design and analysis of experiments. 8th edn. New York: John Wiley Sons, Inc.; 2013.

62. Barker TB. Quality by experimental design. New York: Marcel Dekker, Inc.; 1985.

63. Lewis GA, Mathieu D, Phan-Tan-Luu R. Pharmaceutical experimental design. New York: Marcel Dekker, Inc.; 1999.

64. Montgomery, DC.; Introduction to statistical quality control. 6th edn.; New York: John Wiley Sons Inc; 2009.

CHAPTER - 3

Solubility

Importance, Experimental Determination, Phase- Solubility Analysis, Ph-Solubility Profile, Solubility Techniques to Improve Solubility and Utilisation of Analytical Methods – Cosolvency, Salt Formation, Complexation, Solid Dispersion, Micellar Solubilization and Hydrotropy.

IMPORTANCE

Ingestion through oral route is the most convenient and commonly employed route of drug delivery due to its ease of administration, high patient compliance, cost effectiveness, least sterility constraints, and flexibility in the design of dosage form. As a result, many of the generic drug companies are inclined more to produce bio-equivalent oral drug[1]. However, the major challenge with the design of oral dosage forms lies with their poor bioavailability. The oral bioavailability depends on several factors, such as, aqueous solubility, drug permeability, dissolution rate, first-pass metabolism, pre-systemic metabolism, and susceptibility to efflux mechanisms. The most frequent causes of low oral bioavailability are attributed to poor solubility and low permeability. Solubility also plays a major role for other dosage forms like parenteral formulations as well[2]. Solubility is one of the important parameters to achieve desired concentration of drug in systemic circulation for achieving required pharmacological response[3]. Poorly water-soluble drugs often require high doses in order to reach therapeutic plasma concentrations after oral administration. Low aqueous solubility is the major problem encountered with formulation development of new chemical entities as well as generic development. Any drug to be absorbed must be present in the form of an aqueous solution at the site of absorption. Water is the solvent of choice for liquid pharmaceutical formulations. Most of the drugs are either weakly acidic or weakly basic having poor aqueous solubility. More than 40% NCEs (new chemical entities) developed in pharmaceutical industry are practically insoluble in water. These poorly water-soluble drugs having slow drug absorption leads to inadequate and variable bioavailability and gastrointestinal mucosal toxicity. For orally administered drugs solubility is the most important one rate limiting parameter to achieve their desired concentration in systemic circulation for pharmacological response. Problem of solubility is a major challenge for formulation scientist[4].

The improvement of drug solubility thereby its oral bioavailability remains one of the most challenging aspects of drug development process especially for oral-drug delivery system. There are numerous approaches available and reported in the literature to improve the solubility of poorly water-soluble drugs. The techniques are chosen on the basis of certain aspects such as

- Properties of drug under consideration,
- Nature of excipients to be selected, and
- Nature of intended dosage form.

The poor solubility and low dissolution rate of poorly water-soluble drugs in the aqueous gastrointestinal fluids often cause insufficient bioavailability. Especially for class II (low solubility and high permeability) substances according to the BCS, the bioavailability may be enhanced by increasing the solubility and dissolution rate of the drug in the gastrointestinal fluids. As for BCS class II drugs rate limiting step is drug release from the dosage form and solubility in the gastric fluid and not the absorption, so increasing the solubility in turn increases the bioavailability for BCS class II drugs[5].

The negative effect of compounds with low solubility includes poor absorption and bioavailability, insufficient solubility for IV dosing, development challenges leading to increasing the development cost and time, burden shifted to patient (frequent high-dose administration).

EXPERIMENTAL DETERMINATION OF SOLUBILITY

Solubility is defined as *the amount of substance that passes into solution to achieve a saturated solution at constant temperature and pressure.* Solubility is expressed in terms of maximum volume or mass of the solute that can be dissolved in a given volume or mass of a solvent. Pharmacopoeias refer to the meaning of the term, *solubility* in terms of the number of parts by volume of solvent would be required to dissolve one part by weight of a solid, or one part by volume of a liquid.

The dissolution rate and the release rate of a drug are essential to be known for characterisation of drug. In order to measure the dissolution an instrument called rotating disc is used. It is necessary to investigate with the help of rotating disc method to secure a robust method of dissolution measurements. The benefit of the rotating disc method is that it uses well defined dissolution process and easy to use equipment to achieve good reproducibility. The purpose of this paper is therefore to give a wide introduction to dissolution in the Pharmacopeial area and a make a pre-study of the rotating disc. The focus will be on determining the important factors that might affect the method and then make further analysis of the most important factor. Securing the reliability also means investigating the reproducibility of the method.

Solubility

Solubility is defined as the amount of substance that goes into solution to produce a saturated solution at constant temperature and pressure. Solubility is expressed in terms of maximum volume or mass of the solute that is dissolved in a given volume or mass of a solvent. In Pharmacopoeias the term solubility is defined in terms of the number of parts by volume of solvent required to dissolve one part by weight of a solid, or one part by volume of a liquid.

Intrinsic Solubility

In the pharmaceutical industry, the intrinsic solubility is measured to indicate the solubility of a substance. Intrinsic solubility refers to the equilibrium solubility at thermodynamic equilibrium of the pure uncharged compound/drug. The term intrinsic means that *the species in solution is the same as that of the solid form.* Measurements are taken at two temperatures, at first 4°C it ensures physical and chemical stability for short-term storage. A minimum in aqueous solubility can be observed at 4°C because of a maximum of water density. The second temperature of interest is 37°C, to support biopharmaceutical evaluation.

The hypothetical compound/drug/chemical AB illustrates solubility as follows:

$$AB_{solid} \underset{}{\overset{K_o}{\rightleftharpoons}} AB_{soln} \underset{}{\overset{K_o'}{\rightleftharpoons}} A^+ + B^-$$

Where, $AB_{(solid)}$ refers to a chemical substance in the solid form, $AB_{(soln)}$ refers to the chemical in solution in an undissociated form and (A^+) and (B^-) to ions of the dissociated solute in solution. Salts from strong acids (Cl^-, SO_4^{2-}, NO_3^-) are not protonized, they are neutral. An exception is aluminium salts of strong acids, they are basic in. nature. Salts from weak acids can be pronized. The equilibrium solubility relationship for a non-electrolyte where the equilibrium constant, K_o, is also known as S_o, the intrinsic solubility:

$$K_o = \frac{(AB)_{soln}}{(AB)_{solid}} = S_o$$

The total solubility observed represents the sum of the equilibrium concentrations of all species present. For a non-electrolyte, the total solubility is called the intrinsic solubility. Non-electrolytes, and strong electrolytes where neither A nor B is acidic or basic. They generally do not display solubility characteristics that are directly dependent on pH. But most drugs are weak bases and around 20% are weak acids and only 5% are non-ionic.[6] The Henderson-Hasselbalch equations are used to find the intrinsic solubility for weak bases and acids.

$$pH = pK_a + \log_{10}([B]/[BH^+])$$

$$pH = pK_a + \log_{10}([A^-]/[AH])$$

A saturated aqueous solution of the salt of a weak base has a concentration equal to the intrinsic solubility of the salt, and it will be relatively acidic (it will have a pH usually more that 2 units below the pKa of the weak base). The intrinsic solubility of the weak base is the lowest observed solubility, and it will be observed when pH is more than 2 units above the pKa.

A saturated aqueous solution of the salt of a weak acid has a concentration equal to the intrinsic solubility of the salt, and it will be relatively basic (it will have a pH usually more than 2 units above the pKa of the weak acid). The intrinsic solubility of the weak acid is the lowest observed solubility, and it will be observed when pH is more than 2 units below the pKa.

Measurement of Solubility

In pharmaceutical practice, one important task is to measure the solubility of solids in liquids. The following precautions serve as guidelines when running the solubility tests:

- The solvent and the solute must be pure.
- The sample is removed for analysis after confirmation of saturation.
- Sample separation from saturated solution with un-dissolved solute must be reliable and satisfactory.
- The method used to analyse the solution must be reliable and reproducible.
- Temperature must be adequately controlled.

Traditionally, the equilibrium solubility at a given pH and temperature is determined by the shake flask method. According to this method, the compound is added in surplus to a certain volume of medium and shaken for a predetermined time, usually 24h or longer. The saturation is confirmed by observation of the presence of un-dissolved material in the solution. Saturation can also be reached, if the solvent and excess solute is heated and then allowed to cool to the given temperature. Some solutions can hold a certain amount of excess solute in the solvent, commonly called a supersaturated solution. This often occurs when the saturated solution is cooled slowly. Super saturation for salts can be avoided by slow cooling and continuous shaking of the sample during cool down period. After filtration of the slurry a sample for analysis can be taken. Both filtration and analysis should be performed under the same temperature as the solubility determination and under conditions to minimise loss of volatile components. Often the sample is diluted to prevent crystallisation. The amount of solute contained in the sample is determined by an appropriate method affected by the nature of the solute/solvent and by the concentration. Common methods are;

- Ultraviolet /visible spectroscopy
- Chromatographic methods
- Gravimetric/volumetric

The shake-flask method is the most accurate method to determine solubility but, it is time consuming. Due to the growing need to determine solubility faster new devices[7,8] and automated methods[9,10] have been developed.

1. Miniaturised shake-flask method can be used for almost all compounds. Its precision and throughput was proven greater the potentiometric method. Up to 20 compounds per week can be studied with one set-up. The miniaturised shake-flask method needs more drug to ensure an equilibrium between solid and dissolved drug.[11]
2. Semiautomated potentiometric acid/base titrations method is a very economical method and is able to create a pH/solubility profile with one single determination. Only 100 μg of poorly soluble drug substance is required. Depending on the compound, the time required for a potentiometric titration may vary; whereas the time consumption with a shake-flask method is fixed but generally it requires more time. This method is limited to ionisable compounds.[12]
3. A computational screening model is used for the prediction of intrinsic solubility, which is based on lipophilicity and molecular surface area.[13]
4. Another devise, simply called miniature device, has been developed for measuring aqueous and non-aqueous equilibrium solubility during drug discovery. With only ≈ 1mg of compound, it can be possible to determine the entire pH-solubility profile. This devise can produce similar solubility values compared to other conventional shake-flask methods.[14]

Biopharmaceutics Classification System

The Biopharmaceutics Classification System[15] is used to classify the drug substances on the basis of their aqueous solubility and intestinal permeability. BCS introduces an in vitro-in vivo correlation and is the first step to approve a product based on in vitro dissolution tests rather than bioequivalence studies in human subjects. As a result, the unnecessary human experiments can be avoided. Thus, it lowers the development costs of new drugs. Solubility is based on the highest dose strength and is considered highly soluble, if it is soluble in 250 ml or less of aqueous media over the pH range of 1.0 - 7.5. Otherwise, it is considered to be poorly soluble. Permeability is based indirectly on the measurement of the rate of mass transfer across the human intestinal membrane. Models capable of predicting the extent of intestinal absorption in humans may be used as alternatives. A drug substance is considered highly permeable when its intestinal absorption is determined to be 90% or higher. Otherwise, it is considered to be poorly permeable. Combined with in vitro dissolution characteristics of the drug, BCS takes into account all factors that govern the rate and extent of oral drug absorption for immediate release dosage forms. The theoretical considerations suggested by Amidon in1995 describes a simplified model with three dimensional numbers controlling drug absorption with Dose Number D_o, Dissolution Number D_n and Absorption Number A_n. This model gives a basis to determine when and under what conditions in vitro-in vivo correlations are to be expected. The definitions are shown below.

$$D_o = \frac{M_o / V_o}{C_s}$$

$$D_n = \frac{DC_s}{r_o} \cdot \frac{4\pi r_o^2}{4/3\pi r_o^3 p} \cdot t_{res} = \frac{t_{res}}{t_{diss}}$$

$$A_n = \frac{P_{eff}}{R} \cdot t_{res}$$

$$t_{res} = \frac{\pi R^2 L}{Q}$$

$$t_{diss} = \frac{r_o^2 p}{3DC_s}$$

Where, the dose of the drug administered is M_o, the initial gastric volume V_o, the saturation solubility C_s, the diffusion coefficient D, the initial particle radius r_o, the density ρ, tube length L, fluid flow rate Q, tube radius R, the mean residence time t_{res}, the time required for a particle of the drug to dissolve t_{diss}, the effective permeability P_{eff}, and the segment radius R.

According to solubility and permeability of the drug, the BCS introduces four classes of drug. The permeability of the drug is difficult to obtain and is often derived from the fraction of the drug absorbed. For class I drugs *in vitro-in vivo* correlation may be expected if dissolution rate is slower than gastric emptying rate. For class II drugs an *in vitro-in vivo* correlation is expected if in vivo and in vitro dissolution rates are similar. For class III drugs limited to no *in vitro-in vivo* correlation is expected because the absorption is the rate determine step. Class IV show limited or no in vitro-in vivo correlation.

PHASE-SOLUBILITY ANALYSIS

When two or more substances are mixed together in solution, it must be considered as solubility. Solubility may be defined as *the maximum concentration of a substance that may be completely dissolved in a given volume of solvent at a given temperature and pressure*. When both solute and solvent are liquids, the term miscibility rather than solubility is used to describe the affinity between the liquids. The solubility of a substance may be described in a variety of ways. The USP/NF generally expresses the solubility in terms of the volume of solvent required to dissolve 1 gram of the drug substance at a specified temperature, such as 1 g of acetyl salicylic acid in 300 ml water, 5 ml ethanol at 25°C. Other references may use more subjective terms to describe solubility.

Liquids which form a homogenous system when mixed in any proportion are said to be miscible, such as water and ethanol. Those in which only certain volume ratios produce homogenous mixtures are said to be miscible in certain proportions, such as water and chloroform. Immiscible liquids will not produce a homogenous solution in any proportions such as water and olive oil[16].

Factors Influencing Solubility

Temperature

The solubility of a given solute in a given solvent often depends on temperature. For around 95% of solid solutes, the solubility increases with temperature[17], but gaseous solutes exhibit more complex behaviour. As the temperature is raised gases usually become less soluble in water, but more soluble in organic solvents. The chart shows solubility curves for some typical inorganic salts (all solids). Many salts behave like barium nitrate and disodium hydrogen arsenate and show a large increase in solubility with temperature. Some solutes (e.g. NaCl in water) are fairly independent of temperature. A few, such as cerium (III) sulphate, become less soluble in hot water. Occasionally, a more complex pattern is observed, as with sodium sulphate, where the less soluble decahydrate crystal loses water of crystallisation at 32°C to form a more soluble anhydrous phase. Organic compounds nearly always become soluble as the temperature is raised, in most solvents. The technique of recrystallisation, used for purification of solids, depends on this difference in solubility in hot and cold solvent. There are a few exceptions, such as certain cyclodextrins[18].

There is essentially no detectable heat effect in non-polar substances. The forces holding the particles together are small, and any interaction between solute and solvent is small.

Polar Substances

In polar substances, the energy is required to separate the molecule from surrounding molecules. This energy is supplied in the form of heat, producing a cooling effect. On the other hand, there is the possibility of interaction between the solute and solvent with formation of a dipole-dipole type bond, and this interaction will tend to release heat. Depending on which of the two interactions is greatest one can get an increase or decrease in temperature.

Presence of Multiple Solutes

The aqueous solubility of non-electrolytes is nearly always affected in some way by the addition of an electrolyte. Salting-out is the precipitation of organic solutes from aqueous solution by the addition of an electrolyte or salt. This is attributed to competition between solute molecules for the solvent and is dependent upon the size and valence of the ion. Salting-in is the increase in solubility of an organic solute upon addition of an electrolyte. The mechanism of this phenomenon is poorly understood, and it is rarely encountered. An example is with the group of proteins called globulins which are more soluble in dilute salt solutions than in water. Complex ion formation occurs when an insoluble solute reacts with a soluble substance to form a soluble complex. An example is the addition of the soluble potassium iodide (KI) to the insoluble iodine molecule (I_2) to form a soluble tri-iodide complex (KI_3).

Solute pKa, Solvent pH and Solubility

The Henderson-Hasselbalch equation states the relationship between pH, pka, and relative concentrations of an acid and its salt.

Non-ionisable Substances

Similar to the lack of effect of heat on the solubility of non-polar substances, there is little effect of pH on nonionisable substances. Nonionisable, hydrophobic substances can have improved solubility by changing the dielectric constant of the solvent using cosolvents rather than the pH of the solvent.

Ionisable Substances

For substances that have an ionisable component like a carboxylic acid (HA), solubility is a function of pH. As can be remembered from general chemistry, the pH of a substance is related to its pKa and the concentration of the ionised and unionised forms of the substance by the equation:

$$pH = pKa + \log(A^- /HA)$$

If the substance is brought outside its pKa, the pH value where half the substance is ionised and half is not, then the solubility will be changed because of introducing new intermolecular forces, mainly ionic attraction.

Where $[A^-]$ is the molar concentration of the salt (dissociated species) and [HA] is the concentration of the undissociated acid.

When the concentrations of salt and acid are equal, the pH of the system becomes equal to the pka of the acid. As the pH decreases, the concentration of the molecular acid increases and that of the salt decreases. This has some interesting implications on the aqueous solubility of the acid, since the undissociated form is much less soluble than its salt. It is more interesting, therapeutically, is that it is the undissociated acid (HA) that more readily penetrates biological tissues to exert a therapeutic effect. Thus, in formulating the product, some balance must be struck between the more soluble salt form and the biologically active acid and the factors other than pka and pH must be considered, such as, safety and comfort.

Solute molecules are held together by certain intermolecular forces (dipole-dipole, induced dipole-induced dipole, ion-ion, etc.), as are molecules of solvent. For dissolution to occur, these cohesive forces of like molecules must be broken and adhesive forces between solute and solvent must be formed. The solubility of a drug in a given solvent is largely a function of the polarity of the solvent. Solvents may be considered polar, semipolar or non-polar. Polar solvents will dissolve ionic and other polar solutes, that is, those with an asymmetric charge distribution (like dissolves like), whereas, non-polar solvents will dissolve non-polar molecules. For a substance to dissolve the cohesive energy of the bonds holding the solid or liquid solute together, and the energy cost of disrupting the solvent-to-solvent bonds must be overcome by the cohesive energy released by the formation of the solute-to-solvent bonds. Thus, there are two energy-costs- one is solute/solute and other is solvent/solvent and two energy-gains- two solute/solvent bonds. If these energies are approximately equal, which occurs when the solvent and solute molecules are structurally similar, then the substance will dissolve in the solvent. Hence, the saying: Likes dissolve Likes is justified as shown in Fig.3.1.

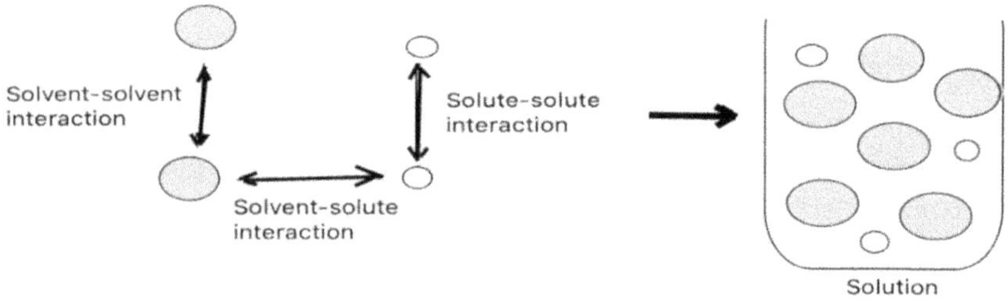

Fig.3.1 Like molecules like solution.

Semi-polar solvents, such as, alcohols and ketones may induce a certain degree of polarity in non-polar molecules and may act to improve the miscibility of polar and non-polar liquids. The relationship between polarity and solubility may be used in practice to alter the solubility of a drug in a pharmaceutical solution. One approach is to alter the polarity of the solute by shifting it between its molecular (undissociated) and ionic (dissociated) states. A shift towards the ionic form improves solubility of the solute in water and other polar solvents. A shift toward the molecular species improves solute solubility in non-polar solvents. Such shifts may be produced by altering the pH of the solution (or using the salt form of the compound). Another approach is to mix solvents of different polarities to form a solvent system of optimum polarity to dissolve the solute. Such solvents must, obviously, be miscible. This method is referred to as solvent blending or co-solvency and uses the dielectric constant as a guide to develop the co-solvent system. If we look at the structure of water, we see it is highly ordered due to hydrogen bonding caused by the dipole nature of the molecule. Due to this bonding with water molecule a good solvent for polar molecules and has a high dielectric constant.

The dielectric constant is a measure of the effect a substance has on the energy required to separate two oppositely charged bodies. A vacuum is arbitrarily given a dielectric constant of 1. If two oppositely charged bodies are put into any medium, the medium should tend to separate or make it more difficult for the two oppositely charged bodies to unite. The energy required to separate two oppositely charged bodies is inversely proportional to the dielectric constant of the medium. The dielectric constant is also a measure of the degree of polarisation in both an induced and permanent dipole. The dipole moment is a function of the charge and the distance between the charges. Associated molecules such as water and alcohol have high dipole moments and therefore, high dielectric constants because of the long-chain pseudo-molecules. Non-polar compounds like benzene do not have a sufficiently high dielectric constant to separate polar molecules. These compounds can only dissolve those molecules held together by very weak intermolecular forces (induced dipole-induced dipole), such as naphthalene. Because there are very weak interactions, that is, London forces between solute-solute, solute-solvent, and solvent-solvent molecules. These types of non-polar solutions behave nearly ideal. It should be remembered that ideal solutions imply there is no interaction between solvent and solute.

The dielectric constant of a compound is an index of its polarity. A series of solvents of increasing polarity shown in Table 3.1 will show a similar increase in dielectric constant.

Table 3.1 Dielectric constant of different solvents.

Solvent	Dielectric constant
Water	80
Sorbitol Solution USP (70% w/w)	62
Syrup USP	56
Glycerol (glycerin)	46
Methanol	33
Propylene glycol	32.1
Ethanol	25
n-Propyl alcohol	22
Acetone	21

Solvents may be classified according to their dielectric constants as polar ($\varepsilon > 50$), semi-polar ($\varepsilon = 20 - 50$), or non-polar ($\varepsilon = 1$ to 20). Water, on the other hand, cannot dissolve things like naphthalene because the attraction of water for naphthalene is much less than that of water for water. The classification of solvents on the basis of polarity is often referred to as the rule of "like dissolves like". In other words, if you want to dissolve a highly polar or ionic compound you should use a solvent that is also highly polar or has a high dielectric constant. If you want to dissolve a compound that is non-polar, you should use a solvent that is relatively non-polar, or, in other words, as a low dielectric constant.

Effect of Pressure

Liquids and solids exhibit practically no change of solubility with changes in pressure. Gases as might be expected increase in solubility with an increase in pressure. Henry's Law states that: *The solubility of a gas in a liquid is directly proportional to the pressure of that gas above the surface of the solution.* If the pressure is increased, the gas molecules are "forced" into the solution since this will best to relieve the pressure that has been applied. The number of gas molecules is decreased. The number of gas molecules dissolved in solution is increased. For example: carbon dioxide is filled in cold drink bottle (such as coca cola, Pepsi, 7up) under pressure.

Effect of Polymorphs

A solid has a rigid form and a definite shape. The shape or habit of a crystal of a given substance may vary but the angles between the faces are always constant. A crystal is made up of atoms, ions, or molecules in a regular geometric arrangement or lattice constantly repeated in three dimensions. This repeating pattern is known as the unit cell. The capacity for a substance to crystallise in more than one crystalline form is polymorphism. It is possible that all crystals can crystallise in different forms or polymorphs. The colour, hardness, solubility, melting point, and other properties of a compound depend on its polymorphic form. If the change from one polymorph to another is reversible, the process is called enantiotropic. If the system is monotonic, there is a transition point above the melting points of both polymorphs. The two polymorphs cannot be converted from one another without undergoing a phase transition. As mentioned, polymorphs can vary in melting point. Since the melting point of the solid is related to solubility, then the polymorphs will most likely have different solubility. If the wrong polymorph is chosen during the formulation process, the detestable (i.e., thermodynamically unstable form) form can convert to the stable form which can result in changes in solubility.

Effect of Molecular Size

Molecular Size will affect the solubility. The larger the molecule or the higher its molecular weight the less soluble the substance will be. Larger molecules are more difficult to surround with solvent molecules in order to solvate the substance. In the case of organic compounds, the amount of carbon "branching" will increase the solubility since more branching will reduce the size (or volume) of the molecule and make it easier to solvate the molecules with solvent.

pH-SOLUBILITY PROFILE

Solubility is one of the most important physico-chemical properties studied during pharmaceutical preformulation and development phase and is also required for formulation optimization and salt selection1. For solid dosage forms, solubility data are important in determining an adequate amount of drug is available for absorption in vivo[19]. If a compound has a low aqueous solubility, it may be subject to dissolution rate-limited or solubility-limited absorption within the gastrointestinal (GI) residence time[20].

The solubility of a drug is defined as *the maximum quantity of a drug dissolved in a given volume of a solvent at particular temperature, pressure and pH.* For ionisable drugs, the solubility can be affected by the pH of the solution, and the intrinsic solubility (S_0) is defined as *the concentration of a saturated solution of the neutral form of the drug, in equilibrium with its solid at constant temperature and pressure.* Nowadays, drug design approaches is based on a combination of chemistry and quantitative structure–activity relationship. This leads to new active substances that are less water soluble and more lipophilic. Very lipophilic drugs show lower solubility in water and faces trouble in crossing membranes. The acidic group of a drug molecule becomes negatively charged by losing a hydrogen ion at pH < 7. Research in pharmaceutical chemistry has devoted little attention to the physicochemical properties of the chemical and has focused mainly on optimization of the in vitro activity[21-23]. *The rate at which a drug goes into the solution when it is dissolved in an acidic or a basic medium is proportional to the solubility of the drug.* Many drugs have different solubilities at different pHs. This pH-dependent solubility difference leads to pH-dependent dissolution profile. The solubility-pH profile of drugs has already been reported by many authors[24-26]. The Henderson-Hasselbalch (HH) equation[25] has been used many times for the mathematical description of the solubility-pH profile of drugs or amines which exist in the solution as a monomer. Aqueous solubility has an essential role in the bioavailability of oral drug formulations. There is an established classification, the biopharmaceutical classification system (BCS). This system divides drugs into four classes in terms of their solubility and permeability[27]. The BCS classification correlates the in vitro solubility and permeability to the in vivo bioavailability.

Recently, the problem of drug-solubility in water has become more acute and more common as pharmaceutical companies have improved drugs for certain therapeutic areas[28]. The accuracy of many predictive methods have been discussed when it is required to compare the calculated and measured solubility[29,30]. A number of useful experimental methods have been reviewed, such as, the miniaturised shake-flask microtitre plate, the micro-solubility self-calibrating direct UV, the potentiometric and micro-dissolution methods as well as the "new shake-flask method"[31-33]. The thermodynamic solubility of the drugs have to be measured as a function of temperature at pH 7 in water, ethanol and n-octanol[34-38]. The results can be used to compare the buffer solutions at the same temperature and pH. The pKa values obtained using the Bates-Schwarzenbach spectrophotometric method can be compared with the pKa values, obtained from the solubility-pH profile measurements. The sigmoidal relationship of solubilities of weak acid drugs and two salts can predict the HH equation. The pKa of an ionisable compound is an important property, describing the charge state of the drug at a certain pH. However, according to Avdeef, it is not recommended to determine pKa values from the solubility-pH measurements (pKa^S). The results show a reasonably good agreement between the results obtained by the two different methods at two temperatures: from the solubility-pH measurements (pKa^S), and with the precise spectrophotometric Bates-Schwarzenbach method ($pKa^{B\text{-}S}$).

Kinetic solubility is a non-equilibrium solubility, which can be used during early drug discovery of new chemical entity and for lead optimization[39]. The usefulness and application of the solubility data from these non-equilibrium methods is questionable for formulation development and dosage form design. The purpose of kinetic solubility measurements is to -

1) identify the compounds that do not have good kinetic solubility even in aqueous buffer containing DMSO,
2) guide modification of structures to improve solubility, and
3) guide formulation selection for animal dosing[40].

As compounds progress to development, typically the most stable crystal form, it is selected, and more detailed thermodynamic solubility studies are to be conducted in various solvents. It is important to remember that kinetic solubility data vary with the conditions of the solution. Small changes in

- pH,
- organic solvent,
- ionic strength,
- ions in solution,
- co-solutes,
- incubation time, and
- temperature can result in large changes in the solubility of a compound.

Dimethyl sulfoxide is widely used in kinetic solubility determination at early drug discovery. Dimethyl sulfoxide can dissolve a wide range of drugs due to its aprotic nature. Kinetic solubility has two distinguishing characteristics:

(a) the compound initially is fully dissolved in an organic solvent (e.g., DMSO) then added to the aqueous buffer, and
(b) equilibrium is not reached between dissolved compound and solid compound.

Here using the basic concept of kinetic solubility, a new solubility determination method has to be designed at laboratory scale. Dimethyl sulfoxide-based method can give a preliminary idea about solubility of a drug. These methods can determine the drug solubility in short time using a little amount of drug[41]. Hydrochlorothiazide is used here as a model drug. It is a BCS class IV drug i.e. is low soluble and low permeable drug[42]. So solubility of such drug can be determined quickly by using DMSO method which will give an estimate solubility value. But the true solubility value can be determined by shake flask method.

The pKa Measurements

The pK_a measurements are performed on the basis of the Bates-Scwarzenbach (BS) method using a suitable UV-Vis spectrophotometer. The UV-Vis spectra for acidity constant measurements at temperature 310.2 K are performed at three conditions: buffer, 0.2 M HCl, and 0.12 M NaOH. The pK_a values are also determined from the solubility-pH profiles and are compared to those obtained with BS method.

Spectrophotometric method

Stock solution of drug in both buffer systems is prepared of concentration 5, 10, 20, 25, and 30 μg/mL in triplicate. The absorbances of above prepared concentrations are taken on UV spectrophotometer at λmax 272 nm and calibration curve is plotted. As process mentioned in titration method, DMSO drug solution added in excess to get precipitate. Precipitate has to be filtered. Filtrate has to be diluted suitably with buffer and absorbance is measured. This process must be repeated three times for each buffer. This absorbance is further converted to concentration with calibration curve equation of drug in that buffer.

Dimethyl Sulfoxide Based Methods

- **Titration method:** Number of drops in 1 mL of pipette has to be counted three times with DMSO. Volume of each drop has to be calculated. 200 mg of drug is to be added to 1 mL of DMSO. Drug solution in DMSO has to be added to 50 mL of buffer solutions. The number of drops required for just opalescence has to be noted three times in each buffer. Opalescence in buffer shows the excess drug, which come out as precipitation. Drug amount is calculated with the number of drops miscible in buffer system. Spectrophotometric method: Stock solution of drug in both buffer systems has to be prepared of concentration 5, 10, 20, 25, and 30 μg/mL in triplicate. The absorbances of above prepared concentrations are taken on

UV spectrophotometer at suitable wavelength and calibration curve is plotted. As the process mentioned in titration method, the DMSO drug solution is added in excess to get precipitate. Precipitate is filtered. Filtrate is diluted suitably with buffer and absorbance is measured. This process is repeated three times for each buffer. This absorbance further converted to concentration with calibration curve equation of drug in that buffer.

- **Shake flask method:** Conical flask is filled with the buffered solutions (50 mL) of pH 1.2 and 6.8. To each solution, excess of drug is added. All the solutions are kept for shaking in Orbital Shaker, the temperature is set to 25°C. From this flask a 100 µL clear supernatant is taken and the volume is made up with respective buffers. The above samples were analysed by previously developed UV spectrophotometric method.

pH-Dependent Solubility Studies

The solubility experiment has been performed with a new small-scale shake flask method at constant temperatures of 298.2 and 310.2 K. The shake-flask method proposed by Higuchi and Connors is the most reliable and widely used solubility measurement method. This method determines thermodynamic solubility and could be carried out in several steps. Each drug has been added in excess to 10 ml of dipotassium hydrogen phosphate (0.15 M) in a test tube. The test tubes have been placed on a plate shaker. Using a pH-meter up to a stable pH (solubility equilibrium), the pH of each drug suspension has been measured and adjusted if necessary, with either diluted 0.2 M HCl, or 0.2 M NaOH to a selected pH value. The experiment was completed when at least three pH measurements performed at an early, an intermediate and a late time-point of the 24 h period resulted in the same pH value. The equilibrium solubility was attained within 24 h. The pH values were also measured for the supernatants obtained after centrifugation, in order to certify that the drug solutions analysed had the same pH value as the suspensions. Measurements were made using pH-meter (CPC-401 Elmetron) with an associated uncertainty of 0.01. The test-tubes were thermostated by a temperature control thermostat (Lauda A3, Germany) through the jacket of the vessel with uncertainty 0.1 K. Samples were withdrawn after 24 h, since a previous study had shown that a majority of drugs reach their solubility equilibrium within this time-scale. Furthermore, this time-scale often is used in drug development settings. Excess solid was equilibrated using a rotating-bottle apparatus (Hettich Zenrifugen, EBA 20) at 300000 rpm for 30 min. Following centrifugation, the supernatant was collected and used for solubility and pH determinations.

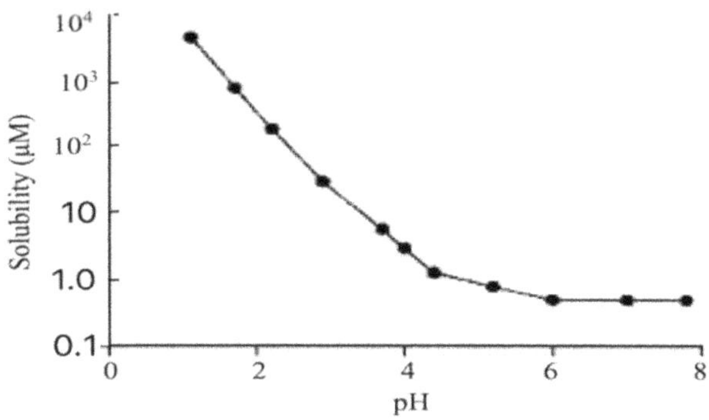

Fig.3.2 Schematic diagram of pH-solubility profile of drug.

The concentration of the drug in the supernatant solution was determined by an HPLC procedure with single-wavelength UV detection. All compounds were analysed in quadruplicates at each investigated pH value, as it was shown in the previous works. The prerequisites in the selection of the buffer system were that the buffer should display an osmotic pressure comparable to the osmotic pressure of the intestinal fluid (278 mOsm/kg) and that it should have an acceptable buffer capacity. Thus, 150 mM K_2HPO_4 (340 mOsm/kg) was chosen as buffer, and this buffer was mixed with pure drug to obtain the desired pH values. For pH below the pKa value the HCl has been added and for the values above the pKa values, the NaOH has been added.

HPLC Analysis

Each sample contained excess of drug and buffer solutions, sodium hydroxide or hydrochloric acid solution. Drug concentration in each sample has been measured using a suitable HPLC-UV-Vis apparatus consisting of: 1200 Series Quat pump, 1200 vacuum degasser, 1200 DAD/ /MWD. A C18 analytical column (4.6 mm×150 mm) with a mean particle size of 5 μm has been used. One buffer was prepared for mobile phase: disodium tetraborate (0.01038 M $Na_2B_4O_7$ and 0.01925 M NaCl). As a mobile phase two solutions have been used: methanol (A) and borate buffer, pH 9 (B). Injection volumes of 5 μl has to be used during the analysis.

TECHNIQUES TO IMPROVE SOLUBILITY

A number of methodologies can be used to improve solubilisation of poorly water-soluble drug and thus, to improve its bioavailability. The techniques generally used for solubilisation of drug includes:

1) Micronisation,
2) Chemical modification,
3) pH adjustment,
4) Solid dispersion,

5) Complexation,
6) Co-solvency,
7) Micellar solubilisation,
8) Hydrotropy etc.

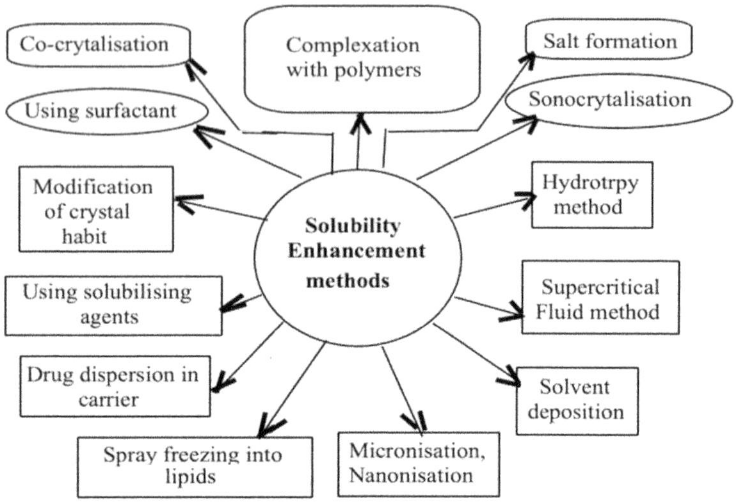

Fig.3.3 Techniques used for enhancement of solubility.

Solubilisation of poorly soluble drugs is a frequently encountered challenge in screening studies of new chemical entities as well as in formulation design and development[43,44]. Any drug to be absorbed must be present in the form of an aqueous solution at the site of absorption[45-48]. As Solubility and permeability is the deciding factor for the in-vivo absorption of the drug, these can be altered or modified by enhancement techniques like. In qualitative terms, solubility may be defined as the spontaneous interaction of two or more substances to form a homogenous molecular dispersion. A saturated solution is one in which the solute is in equilibrium with the solvent. The solubility of a drug is represented through various concentration expression such as parts, percentage, molarity, molality, volume fraction, mole fraction[49,50]. This review thus begins with discussion regarding the traditional approaches to drug solubilisation include pH adjustment, cosolvency and particle size reduction. While micro-emulsion and self-emulsifying systems are novel approaches. Most of drugs are weakly acidic and weakly basic with poor aqueous solubility.

The dissolution rate of a solid in a liquid may be described quantitatively by the Noyes-Whitney equation:

$$dm/dt = ka\ (Cs - C)$$

where,

m = mass of solute that has passed into solution in time t,

dm/dt = rate of dissolution,

A = surface area of undissolved solid in contact with the solvent,

Cs = concentration of solute required to saturate the solvent at the experimental temperature,

C = solute concentration at time t and

ka = intrinsic dissolution rate or simply the dissolution rate constant.

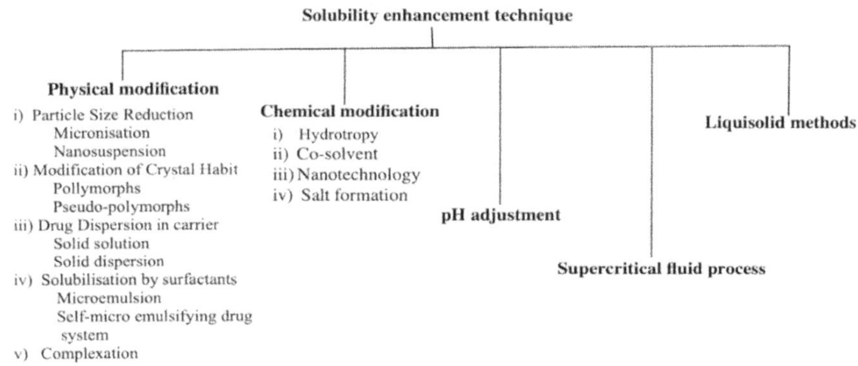

Fig.3.4 Classification of solubility enhancement technique.

The techniques to increase the solubility can be classified in five categories which are shown below in Fig 3.4.

UTILISATION OF ANALYTICAL METHODS

Cyclodextrins belong to a family of cyclic oligosaccharides composed of-(1,4) linked glucopyranose subunits. Cyclodextrins have been used as molecular chelating agents. They contain a cage-like supramolecular structure, similar to the structures formed from cryptands, calixarenes, cyclophanes, spherands and crown ethers. These compounds with their supramolecular structures can perform the chemical reactions that use intramolecular interactions. In these structures the covalent bonds are not formed between interacting molecules, ions or radicals. In most of the cases, all these reactions are of 'host–guest ' type. For this reason, molecular complexation phenomena CDs are used in many industrial products, technologies and analytical methods. Their cytotoxic effects are of negligible; hence, CDs are used as drug carrier, in food and flavours, cosmetics, packing, textiles, separation processes, environment protection, fermentation and catalysis.

Cyclodextrins are of three types: α-cyclodextrin, β-cyclodextrin and γ-cyclodextrin. These cyclodextrins contain six, seven and eight -(1,4)-linked glycosyl units, respectively[51]. β-Cyclodextrin is the most common, the lowest-priced and commonly used. Depending on the type of cyclodextrin and guest compound, cyclodextrins crystallise in two major types of crystal packing- (1) channel structures and (2) cage structures, These crystal structures indicate that cyclodextrins in complexes accept the 'round 'structure with all glucopyranose units in the $^4C_1$ chair conformation. Furthermore, studies with linear maltohexaoses, which form an antiparallel double helix, show that α-cyclodextrin is the form in which the steric strain due to cyclisation is least while γ-cyclodextrin is the most strained[52]. Besides these naturally occurring cyclodextrins, many cyclodextrin derivatives have been synthesised. These derivatives usually are produced by aminations, esterifications or etherifications of primary and secondary hydroxyl groups of the cyclodextrins. Depending on the substituent, the solubility of the cyclodextrin derivatives become different from that of their parent cyclodextrins. Cyclodextrins are occasionally used as building blocks. Up to 20 substituents, have been linked to β-cyclodextrin in a regioselective manner. The synthesis of uniform cyclodextrin derivatives requires regioselective reagents, optimisation of reaction conditions and a good separation of products. The most frequently studied reaction is an electrophilic attack on the OH-groups, the formation of ethers and esters by alkyl halides, epoxides, acyl derivatives, isocyanates, and by inorganic acid derivatives as sulphonic acid chloride cleavage of C–OH bonds has also been studied frequently, involving a nucleophilic attack by compounds such as azide ions, halide ions, thiols, thiourea, and amines; this needs activation of the oxygen atom by an electron-withdrawing group. They are able to link covalently or noncovalently specifically to other cyclodextrins. Cyclodextrins can be used as building blocks for making of supramolecular complexes. They are able to form inclusion complexes with organic host molecules, most probably to build supra molecular threads. Accordingly, the molecular structures such as catenanes, rotaxanes, polyrotaxanes, and tubes, are constructed. Such building blocks cannot be prepared by other methods.

COSOLVENCY

Apart from experimental determinations of solute solubility in water-cosolvent mixtures, there are many mathematical models describing the solute solubility in mixed solvents. By considering chemical theory, some of them are theoretical and some others are semi-theoretical or empirical. Theoretical models provide some evidence for better understanding of solubility behaviour for drugs in mixed solvents, while semi-theoretical or empirical approaches are very useful models for correlating experimental solubilities to the independent variables such as volume fraction of the cosolvent.

From a practical point of view, one can categorise these models into two groups, i.e. predictive and correlative models. The predictive cosolvency model means that the model is capable of predicting the solubility of a drug in mixed solvents by using no experimental solubility data (pure or fully predictive model) and/or using one or two solubility points as input data. The correlative cosolvency model means that the model provides good correlation between the solubility of a drug in mixed solvents and the independent variables like cosolvent concentration or physico-chemical properties of the solutes or cosolvents. The advantage of the predictive models such as universal functional group activity coefficient, UNIFAC, is that these models do not employ any experimental data points. However, the low prediction capability of the UNIFAC model for biphenyl solubilities in several binary mixed solvents (as a simple model system) has been reported. In addition, these methods usually require a number of physico-chemical properties of drugs and relatively complex computations and are not more favourable methods in pharmaceutical area. The correlative equations, such as the general single model, employ the curve-fitting parameters to correlate experimental solubility data with respect to the concentration of the cosolvent. To calculate these curve-fitting parameters, one has to determine a set of experiments in mixed solvents to train the model. From a practical point of view, a model containing a minimum number of the curve-fitting parameters is the best cosolvency model. The final goal of developing cosolvency equations is that it enables researchers to predict the solute solubility in mixed solvents from a minimum number of experiments or even without experimental data. It has been shown that solubility prediction in binary solvents using correlative equations can fail when using insufficient experimental data points and produces unacceptable errors. On the other hand, Bustamante and coworkers employed a modified form of the extended Hildebrand solubility approach to correlate structurally related drugs solubility in binary solvent mixtures. The authors used the solute solubility in water and cosolvent, the solute's solubility parameter, the Hildebrand solubility parameter of the solvent and the basic solubility parameter of the mixed solvent as independent variables. This approach was a useful solution to the solubility problem of similar chemically solutes. The applicability of the Jouyban-Acree model for reproducing solubility data of structurally related drugs in binary solvents was presented. It was also shown that the prediction error of the JouybanAcree model is less than that of the modified form of the extended Hildebrand solubility approach.

The solubility of a poorly water-soluble drug can be increased frequently by the addition of a water miscible solvent in which the drug has good solubility known as cosolvents[53]. Co-solvents are mixtures of water and one or more water miscible solvents used to create a solution with enhanced solubility for poorly soluble compounds. Historically, this is one of the most widely used techniques because it is simple to produce and evaluate. Examples of solvents used in co-solvent mixtures are PEG 300, propylene glycol or ethanol. Co-solvent formulations of poorly soluble drugs can be administered orally and parenterally. Parenteral formulations may require the addition of water or a dilution step with an aqueous media to lower the solvent concentration prior to administration. The pharmaceutical form is always liquid. Poorly soluble compounds which are lipophilic or highly crystalline that have a high solubility in the solvent mixture may be suited to a co-solvent approach. CoSolvents can increase the solubility of poorly soluble compounds several thousand times compared to the aqueous solubility of the drug alone. Very high drug concentrations of poorly soluble compounds can be dissolved compared to other solubilisation approaches. However, the bioavailability may not be dramatically increased because the poorly soluble drug will typically uncontrollably crash out upon dilution into a crystalline or amorphous precipitate. In this case, dissolution of this precipitate is required for oral absorption. Co-solvents may be combined with other solubilisation techniques and pH adjustment to further increase solubility of poorly soluble compounds. The use of co-solvents is a highly effective technique to enhance the solubility of poorly soluble drugs. The most frequently used low toxicity cosolvents for parenteral use are propylene glycol, ethanol, glycerin, and polyethylene glycol. Dimethylsulfoxide (DMSO) and dimethylacetoamide (DMA) have been widely used as cosolvents because of their large solubilisation capacity for poorly soluble drugs and their relatively low toxicity[54].

Advantages

- Simple and rapid to formulate and produce.

Disadvantages

- As with all excipients, the toxicity and tolerability related with the level of solvent administered has to be considered.
- Uncontrolled precipitation occurs upon dilution with aqueous media. The precipitates may be amorphous or crystalline and can vary in size. Many of the insoluble compounds worked are unsuited to co-solvents alone, particularly for intravenous administration. This is because the drugs are extremely insoluble in water and do not readily redissolve after precipitation from the co-solvent mixture. In these situations, there is a potential risk for embolism and local adverse effects at the injection site.
- As with all solubilised forms, the chemical stability of the insoluble drug is worse than in a crystalline state.

SALT FORMATION

Salts formation offer many advantages to the pharmaceutical products as it can improve the solubility, dissolution rate, permeability and efficacy of the drug. In addition, salts can help in the improvement of the hydrolytic and thermal stability[55,56]. Also salts play an important role in targeted drug delivery of dosage form (e.g. in the cases of controlled release dosage forms). Furthermore, the organoleptic properties of the active pharmaceutical ingredients (e.g. taste acceptability can be modified by salt formation). It has been also stated that salts reduce the pain of injection (e.g. Morphine, diethyl-amine, N-methyl glucamine salts of cephalosporin).

Concept of Salt Formation

The process of salt formation is relatively simple and involves, in essence, pairing the parent drug molecule with an appropriate counterion. The essential prerequisite is the presence of ionisable functional groups in the drug's structure that allow sufficient ionic interaction between the drug and the salt former. The charged groups in the structure of the drug and the counterion are attracted by ionic intermolecular forces. At favourable thermodynamic conditions, the salt is precipitated in the crystallised from.

Selection of Salt Former

The choice of the salt forming agent is dictated by a number of criteria that the salt is intended to meet. Formulation (dosage form) type may influence this choice – for solid dosage forms, oral solutions, and injectables, highly soluble hydrochlorides and mesylates can be chosen. Alternatively, for suspensions, relatively insoluble counterions such as embonate, estylate, and tosylate may be preferred[57].

Additionally, the molecular weight of the counterion may also play a role as for high-dose (low-potency) drugs ions of a low molecular weight are preferred, while for low-dose (potent) drugs the molecular weight of the counterion is not usually an issue. Moreover, the immediate drug release profile usually requires hydrochloride and sodium, while slow drug release is usually achieved with large and relatively insoluble counterions such as embonate, estylate, and tosylate. Furthermore, the therapeutic indication of the drug is a limiting factor as the intake of some ions such as sodium is restricted in conditions such as hypertension and diabetes. Importantly, salt formers should also meet regulatory requirements. For example, counterions should not have adverse safety implications as well as they should not be characterised by known of potential toxicity (e.g. lithium). The choice may also be influenced by intellectual property rights as commercial use of previously patented salt forms is restricted. Finally, marketing issues may an impact on the drug formulation choice or change, what may consequently influence the salt former used in order to achieve the desired dosage form presentation. The degree of ionisation is also considered to be a critical parameter for salt selection, where the difference in the pKa values of the drug and counterion are important for successful salt formation. For the synthesis of salt forms of basic drugs, the pKa of the counterion is required to be at least

2 pH units lower than the pKa of the drug. Conversely, for the synthesis of salt forms of acidic drugs, the pKa of the counterion should be at least 2 units higher than the pKa of the drug. This rule of difference in pKa of the ionisable group of the drug molecule and of the salt former (acid or base) is to confirm that the proton transfer is energetically favourable. When that difference is significantly small, a complex may form but it may rapidly dissociate in an aqueous environment back into the drug and salt former components with no desirable influence on the drug properties.

Salt Selection Process

In the pre-formulation stages of drug development multiple salt forms can be prepared for a drug that is to be developed. Those salt forms need to be compared with regard to their physiochemical and biopharmaceutical properties. The main aim of the process is to choose an optimal salt form that will ensure the most desirable properties for processing, storage, and product performance. Morris et al developed a multi-staged approach by allowing effective and efficient salt screening. Every tier of the process is designed to test different physicochemical properties and the analysed salts can be rejected or progressed to the subsequent stages based on their performance. The first stage of salt selection is the crystallinity assessment. Crystalline structure is associated with a higher stability and therefore the properties of a crystalline salt may be expected not to vary extensively during transportation, handling, storage, and use. However, the amorphous salt form may have advantages (e.g. improved solubility profile)[58]. After that, the hygroscopicity profile of the salt form is evaluated to define the degree of variability of the properties in the varying humidity conditions. The salt forms with appropriate hygroscopicity profiles are subsequently evaluated for their solubility. The acceptable salts are tested for their physicochemical stability that includes polymorphic stability and excipient compatibility. Subsequently, polymorphism of the salt forms is investigated and its influence on the variability of salt's properties is assessed. After the stage of polymorphism assessment, the acceptable salt forms are tested for process control, economic feasibility, and processability. At this stage the parameters of corrosiveness, taste, wettability, and flowability are assessed). Finally, the selected salt form is tested in regard to its pharmacological properties (onset and the duration of activity) and drug release profile. These stages may be followed by safety studies. Upon satisfying completion of the tests, the optimal salt form will enter pre-clinical and clinical testing phases.

Effects of Salt Formation

Salt forms of drugs have significant effects on physicochemical properties of the drug influencing its quality, safety, and performance. Importantly, different salt forms rarely change drug's pharmacological properties.

One of the main effects is the drug's increased solubility and dissolution rate. If the drug is a weak base and formulated as a salt, its solubility and dissolution rate will increase in the intestine (pH ca. 7.0) due to the buffering action of the salt. Namely, upon dissolution the salt form will release protons to the medium decreasing the pH of the drug's microenvironment (drug's microclimate or diffusion layer) and increasing the dissolution rate of the basic drug. Conversely, if the drug is a weak acid, upon dissolution in the stomach (pH ca. 1.5), its salt will increase the pH of the drug's microenvironment resulting in a higher dissolution rate of the acidic drug. For example, the sodium salt form of an oral hypoglycaemic agent tolbutamide is known to dissolve 5,000 times faster in acidic media if compared to the free acid. Similarly, the sodium salt of a nonsteroidal anti-inflammatory drug naproxen has a better solubility profile if compared with the free acid form and as a result of that the salt form is absorbed faster. Analogically, strongly acidic salt forms of weakly basic drugs such as chlorpromazine and ranitidine (as hydrochlorides) have enhanced dissolution profiles in gastric and intestinal media if compared to the free base forms.

Other desirable physicochemical effects of salt formation include improved thermal, hydrolytic, and photo-stability, enhanced organoleptic properties, and improved compatibility. Furthermore, salt formation may be used to achieve a controlled release of a drug through the control of the drug microenvironment's pH that is independent of the varying bulk pH (as demonstrated with salicylic acid, benzoic acid, and sulfathiazole). Moreover, targeted drug delivery to the colon can be achieved by forming salts and thus availing the reduced absorption of the ionised drug. Despite the vast application of salts, salt formation may have a number of undesirable effects on the drug's properties and ultimately affect its performance in vivo. Firstly, as counterions are therapeutically inactive, the proportion of the drug in the formulation is decreased resulting in higher powder volumes for capsule loading and tablet compaction. These in turn can result in larger dosage units and consequently pose problems at administration. Moreover, introducing counterions to the drug structure may result in the increased formation of hydrates and polymorphs what ultimately leads to increase in variability of the drug's pharmaceutical properties. Furthermore, salts prepared from strong acids and bases are usually highly hygroscopic posing problems with storage and reducing product's shelf life. In addition, salts may cause problems with corrosiveness resulting in impaired manufacturing process (e.g. hydrochloride salts may cause deterioration of the punch tooling). What is more, hydrochloride salts may experience reduced dissolution rate and solubility in the stomach due to precipitated free acid or base at the surface of the solid dosage form4 Finally, as salt forms are ionised species their partitioning into lipophilic phases may be reduced. This may in turn reduce their permeability through biological membranes (such as gastro-intestinal membranes) and consequently reduce absorption and drug's bioavailability. However, drug's bioavailability may be improved through salt formation, what was achieved with piroxicam (formulated as an ethanolamine salt)[58].

COMPLEXATION

Complexation is the process of complex formation that is the process of characterisation of the covalent or non-covalent interactions between two or more compounds. The ligand is a molecule that interacts with another molecule, the drug, to form a complex. Drug molecules can form complexes with other small molecules or with macromolecules such as proteins. A coordination complex is the product of a Lewis acid-base reaction in which the neutral molecules or anions (called ligands) form bond to a central metal atom (or ion) by coordinate covalent bonds. Simple ligands are water, ammonia and chloride ions.

Once the complexation occurs, the following physical and chemical properties of the complexing species are altered;

- Solubility,
- Stability,
- Partition co-efficient,
- Energy absorption,
- Energy emission.
- Conductance of the drug

***Forces utilised in complex formation are*:**

- Covalent bond.
- Co-ordinate covalent bond.
- Van der Waals force of dispersion.
- Dipole-Dipole interaction.
- Hydrogen bond.

Advantages of Complexation

- Drug complexation, therefore, can lead to beneficial properties such as enhanced aqueous solubility, for example, theophylline complexation with ethylenediamine to form aminophylline and stability, such as, inclusion complexes of labile drugs with cyclodextrins.
- Complexation also can aid in the optimization of delivery systems, for example, ion-exchange resins and affect the distribution in the body after systemic administration as a result of protein binding.

- In some cases, complexation also can lead to poor solubility or decreased absorption of drugs in the body.
- For some drugs, complexation with certain hydrophilic compounds can enhance excretion.

Classification of complex:

- *Metal ion complexes*

  Metal ions are the central atom such as drug. It interacts with a base (electron-pair donor, ligand), forming co-ordination bonds between the species.
- Inorganic type
- Chelates
- Olefin type
- Aromatic type

  o Pi (π) complexes

  o Sigma (σ) complexes

  o "Sandwich" compounds
- *Organic molecular complexes*
- Quinhydrone type
- Picric acid type
- Caffeine and other drug complexes
- Polymer type
- *Non-Bonded or Inclusion/ occlusion compounds*
- Channel lattice type
- Layer type
- Clathrates
- Monomolecular type
- Macromolecular type Metal ion complexes:
- *Metal ion are the central atom as Drug. It interacts with a base (electron-pair donor, ligand), forming co-ordination bonds between the species:*

Inorganic type –

- In inorganic metal complexes, there is only one site for binding with metal which is called ligand.
- The ammonia molecules present in hexamminecobalt (III) chloride, as the compound $[Co(NH_3)_6]^{3+}$ Cl^{3-}, are known as the ligands and are to be coordinated to the cobalt ion. The coordination number of the cobalt ion,

or number of ammonia groups coordinated to the metal ions, is six. Other complex ions belonging to the inorganic group are $[Ag(NH_3)_2]+$, $[Fe(CN)_6]^{4-}$, and $[Cr(H_2O)_6]^{3+}$.

- Each ligand donates a pair of electrons to form a coordinate covalent bond between itself and the central ion having an incomplete electron shell.

$$Co^{3+} + 6NH_3 = [Co(NH_3)_6]^{3+}$$

- Hybridisation plays an important role in formation of coordination compounds in which sufficient bonding orbitals are not ordinarily available in the metal ion.

Chelates -

- The chelates are a group of metal ion complexes. These complexes have a substance (Ligands) with two or more donor groups which can combine with a metal ion.
- Some of the bonds in a chelate may be ionic or of the primary covalent type, whereas others are coordinate covalent bonds.
- When the ligand provides one group for attachment to the central ion, the chelate is called monodentate.
- Pilocarpine behaves as a monodentate ligand for Co(II), Ni(II), and Zn(II) ions to form chelates of pseudotetrahedral geometry.

Olefin type -

- The aqueous solution of certain metal ions like Pt, Fe, Pd, Hg and Ag can absorb olefins such as ethylene to produce water soluble complexes.
- These are used as catalyst in the manufacture of bulk drugs and analysis of drugs.

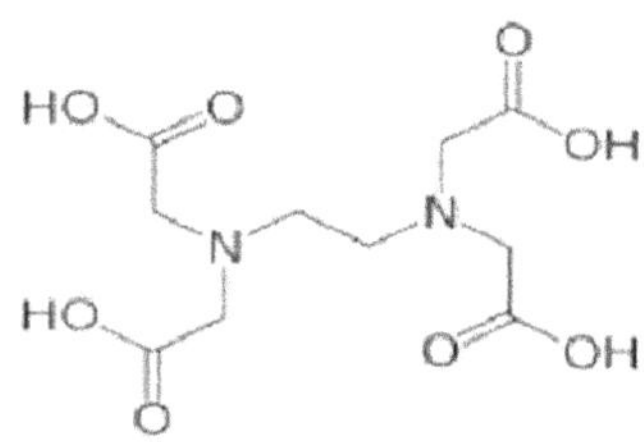

Fig.3.5 Structure of EDTA.

Aromatic type -

- Pi (π) complexes are aromatic bases (such as, benzene, toluene and Xylene) which form pi-bond complexes with metal ions like Ag by Lewis acid-base reactions.
- Sigma (σ) complexes are sigma bond complexes that are involved in the formation of a sigma-bond between ion and a carbon of aromatic ring.
- "Sandwich" compounds – These are relatively stable complexes which are involved in the delocalized covalent bond between the d-orbital of transition metal and a molecular orbit of the aromatic ring.

***Organic molecular complexes*:**

- Many organic complexes are so weak that they cannot be separated from their solutions as definite compounds.
- The energy of attraction between the constituents is probably less than 5 kcal/mole for most organic complexes.
- The bond distance between the components of the complex is usually greater than 3Å, and a covalent bond is not involved.
- An organic coordination compound or molecular complex consists of constituents held together by weak forces of the donor–acceptor type or by hydrogen bonds.
- Donor-Acceptor type – In this type, the bond is between uncharged species which do not have charge transfer. The dipole-dipole interaction and London dispersion forces (Dotted lines) make these complexes stable, for example, the compounds dimethylaniline and 2,4,6-trinitroanisole react in the cold to give a molecular complex as shown below

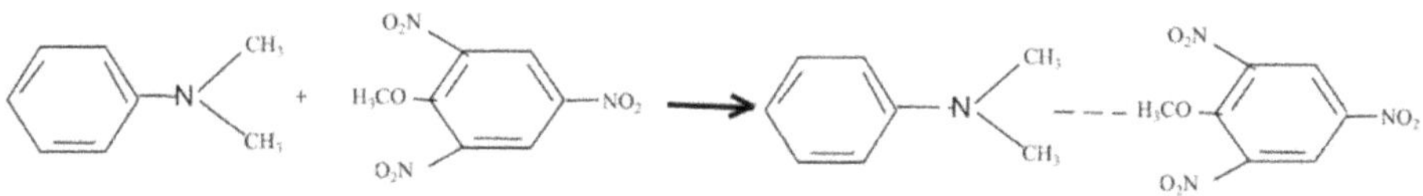

- The charge transfer Complexes - In this case, one molecule polarises the other through a type of ionic interaction or charge transfer. Thus, these molecular complexes are often referred to as charge transfer complexes. The resonance makes the complex more stable. The intermolecular bonding is quite higher compared to donor-acceptor type complexes, for example, the polar nitro groups of trinitrobenzene induce a dipole.

***Caffeine and other drug complexes*:**

- Drugs such as benzocaine, procaine and tetracaine form complexes with caffeine.
- A number of acidic drugs are known to form complexes with caffeine.

***Quinhydrone type*:**

- The molecular complex of this type is obtained by mixing alcoholic solutions of equimolar quantities of hydroquinone and benzoquinone.

***Polymers Type* :**

- Many pharmaceutical additives such as polyethylene glycols (PEGs), carboxymethyl cellulose (CMC) contain nucleophilic oxygen. These can form complexes with various drugs.
- Polymers such as carbowaxes, pluronics etc. can form complexes with drugs such as tannic acid, salicylic acid, phenols etc.

- Carboxy methyl cellulose reacts with amphetamine, a poorly absorbed drugs. Picric acid types
- Picric acid is a strong acid, forms organic molecular complexes with weak bases. It combines with strong bases (anesthetic activity of butesin) to yield salts.

***Inclusion Complexes*:**

- These complexes are also called occlusion compounds in which one of the components is trapped in the open lattice or cage like crystal structure of the other.

***Channel types*:**

- Channels are formed by crystallisation of the host molecules, the guest component is usually limited to long, unbranched straight chain compounds.

***Layer types*:**

- Compounds such as clays, montomorillorite (constituent of bentonite), can entrap hydrocarbons, alcohols and glycols.
- They form alternate monomolecular (monoatomic) layers of guest and host.
- Their uses are currently quite limited; however, these may be useful for catalysis on account of a larger surface area.

***Clathrates*:**

- It is available as white crystalline powder, during crystallisation, certain substances form a cage-like lattice in which the coordinating compound is entrapped.

***Monomolecular types*:**

- Monomolecular inclusion compounds involve the entrapment of a single guest molecule in the cavity of one host molecule.
- Most of the host molecules are cyclodextrins.
- The interior of the cavity is relatively hydrophobic, whereas the entrance of the cavity is hydrophilic in nature.

Applications of Complexation:

***Physical state*:**

- Complexation process improves processing the characteristics by converting liquid to solid complex, for example, β-cyclodextrine complexes with nitroglyerine.

***Volatility*:**

- Complexation process reduces the volatility of drug for following benefits;

- Stabilise the system.
- Overcome the unpleasant odour (I2 complexes with poly vinyl pyrollidone, PVP).

***Solid state stability*:**

- Complexation process enhances solid state stability of drugs.
- β-cyclodextrine forms complexes with vitamin A and D.
- Chemical stability:
- Complex formation inhibits chemical reactivity (mostly inhibit).
- The hydrolysis of Benzocaine is decreased by complexing with caffeine.

***Solubility*:**

- Complexation process improves the solubility of drug.
- Caffeine improves the solubility of PABA (Para Amino Benzoic Acid) by forming the complex.

***Dissolution*:**

- Complexation process improves the dissolution of drug.
- β-cyclodextrine improves the dissolution of phenobarbitone by inclusion complex.

***Partition co-efficient*:**

- Complexation process enhances the partition coefficient of certain drugs.
- Permanganate ion with benzene.

***Absorption and Bioavailability*:**

- Complexation process reduces the absorption of tetracycline by complexing with the cations such as Ca^{+2}, Mg^{+2} and Al^{+3}.
- Complexation process improves the absorption of indomethacin and barbiturates by complexing with β-cyclodextrine.

***Reduced toxicity*:**

- β-cyclodextrine reduces ulcerogenic effects of indomethacine.
- β-cyclodextrine reduces local tissue toxicity of chlorpromazine.

***Antidote for metal poisoning*:**

- BAL (British Anti Lewisite) reduces the toxicity of heavy metals by complexing with As, Hg and Sb.

***Drug acting through metal poisoning*:**

- 8-Hydroxy quinoline forms complexes with Fe and exhibits greataer antimalaria activity.

***Antitubercular activity*:**

- PAS (Para Amino Salicylic acid) forma complexes with cupric ion and exhibits greater antitubercular activity.

***Development of Novel Drug delivery system*:**

- The comlexation of drug with polymers are being used in the formulation of sustained drug delivery device.

***Assay of Drugs*:**

- The complexometric titrations are used for assaying the drug that contains a metal ion.

***As therapeutic tools*:**

- Both citrates and EDTA are used for preservation of blood as anti-coagulant.

***As diagnostic agent*:**

- Ta^{90} forms complexes with citrate and are used for diagnosis of kidney and measurement of glomerular filtration rate.

SOLID DISPERSION

The term solid dispersion refers to a group of solid products containing at least two different components, generally a hydrophilic matrix and a hydrophobic drug. The matrix can be either crystalline or amorphous. The drug can be of the dispersed molecularly, in amorphous particles (clusters) or in crystalline particles. On basis of their molecular arrangement in the drug, six different types of solid dispersions can be obtained.

Although the oral route of administration is of choice, it can be a problematic for many drugs and inefficient mode of delivery too due to various reasons. Limited drug absorption indicates poor bioavailability. This is an important property among the potential problems that can be handled when delivering an active agent through the oral route. Drug absorption from the gastrointestinal (GI) tract can depends on a various factors. These are the most significant contributors for poor aqueous solubility and/or poor membrane permeability of the drug molecule. When delivering an active agent through oral route, the drug must first dissolve in gastric and/or intestinal fluids before it can permeate the membranes of the GI tract to reach systemic circulation. Therefore, a drug with poor aqueous solubility will typically show *dissolution rate limited absorption*, and a drug with poor membrane permeability will typically show *permeation rate limited absorption*. Hence, there are two areas of pharmaceutical research that can attract the interest of the researchers on improving the oral bioavailability of active agents: (i) enhancement of the solubility and dissolution rate of poorly water-soluble drugs, and (ii) improvement of permeability of poorly permeable drugs. In particular, the use of solid dispersion technologies to improve the dissolution characteristics of poorly water-soluble drugs and their oral bioavailability. Numerous solid dispersion systems have been demonstrated in the pharmaceutical literature to improve the dissolution properties of poorly water-soluble drugs. Other methods, such as salt formation, complexation with cyclodextrins, solubilisation of drugs in solvent(s), and particle size reduction have also been used to improve the dissolution properties of poorly water-soluble drugs. However, there are substantial limitations with each of these techniques. On the other hand, formulation of drugs as solid dispersions offers a variety of processing and excipient options that allow for flexibility when formulating oral delivery systems for poorly water-soluble drugs.

Much of the research that has been reported on solid dispersion technologies involves drugs that are poorly water-soluble and highly permeable to biological membranes as with these drugs dissolution is the rate limiting step to absorption. Hence, the hypothesis has been that the rate of absorption in vivo will be concurrently accelerated with an increase in the rate of drug dissolution. In the Biopharmaceutical Classification System (BCS) drugs with low aqueous solubility and high membrane permeability are categorised as Class II drugs. Therefore, solid dispersion technologies are particularly promising for improving the oral absorption and bioavailability of BCS Class II drugs. With recent advances in molecular screening methods for identifying potential drug candidates, an increasing number of poorly water-soluble drugs are being identified as potential therapeutic agents. In fact, it has been estimated that 40% of new chemical entities currently being discovered are poorly water-soluble[59]. Unfortunately, many of these potential drugs are abandoned in the early stages of development due to solubility concerns. It is therefore becoming increasingly more important that methods for overcoming solubility limitations be identified and applied commercially such that the potential therapeutic benefits of these active molecules can be realised.

Advantages of Solid Dispersion

1. Particles with reduced particle size: Molecular dispersions, such as solid dispersions, represent the last state on particle size reduction, and after carrier dissolution the drug is molecularly dispersed in the dissolution medium. Solid dispersions apply this principle to drug release by creating a mixture of a poorly water-soluble drug and highly soluble carriers. A high surface area is formed, resulting in an increased dissolution rate and, consequently, improved bioavailability. Particles with improved wettability A strong contribution to the enhancement of drug solubility is related to the drug wettability improvement verified in solid dispersions. It was observed that even carriers without any surface activity, such as urea improved drug wettability. Carriers with surface activity, such as cholic

acid and bile salts. When used, can significantly increase the wettability property of drug. Moreover, carriers can influence the drug dissolution profile by direct dissolution or co-solvent effects. Particles with higher porosity Particles in solid dispersions have been found to have a higher degree of porosity[60]. The increase in porosity also depends on the carrier properties; for instance, solid dispersions containing linear polymers produce larger and more porous particles than those containing reticular polymers and, therefore, result in a higher dissolution rate. The increased porosity of solid dispersion particles also hastens the drug release profile.

2. Drugs in amorphous state: Poorly water-soluble crystalline drugs, when in the amorphous state tend to have higher solubility. The enhancement of drug release can usually be achieved using the drug in its amorphous state, because no energy is required to break up the crystal lattice during the dissolution process. In solid dispersions, drugs are presented as supersaturated solutions after system dissolution, and it is speculated that, if drugs precipitate, it is as a metastable polymorphic form with higher solubility than the most stable crystal form. For drugs with low crystal energy (low melting temperature or heat of fusion), the amorphous composition is primarily dictated by the difference in melting temperature between drug and carrier. For drugs with high crystal energy, higher amorphous compositions can be obtained by choosing carriers, which exhibit specific interactions with them.

Preparation of Solid Dispersions

- **Fusion Method**
- The fusion method is sometimes referred to as the melt method, which is correct only when the starting materials are crystalline. Therefore, the more general term fusion method is preferred. The first solid dispersions created for pharmaceutical applications were prepared by the fusion method. The dispersion consisted of sulfathiazole and urea as a matrix which were melted using a physical mixture at the eutectic composition, followed by a cooling step. The eutectic composition was chosen to obtain simultaneous crystallisation of drug and matrix during cooling. This procedure resulted in solid dispersions of type I. Poly(ethylene glycol) (PEG) is a hydrophilic polymer often used to prepare solid dispersions with the fusion method. This often results in solid dispersions of type III since many drugs are incorporated as separate molecules in the helical structure present in a crystalline PEG. The helices are aligned in orderly fashion, illustrating that PEG easily crystallises. Another polymer frequently applied as a matrix in the fusion method is poly (vinyl pyrollidone) PVP. PVP, supplied in the amorphous state, is heated to above its Tg (glass transition temperature). The drug has to fuse with or dissolve in the rubbery matrix, which is subsequently cooled to vitrify the solid dispersion. When PVP is used as

matrix, solid dispersions of type V or VI are obtained. The mode of incorporation of the drug depends on the PVP-drug miscibility and the preparation procedure. Grinding is required to obtain the solid dispersion as powder that is easy to handle. Although frequently applied, the fusion method has serious limitations. Firstly, a major disadvantage is that the method can only be applied when drug and matrix are compatible and when they mix well at the heating temperature. When drug and matrix are incompatible two liquid phases or a suspension can be observed in the heated mixture, which results in an inhomogeneous solid dispersion. This can be prevented by using surfactants.

- Secondly, a problem can arise during cooling when the drug-matrix miscibility changes. In this case phase separation can occur. Indeed, it was observed that when the mixture was slowly cooled, crystalline drug occurred, whereas fast cooling yielded amorphous solid dispersions.
- Thirdly, degradation of the drug and or matrix can occur during heating to temperatures necessary to fuse matrix and drug. For example, to get the glassy PVP in the rubbery state a temperature of about 170°C is required. Polyethylene glycols melt at around 70°C and are therefore often used for the preparation of solid dispersions with the fusion method.
- **Hot melt extrusion**

  Melt extrusion is essentially the same as the fusion method except that intense mixing of the components is induced by the extruder. When compared to melting in a vessel, the product stability and dissolution are similar, but melt extrusion offers the potential to shape the heated drug-matrix mixture into implants, ophthalmic inserts, or oral dosage forms. Just like in the traditional fusion process, miscibility of drug and matrix can be a problem. Solubility parameters are investigated to predict the solid-state miscibility and to select matrices suitable for melt extrusion. High shear forces resulting in high local temperatures in the extruder be a problem for heat sensitive materials. However, compared to the traditional fusion method, this technique offers the possibility of continuous production, which makes it suitable for large-scale production. Furthermore, the product is easier to handle because at the outlet of the extruder the shape can be adapted to the next processing step without grinding.
- **Solvent method**

  The first step in the solvent method is the preparation of a solution containing both matrix material and drug. The second step involves the removal of solvent(s) resulting in formation of a solid dispersion. Mixing at the molecular level is preferred, because this leads to optimal dissolution properties. Using the solvent method, the pharmaceutical engineer faces two challenges. The first challenge is to mix both drug and matrix in one solution, which would be difficult when they differ significantly in polarity. To minimise the drug particle size in the solid dispersion, the drug and matrix have to be dispersed in the solvent as fine as possible, preferably drug and matrix material are in the dissolved state in one solution. Various strategies have been applied to dissolve the lipophilic drug and hydrophilic matrix material together in one solution. Low drug concentrations are used to dissolve both drug and matrix material in water, but this requires evaporation of tremendous amounts of solvent, making the process expensive and impractical. Solubilisers like cyclodextrins or surfactants like Tween 80 may increase the aqueous solubility of the drug substantially. However, the amount of solubilisers or surfactants in the final product often remain eminent. This results in solid dispersions that, to a significant extent, may consist of solubilisers or surfactants materials; as a result, this may significantly change the physical properties of the matrix (e.g., decrease of Tg). Moreover, only dosage forms with low drug loads are possible. In addition, they are not always tolerated well in the body or may even be toxic. Chloroform or dichloromethane have been used to dissolve both drug and PVP as matrix simultaneously. These solvents are used also in other preparation methods. However, according to the ICH-Guidelines, these solvents belong to Class I, comprising the most toxic solvents. Therefore, the use of these solvents is unacceptable and impractical because the amount of residual solvent present in the solid dispersion after drying has to be below the detection limits. The last strategy for the dissolution of both drug and matrix is the use of solvent mixtures. Water and ethanol, or dichloromethane and ethanol have been used for this purpose. However, dissolution of drug and matrix in these mixtures is not always possible in the required concentration or ratio.

- The second challenge in the solvent method is to prevent phase separation, e.g. crystallisation of either drug or matrix, during removal of the solvent(s). Drying at high temperatures speeds up the process and reduces the time available for phase separation. On the other hand, at high temperatures the molecular mobility of drug and matrix remains high, favouring phase separation (e.g., crystallisation). To dry the solutions, vacuum drying is often used. The solution is dried by the application of vacuum and moderate heating. Sometimes, the solvent evaporation is accelerated by using a rotary evaporator. Afterwards the formed solid dispersion is often stored in a vacuum desiccator to remove the residual solvent. Vacuum drying at elevated temperature bears the risk of phase separation because the mobility of drug and matrix decreases slowly. Another drying technique is spray drying. The solution is dispersed as fine particles in hot air. Due to the large specific surface area offered by the droplets, the solvent rapidly evaporates, and the solid dispersion is formed within seconds, which may be fast enough to prevent phase separation. Moreover, the solid dispersions prepared by spray drying consist of particles of which the size may be customised by changing the droplet size to meet the requirements for further processing or application (e.g., free flowing particles or particles for inhalation). Spray drying usually yields drug in the amorphous state, however sometimes the drug may have (partially) crystallised during processing. An alternative to these drying techniques is freeze drying. Although it is concluded in literature that this is a promising and suitable technique to incorporate drug substances in stabilising matrices, the technique is poorly exploited for the preparation of solid dispersions. One of the reasons might be the low freezing temperature of most organic solvents. Obviously, sublimation during freeze drying is only possible when the solvent stays frozen. In addition, when the formation of a glass is envisaged, the sample temperature should be kept below the T_g of the maximally freeze concentrated fraction. Therefore, low sample temperatures are required which slows down the process used a condenser temperature of -75°C, to dry a solution with cyclohexanol as the solvent. To obtain a lyophilisation process of acceptable duration, the solvent should have a sufficiently high vapour pressure. Dimethylsulphoxide (DMSO) has a high melting temperature, but it has a very low vapour pressure. Therefore, DMSO is not suitable as a solvent for freeze drying. A suitable solvent that meets both requirements is 2-methyl-2-propanol or tertiary butanol (TBA), because it has a high melting temperature as well as a high vapour pressure. The application of TBA in lyophilisation is discussed by Teagarden. Also, the mixtures of solvents can be considered. For example, while water and DMSO have melting points of 0°C and 19°C, the mixture has eutectic points below -60°C. The sample temperature of such a mixture should be kept below this value, which causes a slow sublimation. An important advantage of freeze drying is that the drug is subjected to minimal thermal stress during the formation of the solid dispersion. However, the most important advantage of freeze drying is that the risk of phase separation is minimised as soon as the solution is vitrified. An even more promising drying technique is spray-freeze drying. The solvent is sprayed into liquid nitrogen or cold dry air and the frozen droplets are subsequently lyophilised. The large surface area and direct contact with the cooling agent result in even faster vitrification, thereby decreasing the risk for phase separation to a minimum. Moreover, spray freeze drying offers the potential to customise the size of the particle to make them suitable for further processing or applications like pulmonary, or nasal administration. In an electrostatic spinning process, a drug-matrix solution is pumped through an orifice and then subjected to an electrical field to form fibres with a diameter of micro- or nanoscale. This process is restricted to a limited number of matrices, because only a few high molecular weight materials are fibre forming materials. The fibre diameter can be adjusted by surface tension, electrical field and dielectric constant. After rapid evaporation of the solvent, the fibres can be directly used or milled and further processed. Evaporative precipitation into aqueous solutions (EPAS) was used to coat a colloidal suspension of carbamazepine with block-copolymers as stabilising surfactants. A solution of drug in dichloromethane was sprayed in an aqueous solution containing polymeric surfactants as stabilisers. The obtained colloidal suspension was spray dried, freeze dried or spray freeze dried, resulting in solid dispersions of type IV/V. It was concluded that the amorphous state of the drug was best preserved with the spray freeze drying process. D. Supercritical fluid methods Supercritical fluid methods are mostly applied with carbon dioxide (CO_2), which is used as either a solvent for drug and matrix or as an anti-solvent. When supercritical CO_2 is used as solvent, matrix and drug are dissolved and sprayed through a nozzle, into an expansion vessel with lower pressure and particles are immediately formed. The adiabatic expansion of the mixture results in rapid cooling. This technique does not require the use of organic solvents and since CO_2 is considered environmentally friendly, this technique is referred to as 'solvent free'. The technique is known as Rapid Expansion of Supercritical Solution (RESS). However, the application of this technique is very limited, because the solubility in CO_2 of most pharmaceutical compounds is very low (<0.01wt-%) and decreases with increasing polarity. Therefore, scaling up this process to kilogram-scale will be impractical. All other supercritical techniques are precipitation methods. Although generally labelled as solvent-free, all these supercritical fluid methods use organic solvents to dissolve drug and matrix and exploit the low solubility of pharmaceutical compounds in CO_2. In fact, these techniques represent alternative methods to remove solvents from a solution containing typically a drug and a polymer. It has been reported their method as solvent-free, but they dissolved PEG and carbamazepine in acetone. They used a technique that is called the Gas-Anti-Solvent technique (GAS) or Precipitation from Gas Saturated Solutions (PGSS). The solution is brought into contact with compressed CO_2. The conditions are chosen so that CO_2 is completely miscible with the solution under supercritical conditions, whereas drug and matrix will precipitate upon expansion of the solution. When the volume of the solution expands the solvent strength (i.e. the ability to dissolve the drug) decreases. This results in precipitation of matrix and drug. Since this technique is often applied with PEG as matrix, this technique results in formation of a solid dispersion with a crystalline matrix. The second type of precipitation technique involves the spraying of a solution containing drug and matrix through a nozzle into a vessel that contains a liquid or supercritical anti-solvent. The supercritical anti-solvent rapidly penetrates into the droplets, in which drug and matrix become supersaturated, crystallise and form particles. The general term for this process is Precipitation with Compressed Anti-Solvent (PCA). More specific examples of PCA are Supercritical AntiSolvent (SAS) when supercritical CO_2 is used, or Aerosol Solvent Extraction System (ASES), and Solution Enhanced Dispersion by Supercritical fluids (SEDS). However, as with the other solvent techniques described in the previous section, the critical step in these precipitation techniques might be the dissolution of drug and matrix in one solution. The use of water is limited, because the water solubility in compressed CO_2 is limited. Usually, organic solvents like dichloromethane or methanol have to be applied to dissolve both drug and matrix. In another process called supercritical fluid impregnation, the drug is dissolved in a supercritical fluid and exposed to solid matrix material that swells and absorbs the supercritical solution. By varying the pressure and the time of exposure, the diffusion process can be controlled. The absorption stops when the pressure is reduced. This process is investigated for poly (methyl methacrylate) but can be applied for other polymers as well.

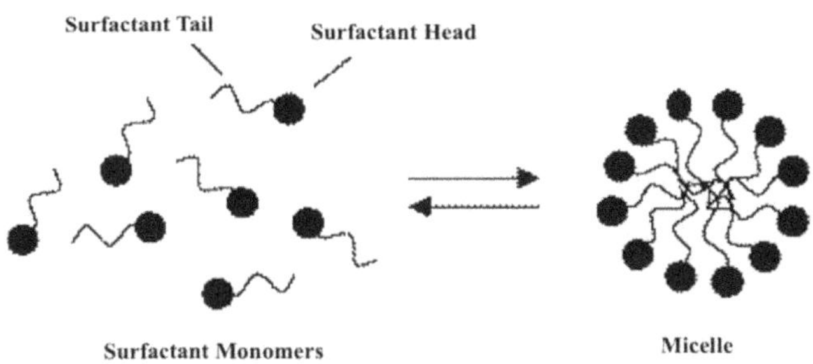

Fig.3.6 Micellar solubilization.

MICELLAR SOLUBILIZATION

Surfactants are known to play a vital role in many processes of interest in both fundamental and applied science. One important property of surfactants is the formation of colloidal-sized clusters in solutions, known as micelles, which have particular significance in pharmacy because of their ability to increase the solubility of sparingly soluble substances in water. Micelles are known to have an anisotropic water distribution within their structure. In other words, the water concentration decreases from the surface towards the core of the micelle, with a completely hydrophobic (water-excluded) core. Consequently, the spatial position of a solubilised drug in a micelle will depend on its polarity: nonpolar molecules will be solubilised in the micellar core, and substances with intermediate polarity will be distributed along the surfactant molecules in certain intermediate positions. On the other hand, numerous drug delivery and drug targeting systems have been studied in an attempt to minimise drug degradation and loss, to prevent harmful side effects, and to increase drug bioavailability. Within this context, the utilisation of micelles as drug carriers presents some advantages when compared to other alternatives such as soluble polymers and liposomes. Micellar systems can solubilise poorly soluble drugs and thus increase their bioavailability, they can stay in the body (blood) long enough to provide gradual accumulation in the required area, and their sizes permit them to accumulate in areas with leaky vasculature. In general, surfactants play an important role in contemporary pharmaceutical biotechnology, since they are largely utilised in various drug dosage forms to control wetting, stability, bioavailability, among other properties. It is important to notice that lyophobic colloids, such as polymers, require certain energy to be applied for their formation, are quite unstable from the thermodynamic point of view, and frequently form large aggregates. Association colloids such as micelles, on the other hand, can form spontaneously under certain conditions (self-assembling systems), and are thermodynamically more stable towards both dissociation and aggregation. Therefore, the study of surfactants and their role in pharmacy is of paramount importance, especially with respect to their ability of solubilising hydrophobic drugs. In this work, we provide a review of micellar solubilisation of drugs in surfactant systems, blending it with basic information on surfactants structure and properties, as well as the applications for drug delivery.

Surfactants and Micelles

Surfactants are amphiphilic molecules composed of a hydrophilic or polar moiety known as head and a hydrophobic or nonpolar moiety known as tail. The surfactant head can be charged to anionic or cationic, dipolar (zwitterionic), or non-charged (nonionic). Sodium dodecyl sulfate (SDS), dodecyltrimethylammonium bromide (DTAB), n-dodecyl tetra (ethylene oxide) (C12E4) and dioctanoyl phosphatidylcholine (C8- lecithin) are typical examples of anionic, cationic, nonionic and zwitterionic surfactants, respectively. The surfactant tail is usually a long chain hydrocarbon residue and less often a halogenated or oxygenated hydrocarbon or siloxane chain. A surfactant, when present at low concentrations in a system, adsorbs onto surfaces or interfaces significantly changing the surface or interfacial free energy. Surfactants usually act to reduce the interfacial free energy, although there are occasions when they are used to increase it. When surfactant molecules are dissolved in water at concentrations above the critical micelle concentration (cmc), they form aggregates known as micelles. In a micelle, the hydrophobic tails flock to the interior in order to minimise their contact with water, and the hydrophilic heads remain on the outer surface in order to maximise their contact with water. The micellisation process in water results from a delicate balance of intermolecular forces, including hydrophobic, steric, electrostatic, hydrogen bonding, and van der Waals interactions. The main attractive force results from the hydrophobic effect associated with the nonpolar surfactant tails, and the main opposing repulsive force results from steric interactions and electrostatic interactions between the surfactant polar heads. Whether micellisation occurs and, if so, at what concentration of monomeric surfactant, depends on the balance of the forces promoting micellisation and those opposing it.

The determination of a surfactant cmc can be made by use of several physical properties, such as surface tension (γ), conductivity (κ) – in case of ionic surfactants, osmotic pressure (π), detergency, etc. When these properties are plotted as a function of surfactant concentration (or its logarithm, in case of surface tension), a sharp break can be observed in the curves obtained evidencing the formation of micelles at that point. Another important parameter that characterises micelles is the aggregation number, Nag, that corresponds to the average number of surfactant monomers in each micelle of a micellar solution. Usually, in a micellar solution the aggregation number is approximately constant for a broad total concentration range (up to about 100 times the cmc), with the number of micelles varying. However, at certain conditions micelles can grow with the aggregation number varying with the surfactant concentration. Micelles are labile entities formed by the noncovalent aggregation of individual surfactant monomers. Therefore, they can be spherical, cylindrical, or planar (discs or bilayers). Micelle shape and size can be controlled by changing the surfactant chemical structure as well as by varying solution conditions such as temperature, overall surfactant concentration, surfactant composition (in the case of mixed surfactant systems), ionic strength and pH. In particular, depending on the surfactant type and on the solution conditions, spherical micelles can grow one-dimensionally into cylindrical micelles or two-dimensionally into bilayers or discoidal micelles. Micelle growth is controlled primarily by the surfactant heads, since both one-dimensional and two-dimensional growth require bringing the surfactant heads closer to each other in order to reduce the available area per surfactant molecule at the micelle surface, and hence the curvature of the micelle surface For all these micellar structures in aqueous media, the surfactant molecules are oriented with their polar heads towards the water phase and their tail away from it. In ionic micelles, the interfacial region between the micelle and the aqueous phase contains the ionic head groups, the Stern Layer of the electrical double layer related to these groups, approximately half of the counter ions associated with the micelle, and water. The remaining counter ions are contained in the Gouy-Chapman portion of the double layer that extends further into the aqueous phase. The length of the double layer is a function of the ionic strength of the solution, and it can be highly compressed in the presence of electrolytes. For the nonionic surfactants having a polyethylene oxide (PEO) head group, the structure is essentially the same, except that the counter ions are not present in the outer region, but rather coils of hydrated polyethylene oxide chains.

The interior of the micelle containing the hydrophobic groups presents a radius of approximately the length of the fully extended hydrophobic chain. Another important characteristic of micelles is that the aqueous phase penetrates into the micelle beyond the hydrophilic head groups, and the first few methylene groups adjacent to the head are considered in the hydration sphere. Therefore, we can divide the interior region of the micelle in an outer core penetrated by water and in an inner core completely water excluded.

Based on the geometry of various micellar shapes and the space occupied by the hydrophilic and hydrophobic groups of the surfactants, it is possible to estimate the structure of a micelle. Accordingly, the parameter VH/lcao can determine the shape of the micelle, with VH corresponding to the volume of the hydrophobic group in the micellar core, lc is the length of the hydrophobic group in the core and ao the cross-sectional area occupied by the hydrophilic group at the micelle-solution interface. Based on Tanford VH = 27.4 + 26.9n Å, where n is the number of carbon atoms in the chain less one, and lc = 1.5 + 1.265n Å, depending upon the extension of the chain. Therefore, for a fully extended chain, lc = 1.5 + 1.265n Å.

Micellar Solubilisation

An important property of micelles that has particular significance in pharmacy is their ability to increase the solubility of sparingly soluble substances in water. In this context, solubilisation can be defined as the spontaneous dissolving of a substance by reversible interaction with the micelles of a surfactant in water to form a thermodynamically stable isotropic solution with reduced thermodynamic activity of the solubilised material. If we plot the solubility of a poorly soluble compound as a function of the concentration of surfactant, usually, what happens is that the solubility is very low until the surfactant concentration reaches the cmc. At surfactant concentrations above the cmc the solubility increases linearly with the concentration of surfactant, indicating that solubilisation is related to micellisation.

From the thermodynamic point of view, the solubilisation can be considered as a normal partitioning of the drug between two phases, micelle and aqueous, and the standard free energy of solubilisation (ΔGS °). Usually, the solubilisation of a molecule by a surfactant can be evaluated based on two descriptors that are the molar solubilisation capacity, χ, and the micelle-water partition coefficient, P. The χ value is defined as *the number of moles of the solute (drug) that can be solubilised by one mol of micellar surfactant and* characterises the ability of the surfactant to solubilise the drug. On the other hand, the micelle-water partition coefficient is the ratio of drug concentration in the micelle to the drug concentration in water for a particular surfactant concentration, as follows:

Combining Equations (2) and (3), we can relate the two solubility descriptors. Accordingly, for a given surfactant concentration:

As can be seen, P is related to the water solubility of the compound, in contrary to χ. In order to eliminate the dependence of P on the surfactant concentration, a molar micelle-water partition coefficient (PM), corresponding to the partition coefficient when Csurf = 1 M, can be defined as follows:

The lower is the cmc value of a given surfactant, the more stable are the micelles. This is especially important from the pharmacological point of view, since upon dilution with a large volume of the blood, considering intravenous administration, only micelles of surfactants with low cmc value still exist, while micelles from surfactants with high cmc value may dissociate into monomers and their content may precipitate in the blood. There are a number of possible loci of solubilisation for a drug in a micelle, Accordingly, hydrophilic drugs can be adsorbed on the surface of the micelle (1), drugs with intermediate solubility should be located in intermediate positions within the micelle such as between the hydrophilic head groups of PEO micelles (2) in the palisade layer between the hydrophilic groups and the first few carbon atoms of the hydrophobic group, that is the outer core, and (3), completely insoluble hydrophobic drugs may be located in the inner core of the micelle. The existence of different sites of solubilisation in the micelle results from the fact that the physical properties, such as micro-viscosity, polarity and hydration degree, are not uniform along the micelle. Mukerjee and Cardinal studied the microenvironments of benzene, some of its derivatives, Triton X100, and naphthalene when solubilized in micelles at low solubilizate to surfactant ratios and proposed the existence of at least two states (loci) of solubilisation with different polarity. According to the authors, the total uptake by micelles could be divided approximately into an "adsorbed" fraction (location at the micelle-water interface) and a "dissolved" fraction (location in the hydrocarbon core). When adsorption takes place, the solubility increases beyond the solubility power of the hydrocarbon core. In fact, numerous studies indicate that the solubility of slightly polar substances and aromatic compounds tend to be considerably higher than the solubility of aliphatic compounds presenting similar molar volumes, despite the fact that the later are expected to be more compatible with the aliphatic hydrocarbon core of most micelles.

The capacity of surfactants in solubilising drugs depends on numerous factors, such as chemical structure of the surfactant, chemical structure of the drug, temperature, pH, ionic strength, etc. Nonionic surfactants usually are better solubilising agents than ionic surfactants for hydrophobic drugs, because of their lower cmc values. For polar drugs it is more complicate to establish a general relationship between the degree of solubilisation and the chemical structure of the surfactant, since solubilisation can be in both the inner and the outer regions of the micelle. Krishna and Flanagan observed that, for the antimalarial drug β-Arteether (an endoperoxide containing a sesquiterpene lactone), nonionic surfactants showed much lower solubilisation power than ionic surfactants. They suggested that the solubilisation of this drug may not only involve incorporation into the micellar interior but may be substantially due to adsorption at the micelle-water interface. Regarding the influence of structure of the drug, crystalline solids generally show less solubility in micelles than do liquids of similar structure. For polar drugs, the depth of penetration into the micelle varies with the structure of the drug. Usually, the less polar the drug (or the weaker its interaction with either the polar head of the surfactant in the micelle or the water molecules at the micelle-water interface) and the longer is the chain length, the smaller its degree of solubilisation, reflecting its deeper penetration into the palisade layer. The extent of solubilisation into a particular micelle depends upon the locus of solubilisation and therefore the shape of the micelle. As described previously, the shape of the micelle is determined by the value of the parameter VH/local and as this parameter increases the micelle becomes more asymmetrical and the volume of the inner core increases relative to that of the outer portion. Therefore, one can expect that the solubilisation of drugs in the core will increase with increase in asymmetry, whereas the solubilisation of drugs in the outer region will decrease. In fact, it was observed that for alkyl sodium sulphites and alkyl trimethylammonium bromides, the solubilization of β-Arteether increases with the increase in the alkyl chain length, due to the larger micellar size.

However, Barry and El Eini while studying the solubilization of non-polar steroidal drugs in aqueous solutions of long-chain polyoxyethylene nonionic surfactants have observed that the molar solubilising efficiency of surfactants increased as the length of the PEO chain increased while micellar sizes are known to decrease with the increase in PEO chain length. The authors suggested that, although the inclusion of nonpolar steroids into the micelles decreases as the PEO hydrophilic chain increases, the number of micelles in equimolar amounts of surfactants increases and consequently the total amount of steroid per mole of surfactant is greater, hence the observed increase in solubilising efficiency with increased hydrophilic chain length when molar concentrations are considered. Ong and Manoukian have studied the solubilization of timobesone acetate, a corticosteroid used in inflammatory therapy, in nonionic surfactants solutions and observed that the solubilization capacity increased with increasing length of the hydrophobic tail of the surfactants. Therefore, timobesone was assumed to be solubilized in the hydrophobic core of the micelles. This observation was also confirmed by the fact that the length of the PEO chain of the surfactants studied did not affect the solubilization capacity, for a given tail length, and thus solubilization should not have occurred in the palisade layer or among the PEO heads. In general, the amount of drug solubilized in a micellar system increases with the increase in temperature. Alkhamis et al., studied the solubilization of the drug gliclazide, a second-generation sulfonylurea used in the treatment of non-insulin dependent diabetes mellitus. The drug solubility was determined as a function of the concentration of different surfactants at 25° and 37°C and, for all the ionic surfactants studied, the solubilization was higher at 37°C than at 25°C. This was attributed to the increase in thermal agitation, which results in an increase in the space available for solubilization in the micelle, in addition to the increase of gliclazide solubility in water at higher temperatures. For the polyoxyethylene nonionic surfactants, the effect of the temperature on the extent of drug solubilization may depend on whether the drug is located inside the hydrophobic core or in the palisade layer. In this same work, the solubility of gliclazide was found to decrease with temperature for the nonionic surfactants studied. Barry and El Eini also observed a significant decrease in the micelle/water molar partition coefficient, PM, obtained for nonpolar steroidal drugs in PEO surfactants solutions when the temperature was increased from 10 to 50°C. The drugs are believed to be located preferentially in the palisade layer, and the increase in temperature causes dehydration of the PEO groups, bringing them closer and consequently reducing the space available for the drugs in this region of the micelle. Nevertheless, the solubility of drugs located preferentially in the inner core of PEO micelles is expected to increase as the temperature is raised, due to micellar growth. The ionic strength can influence significantly the solubilisation of a drug in micellar solutions, especially in case of ionic surfactants. The addition of small amounts of salts decreases the repulsion between the similarly charged ionic surfactant head groups, thereby decreasing the cmc and increasing the aggregation number and volume of the micelles. The increase in aggregation number favours the solubilisation of hydrophobic drugs in the inner core of the micelle. On the other hand, the decrease in mutual repulsion of the ionic head groups causes closer packing of the ionic surfactant molecules in the palisade layer decreasing the volume available for solubilization of polar drugs. The addition of salts to solutions of PEO nonionic surfactants may also increase the extent of solubilization of hydrophobic drugs because of the increase in aggregation number. The pH of micellar solutions can also show significant influence on the extent of solubilization of drugs, since it may change the equilibrium between ionized and molecular forms of some drugs. LI et al. studied the solubility of the ionized and un-ionized forms of flavopiridol in polysorbate solutions at different pH values. This drug is a weakly basic (pKa = 5.68) derivative of rohitukine that has been developed for breast cancer treatment. The authors observed that the highest total drug solubility was achieved at pH 4.3 where most of the drug was ionized. More recently, Li and Zhao studied the solubilization of flurbiprofen, a non-steroidal antiinflamatory drug used in rheumatoid arthritis, in polysorbate solutions at different pH values. This drug is a weak acid, with a pKa of 4.17. It was observed that the drug solubility increases with the increase in pH for pH values over the pKa, due to the increase in the ionized form of the drug. The authors have also proposed an equilibrium-based model to characterise drug-surfactant interactions in pH-controlled systems, reflecting both interactions and interdependence among all drug-containing species: unionised drug in water, ionized drug in water, unionised drug in micelles, and ionized drug in micelles. The model proposed yielded reasonably good estimation when compared to experimental data. Regarding ionic surfactants, a particular kind of behaviour can be observed for the solubility of drugs at different pH values. Enhanced solubility of a drug may be observed at pH values at which the drug is found mostly ionized, when surfactant and drug are oppositely charged. This behaviour is a consequence of the electrostatic interactions between the surfactant molecules and the charged drug that causes a decrease in the repulsive forces between the head groups of the surfactant molecules, contributing to the micellization process and thus decreasing the cmc value. In fact, an early study has demonstrated that the drug chlorpromazine can form mixed monomolecular films with phospholipids such as L-α-dipalmitoyl phosphatidylethanolamine and L-α-dipalmitoyl phosphatidyl-choline. More recently, Caetano et al. observed a comicellization phenomenon for the negatively charged surfactant SDS and trifluoperazine, an amphiphilic cationic drug used as antipsychotic and tranquilizer. The authors demonstrated, based on SAXS (Small Angle Xray Scattering) studies, that the presence of the protonated drug mediates the effect that the counter ion has on the SDS micelle, in such a way that the drug is able to promote micellar surface charge screening. Moreover, the electrostatic interaction between the positively charged drug and the negatively charged SDS must cause a decrease in the repulsive forces between the head groups of the surfactant. One interesting approach is to combine micellar solubilization with other properties that may be improved in a drug solution. In this context, recently Palma et al. combined the solubilization properties of a surfactant with the ascorbic acid antioxidant property that protects drugs from degradation by light, heat, dissolved oxygen and other radical producing species, by means of synthesising an ascorbyl-decanoate surfactant. It was observed that micellar solutions of the surfactant obtained significantly improved the solubility of hydrophobic drugs with respect to pure water, by including these molecules in the hydrophobic micellar core, as well as protected them from degradation. It was also observed that the drug solubilization was more effective for the most hydrophobic drugs (Danthron and Griseofulvin) than for more hydrophilic ones (Phenacetin). A nonionic surfactant that deserves special attention is Cremophor EL (CrEL), which has been used for solubilization of a wide variety of hydrophobic drugs such as anaesthetics, photosensitizers, sedatives, immunosuppressive agents and anticancer drugs. This heterogeneous surfactant is a result of the reaction of castor oil with ethylene oxide, with polyoxyethylene glycerol ricinoleate 35 as the major component identified. Formulations containing CrEL have been shown to present important biological side effects, including severe anaphylactic hypersensitivity reactions, hyperlipidaemia, abnormal lipoprotein patterns, aggregation of erythrocytes and peripheral neuropathy. One of the most recognized applications of CrEL is the pharmaceutical formulation of paclitaxel, a hydrophobic drug active against several murine tumours that has its development suspended for several years due to solubilization problems. Various studies have shown that CrEL influences the pharmacokinetics of many drugs including paclitaxel that presents a nonlinear disposition when formulated with this surfactant. Recently, Sparreboom et al. proposed that the effect of CrEL on paclitaxel pharmacokinetics is associated with micellar solubilization, i.e. encapsulation of the drug within CrEL micelles, with the micelles acting as the principal carrier of paclitaxel in the systemic circulation. In paclitaxel I.V. infusions, an exceptionally large amount of CrEL is necessary, resulting in important biological events that can lead to serious acute hypersensitivity reactions and neurological toxicity. Therefore, large variety CrEL-free formulation vehicles for paclitaxel are currently in (pre)clinical development, including liposomes, nanocapsules and microspheres.

HYDROTROPY

Hydrotrophy is a solubilization procedure, whereby expansion of a lot of the second solute, the hydrotropic operator brings about an expansion in the fluid solvency of first solute. Hydrotropic operators are ionic natural salts, comprises antacid metal salts of different natural acids. Added substances or salts that expansion dissolvability in given dissolvable is said to "salt in" the solute and those salts that lessening solvency "salt out" the solute. A few salts with huge anions or cations that are themselves solvent in water bring about "salting in" of nonelectrolytes called "hydrotropic salts"; a wonder is known as "hydrotropism." Hydrotrophy assigns the expansion in dissolvability in water because of the nearness of enormous measure of added substances. The instrument by which it improves dissolvability is all the more firmly identified with complexation including a powerless connection between the hydrotropic operators such as sodium benzoate, sodium acetic acid derivation, sodium alginate, urea, and the ineffectively solvent medications. Hydrotropy is a developing ground-breaking drug solubilization procedure which has been appeared to fundamentally improve the dissolvability of numerous medications. Hydrotropy alludes to the procedure by which a lot of solute improves the dissolvability of another intensify (the medication). They are as often as possible anionic sweet smelling and non-sweet-smelling mixes and can be once in a while impartial. The hydrotropes are known to self-collect in the arrangement. The order of hydrotropes based on atomic structure is troublesome since a wide assortment of mixes has been accounted for to show hydrotropic conduct. Explicit models may incorporate ethanol, sweet-smelling alcohols such as resorcinol, pyrogallol, catechol, α and β-naphthols and salicylates, and alkaloids such as caffeine and nicotine, and ionic surfactants such as diacids, sodium dodecyl sulfate, and dodecyl oxydibenzene. The fragrant hydrotropes with anionic head gatherings are for the most part contemplated mixes. They are enormous in number in view of isomerism, and their successful hydrotrope activity might be due to the accessibility of intuitive pi (π) orbital.

While recent ultrasound-assisted hydrotropic extraction was used, as a greener approaches for the isolation of geraniol from the leaves of Cymbopogon martini where sodium cumene sulfonate was selected as a suitable hydrotrope for the solubilization studies. It is a clean and green technology, was effectively implemented in extraction of natural products due to advantages like less extraction time, improve in product quality along with reduced processing costs. From the literature survey, it was found that very less work has been done on using natural hydrotropes. The current review focused on advantages and pharmaceutical dosage form using of natural hydrotropes and synthetic hydrotropes. Natural hydrotropes such as caffeine, tannic acid, epigallate, piperazine, and coconut derivatives have been used in few studies. The use of natural hydrotropes is beneficial over synthetic hydrotropes as it is safe for human use. The use of high amount of synthetic hydrotropes is very dangerous for human administration. While using in a combination of natural and synthetic hydrotropes, it has been reported that due to their intermolecular complex formation it helps in enhancing the solubility of drugs. Hydrotropy is given by the scientist Neuberg Carl A. in 1916. Hydrotropes are basically water-soluble and surface-active compounds; they are useful for enhancing the solubility of organic solutes. They have a molecular phenomenon by adding a second solute (hydrotrope) which is actually beneficial for increasing the aqueous solubility of poorly water-soluble drugs. Hydrotropes always follows an important solubilisation technique in which many chemical components said as hydrotropes which used as several-fold to increase in solubility of poorly soluble drugs under normal condition. The hydrotropy acts as increase in the solubility of solutes by the addition of high concentration of alkali metal salts of different organic acids. Which forward by Neuberg, there are several concentrated aqueous hydrotropic agent is available synthetically or naturally. Some of our hydrotropic agents describe as sodium benzoate, niacinamide, citric acid, tannic acid, piperazine, and caffeine have been observed to enhance the aqueous solubility of poorly water-soluble drugs. Hydrotropy is an expansion in water dissolubility brought about by the expansion of a subsequent solute. A few hydrotropic operators, for example, urea, caffeine, sodium benzoate, sodium salicylate, and nicotinamide, have been recognised. The fundamental utilisation of this wonder is to build the water solvency of insoluble or somewhat dissolvable medications; there are no reports of the advancement of a hydrotropic plan containing a percutaneous enhancer for the transdermal definition of a water-solvent medication. Unsaturated fat liquor esters are usually utilised as adjuvants for beautifiers and pharmaceuticals. A few esters have been utilised as pervasion enhancers for medications. The use of a high amount of synthetic hydrotropes is very dangerous for human administration. There has been relatively little work since the introduction of hydrotropy to explore in details and systematic manner the ability of natural hydrotropes to increase the apparent solubility of drug. This research work gives insight to use the natural hydrotropes in solubility enhancement as well as formulation development. Natural hydrotropes can be used in combination of synthetic hydrotropes, and this reduces the concentration of individual hydrotropes using mixed hydrotropy approach.

Characteristics of hydrotropes

- Completely dissolvable in water and essentially insoluble in the framework.
- Hydrotropes are surface dynamic and total in watery arrangement in light of their amphiphilic structure.
- Should not create any temperature when disintegrated in water.
- Cheap and simple accessibility.
- Nonlethal and non-receptive.
- Insensitive to temperature impacts, when disintegrated in water.
- The dissolvable character being free of pH, high selectivity, and the nonappearance of emulsification are the other one of kind points of interest of hydrotropes.

Advantages of Hydrotropes

- Hydrotropy is important tool to the other solubilisation methods, such as micellar solubilisation, salting, and miscibility because of the independent character of solvent.
- Hydrotropes do not require any chemical modification of drugs.
- Hydrotrope should not produce any temperature condition when it dissolved in water.
- It only requires mixing the drug with the hydrotrope in water.
- It does not require chemical modification of hydrophobic drugs, use of organic solvents, or preparation of the emulsion system.
- It provides an efficient, simple, and green platform for various pharmaceutical industries as organic transformations.
- They are easily available and having a low cost.
- Nontoxic and nonreactive.

By use of 'hydrotropic agents', the drug solubility may be changed by pH solution for parenteral administration. The minimum amount of cosolvent is required for the solubility enhancement which should have less toxicity. Parenteral formulation can conduct the problem of reducing injection difficulties and also in blood compatibilities due to increase in viscosity using of cosolvent. These vehicles should contain a less amount and low concentration of cosolvent.

Mechanism of Hydrotropy

Each hydrotrope has specific capacity toward a specific segment in the blend, which encourages simple recuperation of the hydrotrope arrangement by controlled weakening with water. Dissolvability does not demonstrate any apparent increment even after the expansion of hydrotrope in the fluid stage, however on ensuing increment in the centralization of hydrotrope, the solvency of the natural compound present in watery stage increments essentially. This solvency increments in the natural compound when present in water could be because of the development of sorted out gatherings of hydrotrope particles at basic focuses. The basic convergence of hydrotrope is named as the base hydrotrope fixation minimum hydrotropic concentration (MHC) which is the base required hydrotrope focus on the watery stage above which the dissolvability of the natural compound in fluid stage increments altogether. This expansion is apparently through a self-collection process due to their amphiphilic nature and differs with the idea of the natural compound. The expanding pattern is kept up just up to a specific grouping of hydrotrope past which there is no calculable increment in the dissolvability of natural compound in the watery stage. This convergence of hydrotrope is named as the greatest hydrotrope focus. Barely any models important to the system of hydrotropy are exhibited beneath: The plant cell divider is comprised of phospholipid bilayers. The hydrotrope demolishes the phospholipid bilayer and infiltrates through the cell divider into the inward structures. The water drenching indicates exceptionally less impact on stopper cells. The cellulose and suberin (an inert impermeable waxy substance present in the cell walls of corky tissues) lamellae are the cell divider part of plug cells. The suberin lamella makes the plug cell impermeable to water. In any case, the hydrotrope arrangements tear open the water-impermeable suberin lamella and after that the develop stopper cells. The plug cell layers are bothered by the hydrotrope, and the watery arrangement enters through the cell divider. At the point when the inward part is presented to the hydrotrope arrangement, the cell swells and liberates the cells from firmly bound structures. Hydrotropic arrangements accelerated the solutes; out of the arrangement on weakening with water in this manner empower the prepared recuperation of the disintegrated solutes. Hydrotropic operators can make the O/W and W/O microemulsion and the lamellar fluid precious stone destabilised, which results in the "stage change" from lamellar fluid gem stage to bi-constant structure this is called as hydrotrope-solubilization activity. Nutrient C demonstrates hydrotrope-solubilization activity. Hydrotropes are known as "coupling specialists.". At the point when hydrotropes are added to a turbid fluid with generally high-water substance makes the fluid straightforward in light of stage change.

Exercise

Multiple Choice Questions

1. The oral bioavailability does NOT depend on several factors such as............
   a) First-pass metabolism,
   b) Aqueous solubility
   c) Dissolution rate
   d) Permeability through skin
2. Fill in the blank with appropriate words or phrase of words given below:

   The ....and the release rate of a drug are essential to be known for characterisation of drug.
   a) Disintegration time
   b) Dissolution rate
   c) Rate of permeation
   d) Rate of absorption
3. Which of the following precautions should be treated as guidelines when running the solubility tests?
   a) The solvent and the solute must be pure.
   b) The sample is removed for analysis after confirmation of saturation.
   c) All the above
   d) None of the above
4. Fill in the blank with appropriate words or phrase of words given below:

   Semiautomated potentiometric acid/base titrations method is a very ....method.

   and can create a pH/solubility profile with one single determination.
   a) Economical
   b) Costlier
   c) Non-convenient
   d) Hazardous
5. Fill in the blank with appropriate words or phrase of words given below:

   Solubility is based on the ....dose strength.
   a) Lowest
   b) Medium
   c) Highest
   d) None of the above

6. Fill in the blank with appropriate words or phrase of words given below:

   The solubility of a drug in a given solvent is largely a function of the ....of the solvent.

   a) Polarity
   b) pH
   c) Both
   d) None

7. Fill in the blank with appropriate words or phrase of words given below:

   The relationship between polarity and solubility may be used in practice ....

   a) As the solubility of a drug in a pharmaceutical solution.
   b) To alter the solubility of a drug in a pharmaceutical solution.
   c) To make the solution of a drug in a pharmaceutical solution.
   d) None of the above

8. Fill in the blank with appropriate words or phrase of words given below:

   Liquids and solids exhibit practically no change of solubility with changes in ....

   a) Polarity
   b) Temperature
   c) Pressure
   d) pH

9. Fill in the blank with appropriate words or phrase of words given below:

   .... is one of the most important physico-chemical properties studied during pharmaceutical preformulation.

   a) Polarity
   b) pH
   c) Cosolvency
   d) Solubility

10. Which of the following conditions can vary the kinetic solubility data of a solute?

    a) Ionic strength
    b) Ions in solution
    c) Co-solutes
    d) All the above

11. The inorganic metal complexes contain only one site for binding with metal which is called?

    a) Chelate
    b) Ligand
    c) All the above
    d) None of the above

12. Which is used as catalyst in the manufacture of bulk drugs and analysis of drugs?

    a) Olefinic complex
    b) Channel type complex
    c) Clathrates
    d) Layer type complex.

13. Fill in the blank with appropriate words or phrase of words given below:

    The bond distance between the components of the complex is usually greater than …….. and a covalent bond is not involved.

    a) 5Å,
    b) 6Å,
    c) 3Å,
    d) 10Å,

14. Fill in the blank with appropriate words or phrase of words given below:

    Sodium dodecyl sulphate is a typical examples of ……………….. surfactants,

    a) Cationic,
    b) Non-ionic
    c) Zwitterionic
    d) Anionic

15. Fill in the blank with appropriate words or phrase of words given below.

    If the cmc value is lowered, the stability of the ……….. would be found more.

    a) Surfactant
    b) Micelles
    c) All the above
    d) None of the above

16. A non-ionic surfactant deserves special attention, which has been used for solubilization of a wide variety of hydrophobic drugs such as …..

    a) Anaesthetics, photosensitizers, sedatives,
    b) Anti-hypertensive drugs
    c) Antipyretic drug
    d) Analgesic drugs

17. Fill in the blank with appropriate words or phrase of words given below.

    Natural ……………… such as caffeine, tannic acid, epigallate, piperazine, and coconut derivatives have been used in few studies.

    a) Hydrotropes
    b) Allotrope
    c) All the above
    d) None of the above

18. Which of the following is an advantage of hydrotrope?

    a) Hydrotropes require some chemical modification of drugs.
    b) They are easily available and having a low cost.
    c) Toxic
    d) Reactive

19. Fill in the blank with an appropriate word given below.

    The large variety of formulation vehicles for paclitaxel are currently in (pre) clinical development, including ………………

    a) Nano particles,

b) Nanospheres,

c) Liposomes,

d) Nanosomes

20. Fill in the blank with an appropriate word given below.

    The study of ....and their role in pharmacy is of paramount importance, especially with respect to their ability of solubilising hydrophobic drugs.

    a) Micelles
    b) Solubiliser
    c) Enzyme
    d) Surfactants

Short Questions

1. What is meant by 'intrinsic solubility'?
2. What is biopharmaceutical classification system? Why such classification has been done?
3. What is meant by the term 'Phase solubility analyses?
4. How can the pressure, molecular size and polymorph influence the solubility of a drug substance?
5. Explain briefly the methods used for improvement of solubility.
6. What is cosolvency? Give two examples of cosolvent. Explain with relevant example how the salt-formation technique be used to improve the solubility.
7. What is a complex? Give three examples. Once a complex is formed what are the chemical properties of complexing ion that change?
8. Classify the complexes. What is solid dispersion? Give the relevant example. What for 'hot melt extrusion 'is used?
9. Write about fusion method used for making solid dispersion.
10. Write in short about hydrotropy.

Long Questions

1. 'The improvement of drug solubility thereby its oral bioavailability remains one of the most challenging aspects of drug development process. – 'Justify the statement.
2. Define term 'solubility'. How can the solubility of a drug be measured?
3. Briefly write down the factors that can influence the solubility of a substance.
4. 'If a compound has a low aqueous solubility, it may be subject to dissolution rate-limited or solubility-limited absorption within the gastrointestinal (GI) residence time. – 'justify the statement.

5. What are the techniques used to improve the solubility? How can the analytical methods be used to improve the solubility?
6. Describe the phenomenon of cosolvency in context to pharmaceutical formulation development.
7. 'Hydrotropic operators are ionic natural salts, comprises antacid metal salts of different natural acids. – 'explain the statement.
8. Write down the advantages of hydrotropy. What is the mechanism of hydrotropy?
9. What is meant by micellar solubilization?
10. Write about application of complexation.

Answers

1	2	3	4	5	6	7	8	9	10	11	12	13	14	15	16	17	18	19	20
d	b	c	a	c	a	b	c	d	d	b	a	c	d	b	a	a	b	c	d

References

1. S. R. K. Yellela, "Pharmaceutical technologies for enhancing oral bioavailability of poorly soluble drugs," Journal of Bioequivalence & Bioavailability, vol. 2, no. 2, pp. 28–36, 2010
2. K. H. Edward and D. Li, "Solubility," in Drug Like Properties: Concept, Structure, Design and Methods, from ADME to Toxicity Optimization, p. 56, Elsevier, 2008.
3. V. R. Vemula, V. Lagishetty, and S. Lingala, "Solubility enhancement techniques," International Journal of Pharmaceutical Sciences Review and Research, vol. 5, no. 1, pp. 41–51, 2010.
4. D. Sharma, M. Soni, S. Kumar, and G. D. Gupta, "Solubility enhancement eminent role in poorly soluble drugs," Research Journal of Pharmacy and Technology, vol. 2, no. 2, pp. 220–224, 2009.
5. A. Kumar, S. K. Sahoo, K. Padhee, P. S. Kochar, A. Sathapathy, and N. Pathak, "Review on solubility enhancement techniques for hydrophobic drugs," Pharmacie Globale, vol. 3, no. 3, pp. 001–007, 2011.
6. Pharmaceutics: The Science of Dosage Form Design Authors: M.E Aulton. Publisher: Pharmaceutics, 2002.
7. Experimental and computational screening models for prediction of aqueous drug solubility. Authors: Christel A.S Bergström, Ulf Norinder, Kristina Luthman and Per Artursson. Publisher: Pharmaceutical Research, vol 19, No 2, February 2002.

8. Miniature device for aqueous and non-aqueous solubility measurements during drug discovery. Authors: Xue-Qing Chen and Srini Venkatesh. Publisher: Pharmaceutical Research, vol 21, No 10, October 2004.
9. Comparison of a miniaturized shake-flask solubility method with automated potentiometric acid/base titrations and calculated solubilities. Authors: A Glomme, J März and J.B Dressman. Publisher: Journal of Pharmaceutical sciences, vol 94, No 1, January 2005.
10. Development of a small-scale automated solubility measurement apparatus. A Avdeef, C.M Berger. Publisher: XXX 2001. Ännu en till. Authors: Yongjin Yi, Dimitri Hatziavramidis, Allan S Myerson, Michael Waldo, Vladimir G Beylin and Jason Mustakis. Publisher: American Chemical Society, 10.1021/ie049215y, 2005.
11. Comparison of a miniaturized shake-flask solubility method with automated potentiometric acid/base titrations and calculated solubilities. Authors: A Glomme, J März and J.B Dressman. Publisher: Journal of Pharmaceutical sciences, vol 94, No 1, January 2005.
12. Comparison of a miniaturized shake-flask solubility method with automated potentiometric acid/base titrations and calculated solubilities. Authors: A Glomme, J März and J.B Dressman. Publisher: Journal of Pharmaceutical sciences, vol 94, No 1, January 2005.
13. 13. Experimental and computational sceening models for prediction of aqueous drug solubility. Authors: Christel A.S Bergström, Ulf Norinder, Kristina Luthman and Per Artursson. Publisher: Pharmaceutical Research, vol 19, No 2, February 2002.
14. Miniature device for aqueous and non-aqueous solubility measurements during drug discovery. Authors: Xue-Qing Chen and Srini Venkatesh. Publisher: Pharmaceutical Research, vol 21, No 10, October 2004.
15. A theoretical basis for a biopharmaceutic drug classification: the correlation of in Vitro drug product dissolution and in Vivo bioavailability. Authors: Gordon L Amidon, Hans Lennernas, Vinod P Shah, John R Crison. Publisher: Pharmaceutical Research, vol 12, No 3, 413-420, 1995.
16. Sokoloski T.D. Remington: The Science and Practice of Pharmacy, 19th ed., 194-200, 2006.
17. Hill J.W., Retrucci R.H.; General Chemistry, 2nd ed.; 524 -527, 1999.
18. Filippone S., Heimann F., Rassat A.; Chem. Commun.; (14), 1508-1509, 2002.
19. C. Lipinski, F. Lombardo, B.W. Dominy and P.J. Feeney, Adv. Drug Deliv. Rev., 23, 3 (1997).
20. X.Q. Chen and S. Venkatesh, Pharm. Res., 21, 1758 (2004).

21. J. Devane, Pharm. Technol. 22 (1998) 68-80 [A.J. Humberstone, W.N Charman, Adv. Drug Deliv. Rev. 25 (1997) 103-128
22. F. De Jaeghere, E. Allémann, R. Cerny, B. Galli, A.F. Steulet, I. Müller, H. Schütz, E. Doelker, R. Gurny, Pharm. Technol. 3 (2001) 1-8
23. G. Völgyi, E. Baka, K.J. Box, J.E.A. Comer, K. TakácsNovák, Anal. Chim. Acta 673 (2010), 40-46
24. A. Avdeef, S. Bendels, O. Tsinman, K. Tsinman, M. Kansy, Pharm. Res. 24 (2007) 530-545
25. A. Avdeef, Adv. Drug Deliv. Rev. 59 (2007) 568-590
26. K.A. Hasselbalch, Z. Die Biochem. 78 (1916) 112-144
27. G.L. Amidon, H. Lennernas, V.P. Shah, J.R. Crison, Pharm. Res. 12 (1995) 413-420
28. J. Dressman, Ch. Repass, Adv. Drug Deliv. Rev. 59 (2007) 603-616
29. J. Dressman, Ch. Repass, Adv. Drug Deliv. Rev. 59 (2007) 603-616
30. L. Du-Cuny, J. Huwyler, M. Wiese, M. Kansy, Eur. J. Med. Chem. 43 (2008) 501-512
31. E. Baka, J.E.A. Comer, K. Takács-Novák, J. Pharm. Biomed. Anal. 46 (2008) 335-341
32. U. Domańska, A. Pobudkowska, A. Pelczarska, J. Phys. Chem., B 115 (2011) 2547-2554
33. U. Domańska, A. Pobudkowska, A. Pelczarska, M. Winiarska-Tusznio, P. Gierycz, J. Chem. Thermodyn. 42 (2010) 1465-1472
34. 35. U. Domańska, A. Pobudkowska, A. Pelczarska, P. Gierycz, J. Phys. Chem., B 113 (2009) 8941-8947
35. C.A.S. Bergström, U. Norinder, K. Luthman, P. Artursson, Pharm. Res. 19 (2002) 182-188
36. M. Mizutani, Z. Phys. Chem. 119 (1925) 318-326
37. A. Li, S.H. Yalkowsky, J. Pharm. Sci. 83 (1994) 1735- –1740
38. C.D. Bevan, and R.S. Lloyd, Anal. Chem., 72, 1781 (2000)
39. A. Avdeef, High-throughput Measurements of Solubility Profiles. Pharmacokinetic Optimization In Drug Research: Biological, Physicochemical and Computational Strategies, [LogP2000, Lipophilicity Symposium], 2nd, Lausanne, Switzerland, Mar. 5-9, (2000), pp. 305-325 (2001).
40. E.H. Kerns and L. Di, Drug-Like Properties: Concepts, Structure Design and Methods: from ADME to Toxicity Optimization, Academic Press (2008).
41. E. Baka, J.E.A. Comer and K. Takács-Novák, J. Pharm. Biomed. Anal., 46, 335 (2008).

42. Bittner B, Mountfield R.J. Formulations and related activities for the oral administration of poorly water soluble compounds in early discovery animal studies. Pharm. Ind. 2002; 64: 800–807

43. Bittner B, Mountfield R.J. Intravenous administration of poorly soluble new drug entities in early drug discovery: the potential impact of formulation on pharmacokinetic parameters. Current opinion in drug discovery & development. 2002; 5: 59–71.

44. Meyer, M, C. "Bioavailability of drugs and bioequivalence In: Encyclopedia of Pharmaceutical Technology" New York. Marcel Dekker Inc.; 1998; 2, 33-58.

45. Shargil, L, & Yu, "Applied Biopharmaceuitcs" Appleton-Century Crofts, Norwalk, C.T, 1985; 2, 193-203

46. Martin, A, "Physical pharmacy," Lippincott Williams & Wilkins, A. Walters Kluwer Co, Philadelphia, 2003; 5, 410-418.

47. Carstensen, J, T, "Pharmaceutical Preformulation" Teelinomoc Publishing Co. Inc, 1998; 14-47.

48. Martin, A, Bustamanate, P, and Chun, A, H, C, "Physical Pharmacy" B.I. Wavely Pvt. Ltd, New Delhi, 1994; 4, 223

49. Osol, A, (Eds.) in: "Remington's Pharmaceutical sciences" Mack Publishing Company, Eastern Pennsylvania, 1990; 18, 203.

50. Dass CR, Jessup W, Apolipo protiens A-I. Cyclodextrins and liposomes as potential drugs for the reversal of atherosclerosis. J Pharm Pharmacol 2000; 52:731–61.

51. Szetjli J. Introduction and general overview of cyclodextrin chemistry. Chem Rev 1998; 98:1743–53.

52. Strickley, R.G, Solubilizing excipients in oral and injectable formulations. Pharmaceutical Research, 2004; 21, 201–230

53. Seedher, N, Bhatia S, Solubility enhancement of Cox-2 inhibitors using various solvent systems. AAPS Pharm Sci Tech, 2003; 4, 33.

54. Berge, S.M, Bighley L.D, Monkhouse, D.C.; Pharmaceutical salts.; J Pharm Sci.; 1977; 66(1): 1-19

55. Stahl, P.H, Nakano M. Pharmaceutical aspects of the drug salt form.; Handb Pharm Salts. 2008:83-116.

56. Kumar, L, Amin, A., Bansal, A.K.; Salt selection in drug development.; Pharm Technol. 2008; 3(32).

57. Hilfiker R. Polymorphism: in the pharmaceutical industry. Chem Today. 2006; 21(1):41-44.

58. Lipinski CA (2001). Avoiding investment in doomed drugs, is poor solubility an industry wide problem?

59. Curr Drug Dis., 4: 17-19.

60. Vasconcelos T and Costa P (2007). Development of a rapid dissolving ibuprofen solid dispersion.

61. In: PSWC – Pharmaceutical Sciences World Conference, DD-W103

CHAPTER - 4

Dissolution

Theories, Mechanisms of Dissolution, In-Vitro Dissolution Testing Models – Sink and Non-Sink. Factors Influencing Dissolution and Intrinsic Dissolution Studies. Dissolution Test Apparatus – Designs, Dissolution Testing for Conventional and Controlled Release Products. Data Handling and Correction Factor. Bio-Relevant Media, *In-Vitro* and *In-Vivo* Correlations, Levels of Correlations.

THEORIES OF DISSOLUTION

The term, dissolution can be defined as "*the process by which a known amount of solid substance goes into solution per unit of time under standardised conditions.*" In other words, *dissolution is the process of dissolving a solid substance by a liquid (water).* The process of dissolution is principally controlled by the affinity between the solid substance and the solvent. The factors that influence the dissolution characteristics of drugs are:

- Physical characteristics of the dosage form.
- Wettability of the dosage form,
- Ability of the dissolution medium to penetrate,
- Swelling process,
- Disintegration of the dosage form,
- Deaggregation of the dosage form.

The term is used to characterise the biopharmaceutical quality of a product at various stages in its lifecycle. For further development, it is used to select alternative formulations. Dissolution testing is an official or compendial test recommended by all Pharmacopoeias for evaluation of drug release from its solid or semi-solid dosage forms.

Particularly, in the United States, various studies have been conducted to establish the significance of relationship between dissolution and bioavailability of the pharmaceutical product. After making considerable efforts the *in vitro/in vivo* correlation has been established, that is, the release of drug from the dosage form and absorption of drug. However, there is limited knowledge about the complex composition and hydrodynamics of the gastrointestinal fluids remains an actual barrier. Although various studies have been found successful in establishing *in vitro/in vivo* correlation, to predict the therapeutic efficacy of a dosage form, the test for dissolution could not be accepted as a predictor. It had been considered as a qualitative tool to provide valuable information about the biological availability of a drug, and batch-to-batch consistency. Another problem is the accuracy and precision of the testing procedure. This depends largely on the strict observance of so many subtle parameters and detailed control of the operation. Presently, dissolution is considered as one of the most important quality procedures which is performed on every pharmaceutical formulation, and dissolution studies have become an essential part of drug applications to regulatory bodies throughout the world.

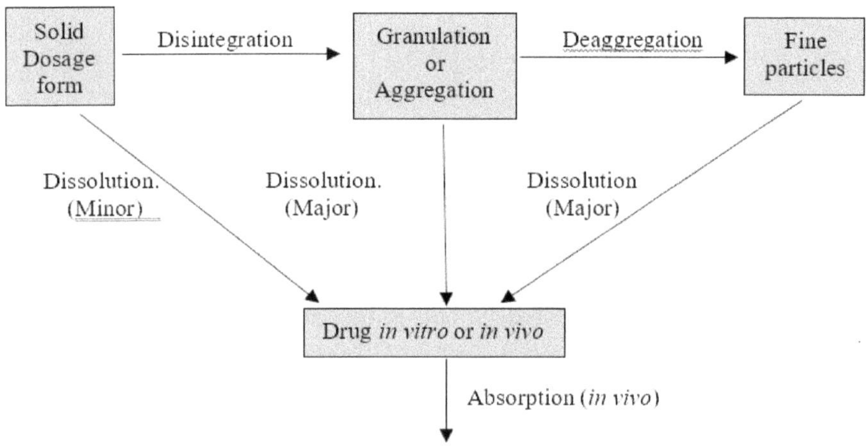

Fig.4.1 Processes involved in dissolution.

Whether or not the dissolution has been correlated with therapeutic effectiveness, the standard dissolution test is considered as a simple and inexpensive indicator of the physical consistency of a product. If the dissolution characteristics of one batch is found different from the subsequent batch or if the dissolution profiles of the batches produced show a consistent trend upwards or downwards, it is considered that some factor in the raw material used, formulation, or process of manufacturing is out of control. It gives a warning situation. In the early stages of drug development and molecular manipulation the dissolution data seems to be a useful tool.

Carstensen proposed a scheme incorporating the following sequences:

1) Initial mechanical lag,
2) Wetting of the dosage form,
3) Penetration of the dissolution medium into the dosage form,
4) Disintegration,
5) Deaggregation of the dosage form,
6) Dislodgement of the granules, and
7) Dissolution and occlusion of some particles of the drug.

According to the explanation proposed by Carstensen the wetting of the solid dosage form surface controls the liquid access to the solid surface and is the limiting factor in the dissolution process many times. The rate of wetting directly depends on the surface tension at the interface (interfacial tension) and upon the contact angle between the solid surface and the liquid.

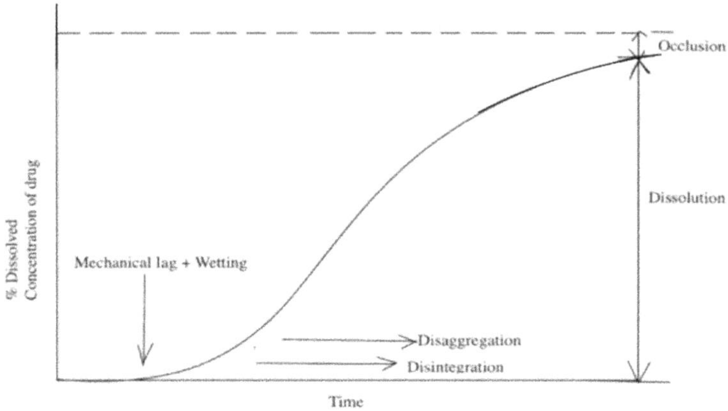

Fig.4.2 Model proposed by Carstensen.

Usually, contact angle of more than 90° indicates poor wettability. Addition of a surfactant, either to the dissolution medium or to the formulation, reduces the contact angle and improve the dissolution. If the air remains present in the dissolution medium, the air bubbles are entrapped in the tablet pores and act as a barrier at the interface. In case of capsule, the gelatine shell being extremely hydrophilic, it creates no problem of wettability for the dosage form, although it may exist for the powders inside the shell. Once the solid dosage form disintegrates into granules or aggregates, penetration characteristics play an important role in the deaggregation process. Hydrophobic lubricants such as talcum and magnesium stearate, commonly used in tablet and capsule formulations, slow the penetration rate and, hence, the deaggregation process. If the pore size is large, it facilitates the penetration. If the pore size is too large, it may inhibit penetration by decreasing the internal strain caused by the swelling of the disintegrant. After deaggregation and dislodgment occur, the drug particles become exposed to the dissolution medium and dissolution proceeds. The Fig 4.2 graphically represents the model proposed by Carstensen. The figure says that the rate of dissolution of the drug can become a rate limiting step before it appears in the blood. When the dosage form is placed into the gastrointestinal tract in solid form, there are two possibilities for the rate-limiting step.

Firstly, the solid must dissolve, and the drug in solution state must then pass through the gastrointestinal membrane. The drugs which are freely soluble in water tend to dissolve rapidly, passive diffusion of the drug takes place, or the active transport of the drug becomes rate-limiting step for absorption through the GI membrane. On the other hand, the rate of absorption of poorly soluble in water will be limited by the rate of dissolution of the undissolved drug or disintegration of the dosage form.

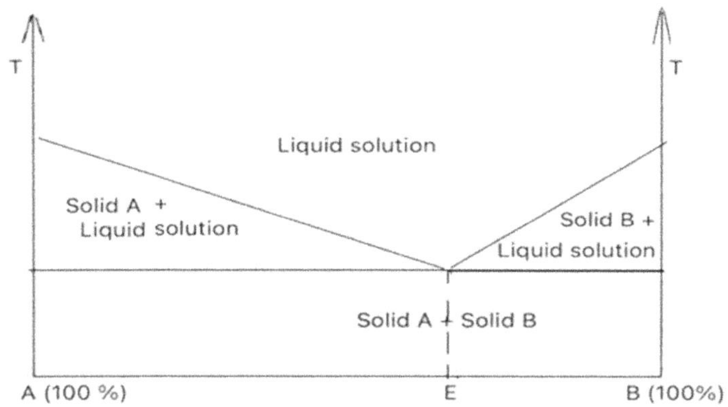

Fig.4.3 Phase diagram for a eutectic system.

The rate of dissolution of the drug substance is determined by the rate at which solvent-solute forces of attraction overcome the cohesive forces present in solid. This process is rate limiting, when the release of solute into the solution is slow and the transport into the bulk solution becomes fast. In this case, the dissolution is said to be controlled. Dissolution may also be diffusion controlled, where the solvent-solute interaction is fast, compared to transport of solute into the bulk solution. In diffusion-controlled process, a stationary layer of solute adjacent to the solid/liquid interface is postulated and is commonly referred to as the diffusion layer. The saturation concentration of solute develops at the interface and decreases with distance across the diffusion layer.

Since long it has been recognized that the release of the active substance (drug) from a dosage form may be extensively influenced by the physicochemical properties of the drug and its dosage form. By the rate of release of the drug from the dosage form, the bioavailability of the drug is usually determined. The release of the drug from its dosage form is generally estimated by the rate at which it dissolves in the surrounding medium. The rate of dissolution of a compound (drug) from the solid state is defined as the amount of drug substance that goes into solution per unit time under standardized condition of liquid/ solid interface, temperature, and composition of solvent. In biopharmaceutics, the rate of dissolution commonly known as the rate at which the drug dissolves from an intact dosage form or from fragments or particles from the dosage form during the test.

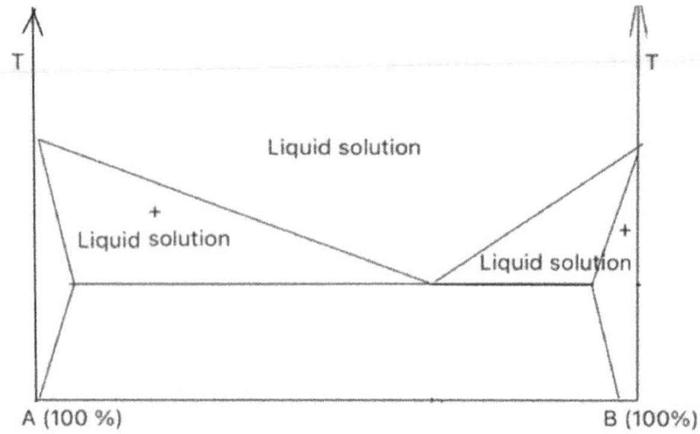

Fig.4.4 Phase diagram for a solid solution.

MECHANISMS OF DISSOLUTION

Till now numbers of theories have been proposed. But the mechanism by which the improvement of dissolution rate can be made- is not fully understood. Currently, accepted range of possible mechanisms of effectively increased dissolution includes that by reducing the particle size and by reducing agglomeration, the eutectic mixture will consist of poorly soluble drug and highly soluble carrier if exposed to gastrointestinal fluid or water, the soluble carrier dissolves and leave the drug in very fine crystalline state to go into solution rapidly. Due to increased surface area of insoluble solid or compound, the rate of dissolution will increase and hence, absorption through oral route would increase. This can be calculated using Noyes-Whitney equation[1] (Fig 4.3). Simple eutectic mixture can be obtained from the rapid solidification of the fused liquid of two components that show complete liquid miscibility and negligible solid-solid solubility. On cooling, the molten mixture forms a microfine dispersion of the two components with a concomitant decrease in the melting points of two components[2]. Various solid dispersions have been described using poorly water-soluble drugs, such as sulphathiazole, paracetamol and chloramphenicol using urea as high-water soluble carrier. These solid dispersions yielded faster release and higher bioavailability than traditional formulations of the same drugs. The small particle sizes of the drug had been the main reasons for the observed improvements in bioavailability[3,4]. Similarly, the solid solution of poorly soluble drugs in rapidly dissolving carrier achieves a faster rate of dissolution than the eutectic mixture, because the drug particle size is reduced to its absolute minimum as it is molecularly dispersed in the carrier in a solid solution (Fig 4.4). Levy and Kanig prepared solid dispersion systems using mannitol as carrier, by preparing solid solutions through molecular dispersions instead of using eutectic mixtures[5,6]. The improvements observed were due to faster carrier dissolution, releasing microcrystals or drug particles[7]. For example, dispersion of digitoxin, hydrocortisone acetate and prednisolone in polyethylene glycol 6000. Amorphous structure can be formed by replacing crystalline structure, for example, poorly water-soluble crystalline drugs are less soluble than the amorphous state, which have higher solubility.

From the thermodynamic point of view, amorphous solids, compared with corresponding crystalline solids, show higher free energy, entropy and specific volume. Thus, amorphous solids show higher transient solubility, dissolution rate, vapour pressure and molecular mobility. Usually, to dissolve a crystalline drug, energy is required to break up the crystalline lattice. This required energy is frequently considered as a barrier for dissolution of the drug substance. In solid molecular dispersion, long-range crystalline structure is absent and the drug is dissolved or molecularly dispersed in a polymeric carrier. The drug exists. in an amorphous state which exhibits a higher kinetic solubility, up to a few orders of magnitude, and dissolution rate than that of the crystalline drug[8,9]. Solid molecular dispersion of naproxen, diclofenac sodium, and piraxicam using poly (2-hydroxy-ethyl methacrylate) (PHEMA) hydrogel as carrier have been prepared by solvent evaporation method in which crystalline drug is converted into amorphous form takes place with higher aqueous solubility[10]. The local solubility and wettability of the poorly soluble drug in the solid dispersion matrix can be improved by improving the solubility and dissolution rate of poorly water-soluble drugs. This is related to the ability of matrix carrier to improve the local solubility and wettability of the drug. The effect of hydrophilic carrier, such as urea, on the solubility of chloramphenicol has been reported where the physical mixture of chloramphenicol and urea was melted, mixed thoroughly and solidified for subsequent solubility and dissolution rate studies. It was observed that as the concentration of urea was increased from 0% (w/v) to slightly more than 60% (w/v), the solubility of chloramphenicol in the presence of urea increased by greater than sevenfold. Moreover, it has been reported the observed solvent effect of PEG 6000 on the solubility of diazepam and temazepam were showed 3.5 fold and 2.5 fold increases in solubility, respectively, in the presence of 15% (w/w) PEG 6000 at 30°C. In addition, it has been suggested that the mechanism of improved solubility and rate of dissolution of diazepam and temazepam in PEG 6000 matrix involves increased wettability of the drug in a polymer-rich microenvironment as the polymer dissolves[11,12]. Interactions of the drug with the functional groups of the carrier can be explained that the ability of the carrier matrix can improve the local solubility and wettability of the drug. They can also contribute to improve aqueous solubility and rate of dissolution of the drug through specific interactions with the drug[13].

a) The intermolecular hydrogen bonding

It has been reported that hydrogen bonding interactions remained in felodipine solid dispersion with polyvinyl pyrrolidone (PVP), hydroxypropyl methylcellulose acetate succinate (HPMCAS), and hydroxypropyl methylcellulose (HPMC) where all polymers were able to maintain the amorphous state of the drug even at low excipient concentrations. The intermolecular hydrogen bonding between piroxicam and PVP in their solid dispersions was confirmed by FTIR. Solid dispersions of piroxicam were prepared using polyvinyl pyrrolidone K-30 by solvent evaporation method. The dissolution of the drug in solid dispersion depends on the ratio of drug to polyvinyl pyrrolidone. At the ratio of 1:4 (drug: PVP), the solid dispersion provide the highest rate of dissolution of about a 38-fold higher than that of pure drug.

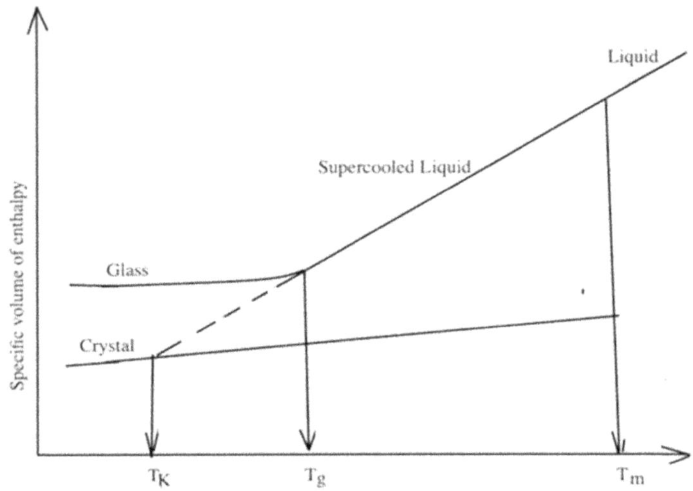

Fig.4.5 Schematic diagram of enthalpy or volume change from crystalline to the glassy state. T_K is the Kauzman temperature.

b) By elevating the T_g of the solid dispersion mixtures

In addition to forming molecular interactions with the drug molecule, polymeric carriers have been shown to reduce the amorphous drug crystallisation by increasing the viscosity and glass transition temperature (T_g) of the polymer-drug mixtures. Glass transition temperature is *the temperature below which the amorphous mixture exists in a glassy state where coordinated molecular motion becomes very slow and restricted*[14]. The Fig 4.5 shows the relationship between temperature (T) and volume (V) or enthalpy (H) for liquid, glassy and crystalline state of a material. It is desirable to elevate the T_g of the solid dispersion mixture to restrict the mobility of drug molecules in the carrier matrix and to prevent subsequent recrystallisation. In principle, such stability can be maintained by storage at a temperature well below T_g.

c) **Inhibited drug precipitation from supersaturated solution**

Owing to the increased kinetic solubility of the amorphous form of the drug, it is possible to generate a supersaturated solution with the drug concentration well above the solubility of the crystalline drug. Over time, the drug tends to precipitate out to reach much lower equilibrium solubility. The presence of dissolved carrier. may also inhibit the precipitation of the drug from the supersaturated solution.

d) **By formation of metastable drug polymorphous with higher solubility and dissolution rate**

In cases where polymeric carriers fail to generate complete amorphous state of the drug, they may still be able to improve the solubility and dissolution rate of the drug by forming metastable crystalline polymorphs of the drug substance which shows higher solubility than that of the crystalline drug alone. The presence of polymorphs 1, 3, and 4 were observed in the solid dispersion products[15].

Complex Formation

In this solid dispersion, a drug forms a complex with an inert soluble carrier in solid state. The availability of the drug depends on (1) the solubility and stability constant of the compound or complex, and (2) the absorption rate of the drug. It is suggested that the rate of dissolution and oral absorption can be increased by formation of water-soluble complex with high dissolution constant. For example, solid dispersions of carbamazepine/PEG 4000 and PEG 6000 have been prepared by fusion method. Dissolution studies suggested that due to complex formation between carbamazepine and PEG 6000, the rate of dissolution has been increased[16]. Cyclodextrins (CD) are cyclic oligomers typically composed of 6 – 8 glucose units. Cyclodextrins represent a class of solubilising agents that form non-covalent, dynamic complexes with lipophilic molecules by a process known as inclusion. The inclusion complex modifies temporarily the physical properties of the substance. Governed by the equilibrium constant between the free drug, free CDs and the drug-CD complex, the drug will be released constantly and rapidly on dilution. CDs have been demonstrated to improve the stability of substances like proteins or peptides. The CDs, approved for pharmaceutical products, can be classified into three major types which are different only in their molecular weight and respective central cavity diameter. α-cyclodextrin $(\alpha - CD)$ has a molecular weight of 972 and a central cavity diameter of around 5A', these increases to MW 1135 and 6.2A 'for β-CD and 8A 'for γ-CD with MW 1297 respectively[17].

- **Swelling and capillary action of carrier**

  Dissolution of poorly water soluble drugs can be improved by using super disintegrants such as sodium starch glycolate, cross-povidone, cross linked polyvinyl pyrrolidone, and cross linked alginic acid etc[18]. Sodium starch glycolate swells 7- to 12-fold in less than 30 sec. uniformly in all three dimensions while croscarmellose swells 4- to 8-fold in less than 10 sec in two dimensions leaving the fibre length similar. This indicates that rate and extent of swelling have an important role in disintegrants that work by swelling. Cross-linked PVP swells little, due to absence of cation-genic groups in the molecule, but returns to its original boundaries quickly after compression. Wicking or capillary action is postulated to be a major factor in the ability of crosslinked PVP to work as. super disintegrant[19]. Gellan gum and xanthan gum have extensive swelling properties for faster disintegration. Calcium silicate is highly porous super disintegrant which acts by wicking action. Cross-linked alginic acid is a hydrophilic colloidal substance with high capacity of sorption and acts by swelling or wicking action.

- **Surface activity and micellar solubilisation**

  Various surfactants such as polyglycolized glyceride, Tweens, Spans, Polyoxyethylene stearates and synthetic block copolymers such as poly (propylene oxide)-poly (ethylene oxide) – poly (propylene oxide), an example of poloxamers based micelles, Poly (β-benzyl-lasparate) – b – poly (caprolactone) – b – poly (ethylene oxide) etc are used as carrier for dissolution enhancement. Improvement of drug solubility by using the amphiphilic surfactants is due to lowering surface tension between drug and solvent, improvement of wetting characteristics and micellar solubilisation of the drug. Micelles are supramolecular self-assemblies of macromolecules where unimers are held by non-covalent interactions. The core of the micelles solubilises drugs whereas the corona/shell allows for their suspension in aqueous media.

- **By increasing porosity of the product**

  Particles in solid dosage forms have been found to have a higher degree of porosity. The increase in porosity depends on the carrier properties, for example, solid dosage forms containing linear polymers produce larger and more porous particles than those containing reticular polymers and, thus, result in a higher dissolution rate. The increased porosity of solid dosage form particles hastens the drug release profile[20,21].

- **Combination and miscellaneous mechanisms**

  Often a solid dispersion does not entirely belong to any of previous classes. For example, in solid dispersion system, the drug can exist in amorphous state and the crystalline state in a carrier. Thus, the observed increased in dissolution and absorption may be due to combination of various mechanisms.

IN VITRO DISSOLUTION TESTING MODELS – SINK and NON-SINK

Dissolution is *a process in which a solid substance solubilises in a given solvent at a particular temperature* i.e. mass transfer from the solid state to the liquid state.

Adequate absorption of orally administered medications involves *solubilisation of drug molecules in the gastrointestinal (GI) fluid and transport across the membrane of the epithelial cells in the human GI tract.* Poorly water-soluble therapeutic candidates require enabling formulation approaches to develop oral solid dosage forms with enhanced solubility to reach the systemic circulation. Hence, Biopharmaceutics Classification System class II and IV drugs may be formulated as supersaturating drug delivery systems (amorphous solid dispersions [ASDs]) that are capable of generating a supersaturated drug solution during GI transit. Considering the strong dependency of the dissolution performance on the formulation, coupled with the complexity of solid-state characterisation for these supersaturating systems, it is necessary to conduct both discriminatory *in vitro* dissolution testing and comprehensive physico-chemical characterisation (X-ray diffraction for determining drug crystallinity) to ensure product quality and *in vivo* performance. The dissolution methods under non-sink conditions have become an increasingly important strategy in measuring the true performance of supersaturating formulations and drug products by assessing the extent of supersaturation that is generated as well as the associated crystal nucleation and growth kinetics. For this reason, concentration–time profiles generated from supersaturated drug delivery systems under non-sink conditions are generally recognised as a direct evaluation of their ability to achieve and maintain drug supersaturation. Drug release kinetics based on diffusion, swelling, dissolution, or combination of aforementioned mechanisms have been well predicted[22,23]

The dissolution process can be performed by two methods - sink and non-sink.

The term sink is related to the volume of solvent. The solvent used is commonly 5 to 10 times greater than the volume present in the saturated solution of the concerned chemical substance, generally API, and sometimes the excipients contained in the dosage form under test. During dissolution testing, maintenance of the sink condition is mandatory. Because when the concentration begins to get too close to the saturation point, even though the total soluble amount still remains constant, the dissolution rate will gradually begin to reduce in significant amounts, sufficient to corrupt the test results.

With respect to both crystalline and amorphous solubility non-sink dissolution test is performed. The volume of dissolution medium used in this method is less than that required to dissolve the solid in its amorphous form, ASDs may dissolve in two patterns.

The sink method for dissolution testing is generally performed by:

Using forced convection sink devices:

i) Wurster pollos adsorption method
ii) Partition method
iii) Dialysis method
iv) Rotating disk apparatus

Using Continuous flow/Flow through method

i) Pernaowski method
ii) Langenbucher method
iii) Baun and Walker method
iv) Tingstad and Reigelman method
v) Teknaka method
vi) Modified Column apparatus

The non-sink method for dissolution testing is generally performed by:

Using Natural convection non-sink methods

i) Klein solvmeter method
ii) Nelson hanging pellet method
iii) Levy static disk method

Using forced convection non-sink methods

i) Tumbling method
ii) Levy or Beaker method
iii) Rotating disk method
iv) Particle size method
v) USP Rotating basket apparatus
vi) USP Paddle apparatus

FACTORS INFLUENCING DISSOLUTION

The dissolution rate data can be used meaningfully, only if the results of successive test on the same dosage form are consistent within reason. The dissolution test should yield reproducible result, even it is performed in different laboratories or with different personnel.

To achieve high reproducibility, all variables that influence the test should be clearly understood and possibly controlled.

The factors that affect the rate of dissolution of drugs from a dosage form are:

1) Physicochemical properties of the drug
2) Drug product formulation factors
3) Processing factors
4) Dissolution test parameters
5) Dissolution test apparatus

1) Physicochemical Properties of the drug

a) Solubility of drug

The physicochemical properties of the drug substance play an important role in controlling its dissolution from the dosage form. The modified Noyes-Whitney equation shows that the aqueous solubility of the drug is the major factor determining its dissolution rate. In fact, some studies show that drug-solubility data could be used as rough proctor of the possibility of any future problems with bioavailability, a factor that should be taken into consideration in the formulation design. At least the drug should have the aqueous solubility of 1% in water to avoid problem in absorption.

Studies of 45 drug compounds of different classes and a wide range of solubilities showed that their initial rate of dissolution is directly proportional to their respective solubility.

b) Salt formation

It is one of the common methods used to increase the solubility of drug and dissolution rate. It has always been assumed that sodium salts dissolve faster than their corresponding insoluble acids. For example, sodium and potassium salts of Penicillin G, sulpha drugs, phenytoin, barbiturates etc. While in case of phenobarbital dissolution of sodium salt was slower than that of weak acid. Same is the case for weak base drug, strong acid salts, such as hydrochlorides and sulphates of weak bases such as epinephrine, tetracycline are commonly used due to high solubility. However, free bases of chlortetracycline, metacycline were more soluble than corresponding hydrochloride salt at gastric pH values, due to common ion suppression.

c) Particle size

The rate of dissolution is directly proportional to the surface area of the drug. Since the surface area increases with the decreasing particle size, higher dissolution rates may be achieved through the micronisation (reduction of the particle size) of sparingly soluble drugs. The micronisation guarantees the better dissolution as well as bioavailability. It can increase the effective surface area. The effective surface area is the surface area available to the dissolution fluid. If the drug is hydrophobic in. nature, micronisation can lead to aggregation and floatation when dispersed into dissolution medium. So, simply by increasing the surface area of the drug does not always guarantee an equivalent increase in dissolution rate. The dissolution medium has poor wetting properties, reduction of particle size may lead to decreased effective surface area and, hence, a "slower" rate of dissolution. Hydrophobic drugs such as phenacetin, aspirin shows decrease in dissolution rate as they tend to adsorb air at the surface and inhibit the wettability. Problem can be eliminated by evacuating the surface from adsorbed air or by use of surfactants. Hence, these drugs *in-vivo* exhibit excellent wetting due to presence of natural surfactants such as bile salts.

d) Co-precipitation

Dissolution rate of sulfathiazole could be significantly increased by co-precipitating the drug with povidone.

e) Shape of the tablet

In some cases, the shape of a tablet can affect the dissolution. For example, in case of controlled release tablets high rpm should be applied to check for robustness and dose dumping.

f) Solid state of the drug

Solid phase characteristics of drug, such as amorphicity and crystallinity, the state of hydration have significant influence on dissolution rate. These are two important solid phase characteristics of drugs that can affect the dissolution profile. Various studies have shown that the amorphous form of a drug usually shows greater solubility and higher rate of dissolution, as compared to that exhibited by the crystalline form. For example, anhydrous ampicillin can dissolve in water more quickly than ampicillin trihydrate, similarly, novobiocin and griseofulvin. show faster dissolution. However, there are some deviations of this rule, dissolution rate of amorphous erythromycin estolate is markedly lower than the crystalline form of erythromycin estolate.

g) Polymorphism

Polymorphic forms of drugs have been demonstrated to influence changes in solubilising characteristics and, thus the rate of dissolution of the concerned drug. Various reports shave been published to show that the polymorphism and the state of hydration, solvation, and/ or complexation markedly influence the dissolution characteristics of the drug. For example, tolbutamide, chloramphenicol, and others are the drugs that can influence the dissolution behaviour. Metastable (high activation energy) polymorphic forms show better dissolution than stable forms. For example, chloramphenicol palmitate exists in at least two polymorphs, α and β . The β form is apparently more bioavailable. Therefore, the manufacturer must be recommended to use the polymorph β only for maximum absorption.

2) Drug product formulation factors

Rate of dissolution of pure drug can be changed significantly when it is mixed with various additives (excipients) during manufacturing process of a product. These additives may be diluents, dyes, binders, granulating agents, disintegrants and lubricants. For this reason, the rate of dissolution of tablets or capsule of the same drug may be found different.

a) Diluents

Diluent in capsule and/ or tablet can influence the dissolution rate of drug. Studies of starch on dissolution rate of salicylic acid tablet by dry double compression process shows three times increase in dissolution rate when the starch content increase from the 5 – 20 %. The starch particles form a layer on the outer surface of hydrophobic drug particles, as a result, impart hydrophilic character to granules and thus, increase in effective surface area and rate of dissolution. Different types of dissolution apparatus utilised affect ranking of different varieties of starch. With stirring type of agitation, order was potato starch>corn starch>arrowroot starch>rice starch. With oscillating type, a different order observed.

Corn>rice>arrowroot>potato. The dissolution rate is not only affected by nature of the diluent but also affected by excipient dilution (drug/excipient ratio). For example, in quinazoline comp. dissolution rate increases as the excipient /drug ratio increases from 3:1 to 7:1 to 11:1.

b) Disintegrants

Disintegrating agent when added before and after the granulation can affect the dissolution rate. Studies of various disintegrating agents on phenobarbital tablet showed that when copa gel (low viscosity grade of Na CMC) is added before granulation decreased dissolution rate but if added after did not have any effect on dissolution rate. Microcrystalline cellulose is a very good disintegrating agent but at high compression force, it may reduce drug dissolution. Starch is not only an excellent diluent but also superior disintegrant due to its hydrophilicity and swelling property. Disintegration and dissolution rate of disintegrants with moderate swelling capacity depend largely on mixing time of drug and excipient pre-blended with lubricant. On other hand, disintegrants with strong swelling capacity such as sodium starch glycolate were hardly affected by mixing time with lubricant.

c) Binders and granulating agents

The hydrophilic binder increases dissolution rate of poorly wettable drug. Large amount of binder increases hardness and decrease disintegration /dissolution rate of tablet. Non aqueous binders such as ethyl cellulose also reduce the drug dissolution. Phenobarbital tablet granulated with gelatine solution (10%) provide a faster dissolution rate in human gastric juice whereas dissolution rate decreases with 20% gelatine. This was due to higher concentration which formed a thick film around tablet. Water soluble granulating agent plasdone gives faster dissolution rate compared to gelatine than those prepared using sodium carboxymethyl cellulose or polyethylene glycol 6000 as binder. Gelatine imparts hydrophilic character to hydrophobic drug surface area.

d) Lubricants

Primarily, lubricants are hydrophobic in nature (metallic stearates) and thus, prolong tablet disintegration time by forming water repellent coat around individual granules. This retarding effect is the most important factor in influencing the rate of dissolution of solid dosage forms. Both amount and method of addition affect the property. It should be added in small amount (1% or less) and should be tumbled or mixed gently for only very short time. Prolonged mixing can increase the dissolution time. However, if an enhancing effect in dissolution of hydrophobic granules is desired, water soluble lubricant such as SLS or carbowaxes may be used.

e) Surfactants

These enhance the dissolution rate of poorly soluble drug. This is due to lowering of interfacial tension and increasing effective surface area. This in turn can cause faster dissolution rate. For example, non-ionic surfactant such as polysorbate 80 increases the dissolution rate of phenacetin granules. Such an increase has been more pronounced when the surfactant was sprayed on granules than when it was dissolved in granulating agent.

f) Water-soluble dyes

Dissolution rate of single crystal of sulphathiazole has been found to decrease significantly in presence of FD & C Blue No.1. The inhibiting effect was related to preferential adsorption of dye molecules on primary dissolution sources of crystal surfaces. These inhibit the micellar solubilisation effect of bile salts on drug. Cationic dyes are more reactive in lower concentration than are anionic dyes.

g) Coating polymer

Tablets with methylcellulose (MC) coating have been found to show lower dissolution profiles than those coated with HPMC at 37°C. The differences may be due to thermal gelation of MC at temperature near 37°C, which creates a barrier to dissolution process and primarily changes the dissolution medium. This mechanism is substantiated by the fact that at the temperature below the gel point and at increased agitation, the effect disappears.

3) Processing factors

a) Method of granulation

Generally, the granulation process can enhance dissolution rate of poorly soluble drug. Wet granulation is traditionally considered superior. But exception is the dissolution profile of sodium salicylate tablets prepared by both wet granulation and direct compression where the dissolution was found more complete and rapid in latter case. A newer technology called as APOC "Agglomerative Phase of Comminution" has been found to produce mechanically stronger tablets with higher dissolution rates than those made by wet granulation. A possible mechanism is increased internal surface area of granules produced by APOC method.

b) Compression force

The compression process influences density, porosity, hardness, disintegration time and dissolution of tablet. Firstly, higher compression force increases the density and hardness of tablet, decreases porosity and hence, penetrability of solvent into the tablet that can retard the wettability by forming a firmer and more effective sealing layer by the lubricant. In many cases, tight bonding between the particles can decrease dissolution rate of tablet. Secondly, higher compression force causes deformation, crushing or fracture of drug particles into smaller ones or convert spherical granules into disc shaped particles with a large increase in the effective surface area so increase in dissolution rate. Combination of both conditions can occur. In short, rate of dissolution decreases at lower pressure (better bonding), then increase at higher pressure (crushing effect) and decrease again with further increase in pressure of extra rebonding and formation of denser tablets with poorer dissolution characteristics.

c) Unit operations involved

These interactions take place during any unit operation such as mixing, milling, blending, drying, and/or granulating result change in dissolution. The dissolution of prednisolone is found to depend on the length of mixing time with Magnesium stearate. Similarly, an increase in mixing time of the formulation containing 97 to 99% microcrystalline cellulose or another slightly swelling disintegrant result in enhance dissolution rate. Polysorbate-80 has been used as excipient in capsules. It causes the formation of formaldehyde by autoxidation which causes film formation by denaturing the inner surface of capsule. This causes decrease in dissolution rate of capsules.

d) Storage conditions

Rate of dissolution of Hydrochlorthiazide tablets granulated with acacia showed a decrease during 1 y of aging at room temperature (R.T.) A similar decrease has been observed in tablets stored for 14 days at 50-80°C or for 4 weeks at 37°C. For tablets granulated with PVP there was no change at elevated temperature but slight decrease at R.T. Tablets with starch gave no change in dissolution rate either at R.T. or at elevated temperature.

4) Dissolution test parameters

a) Temperature

Drug solubility is temperature dependent. Therefore, careful control of temperature during dissolution testing process is extremely important. Generally, a temperature of 37°C ± 0.5 is to be maintained during dissolution rate determination of oral dosage forms and suppositories. However, for topical preparations temp as low as 30°C and 25°C have been used.

b) Dissolution medium

It is very important factor affecting dissolution and is itself affected by number of factors such as (1) Effect of pH - Weak acids, dissolution rate increases with increase in pH whereas for weak bases, increase with decrease in pH.

(2) Volume of dissolution medium and sink conditions - If the drug is poorly soluble, a relatively large amount of fluid should be used, if complete dissolution is to be expected. To minimise the effect of concentration gradient and to maintain sink conditions, the concentration of the drug should not exceed 10 -15% of its maximum solubility in dissolution medium selected. For most of the drugs about 1 L is more than sufficient to maintain sink conditions. However, some

insoluble drug causes a problem to handling of huge volume of dissolution medium that would be required to maintain the sink conditions. For these reasons, different approaches have been tried like:

1) Continuous flow method where fresh solvent is pumped continuously into dissolution flask at a fixed flow rate while maintaining a constant volume.
2) Use of non-ionic surfactant in concentration above critical micelle concentration **(CMC)**.
3) Use of alcoholic solution (10 -30%)

c) Deaeration of dissolution medium

Dissolved air in distilled water could significantly lower its pH and consequently affect the dissolution rate of drugs that are sensitive to pH changes, weak acids. Another effect is to be removed from the medium in form of tiny air bubbles. These bubbles are collected at the surface of the dosage forms, and hence, act as a hydrophobic barrier between solvent and solid surface. This inhibits wetting and reduction of S.A. and lower dissolution rate.

5) Dissolution test apparatus

a) Agitation

Relationship between intensity of agitation and rate of dissolution varies considerably according to type of agitation used, the degree of laminar and turbulent flow in system, the shape and design of stirrer and physicochemical properties of solid. Speed of agitation generates a flow that continuously changes the liquid/solid interface between solvent and drug. In order to prevent turbulence and sustain a reproducible laminar flow, which is essential for obtaining reliable results, agitation should be maintained at a relatively low rate. Thus, in general relatively low agitation should be applied.

1) BASKET METHOD - 100 rpm

The USP/NF rotating basket method of dissolution testing essentially consists of a 25mm × 37mm high stainless steel 40-mesh wire basket, rotated at a constant speed ranging from 25 to 150 rpm. It is immersed in 900 ml of dissolution medium in a vessel of 1000 ml capacity. The medium in the vessel is maintained at a constant temperature of 37°C by means of a suitable water bath. The environment in which the apparatus is placed should not contribute significant motion, agitation, or vibration to the assembly. A fitted cover may be used to retard evaporation. The shaft is positioned so that its axis is not more than 2 mm at any point from the vertical axis of the vessel and rotates smoothly without any significant wobble. In case of non-disintegrating dosage forms, this apparatus is superior to Apparatus 2, since it constrains the dosage form in steady state fluid flow. This method may seem inferior for testing of dosage forms, which contain gums, due to the clogging of screen matrix. In case of floating dosage forms, this method performs well, but care should be taken that excipients do not clog the basket mesh.

2) PADDLE METHOD – 50 -75 rpm

1) USP/NF Method 2 (Rotating Paddle Method)

For all practical purposes, the compendial specifications outlined for this method are identical to method 1, except that the paddle is substituted for the rotating basket. The metallic or suitably inert, rigid blade and shaft comprise a single entity. The paddle and blade shaft may be coated with suitable inert coating. The dosage form is allowed to sink to the bottom of the vessel before rotation of the blade is started. This apparatus is frequently used for both disintegrating and non-disintegrating dosage form at 50 rpm.

2) USP/ NF Method 3 (Reciprocating Cylinder)
3) USP Apparatus 4 (Flow-Through Cell)
4) USP Apparatus 5 (Paddle Over Disk)
5) USP Apparatus 6 (Rotating Cylinder)
6) USP Apparatus 7 (Reciprocating Cylinder

a) Stirring element alignment

The USP / NF XV states that the axis of the stirring element must not deviate more than 0.2 mm from the axis of the dissolution vessel which defines centering of stirring shaft to within ±2 mm. Studies indicating that significant increase in dissolution rate up to 13% occurs, if the shaft is offset 2-6 mm from the central axis of the flask. Tilt in excess of 1.5 mm may increase dissolution rate from 2 to 25%.

b) Sampling probe position and filter

Sampling probe can affect the hydrodynamics of the system and so that no appreciable change in dissolution rate occurs. For position of sampling, USP / NF states that the sample should be removed at approximately half of the distance from the basket or paddle to the dissolution medium and not closer than 1 cm to the side of the flask. Filter material must be saturated with the drug by repeated passage to avoid losses that might remain undetected during the test sampling. Accumulation of the particulate matter on the surface may cause significant error in the dissolution testing.

INTRINSIC DISSOLUTION STUDIES

The intrinsic dissolution rate (IDR) can be defined as the rate of dissolution of a pure pharmaceutical active ingredient (API), where the conditions of surface area, temperature, agitation or stirring speed, pH and ionic strength of the dissolution medium are kept constant[24]. Commercially, the APIs are manufactured by different manufacturers by different processes, as a result, they are manufactured with varying characteristics such as particle size, degree of hydration, and crystalline form. This is true for the pharmaceutical excipients. Thus, by use of the intrinsic dissolution testing, the data on the chemical purity and bioequivalence of the available APIs can be obtained[25-28]. The rate at which a substance dissolves in a liquid (water) to form a solution is controlled by the physical parameters, such as surface area of the substance at a particular temperature during the dissolution process, the shape of the substance, the characteristics of the solid/ liquid interface, and the solubility of the substance in the liquid. During the process of development of new molecules, this parameter is an important one to screen the drug candidates and helps in understanding their solution behaviours under different bio-physiological conditions. The test can be performed with a small quantity and can predict the potential dissolution problems[29]. The intrinsic dissolution rate should be performed by using a particular device, where the compressed drug is exposed to a dissolution medium over a constant surface area and its value is expressed in $mg/cm^2.min$[30]. The USP recommends two methods for determination of the intrinsic dissolution rate:

1) *Rotating disk method:* In this method, the powder compact is prepared and rotated in dissolution media and at a specified rotating speed.
2) *Stationary disk method:* In this method, the disk is kept stationary in the dissolution media and agitation is to be done by a paddle rotated at a specified speed.

Both the methods maintain a constant surface area. The release from the disk is known as a diffusion-controlled process, thus any change in hydrodynamics caused by varying the rotation speed influences the thickness o the diffusion layer and hence, the dissolution rate[31]. However, there are some inherent problems with intrinsic dissolution testing:

- Preparation of the disk by compression can produce changes in solid structure that may influence the dissolution behaviour.
- The assumption of a constant surface area is valid only in the beginning of the determination.

  Since the disk disintegrates or erodes, the surface area cannot be kept constant, so the disk should be compacted properly to prevent its erosion and disintegration. Moreover, test should be stopped when eroded particles are observed in dissolution media.
- Measurement of the rate of dissolution on suspended materials does not normally include an assessment or measurement of inherent changes in surface area.

Intrinsic dissolution testing can be applied as an alternative for determining solubility, since it requires a small amount of material[32]. Recently, studies have indicated its usefulness in the area of the Biopharmaceutic Classification System (BCS) because rather than equilibrium, intrinsic dissolution testing determines the rate and better correlation is expected. In a traditional solubility test, a suitable quantity of a drug is kept under constant agitation and temperature till the solution is saturated, any determination of the actual solubility of the material may be compromised due to recrystallisation, this results in alteration of the crystalline form and hydrate or solvate formation. During manufacturing of solid dosage forms (tablets/ capsules). APIs must be processed to improve rheological characteristics and mechanical strength to get the final product with uniform characteristics. Most of the APIs have poor flow and mechanical strength, which are improved by processing with other excipients, commonly by granulation method (dry and wet granulation). Nature and level of processing can adversely affect dissolution characteristics of the product[33]. The effect of processing parameters on drug release can be evaluated by dissolution testing of the manufactured dosage form, tablets or capsules, and the drug release is estimated. It is a tedious job; it involves further processing. That is, the materials are converted to dosage forms. This method requires resources and time, particularly if desirable results are not obtained. To accelerate the process of formulation development and to reduce the cost and experimentation, a reliable method for estimating the effect of processing parameters on dissolution rate is required. Hence, intrinsic dissolution testing has been extensively applied to measure the dissolution behaviour of pure APIs in different crystalline states and dissolution media. In fact, no data are available on the application of intrinsic dissolution testing in evaluating dissolution behaviour of processed. APIs. The objective of this study should be to apply intrinsic dissolution testing to assess the effect of processing parameters on the dissolution rate of the drug.

Mathematically, the process of dissolution testing can be simply described as:

$$\frac{dM}{dt} = \mathrm{KA}(C_S - \mathrm{C})$$

Where,
M = the mass of the substance remaining to be dissolved,

A = the surface area exposed to the dissolution medium

Cs = the saturation concentration referred to as solubility in the dissolution medium,

C = the amount dissolved or the concentration of the drug in solution at time t, and K is the dissolution rate constant.

This equation is commonly referred to as a sink-condition equation, which implies that sink conditions exist during the process of dissolution. When the process of dissolution takes place under sink conditions, a stagnant film of liquid (dissolution medium) is adsorbed onto the solid, the thickness of this film being 1 cm. The liquid in the film in direct contact with the solid is saturated with drug in solution. The concentration of the drug in solution, then drops as the distance from the dissolving solid surface increases.

At the end of the film, 1 cm from the surface, the concentration in the film is the same as that in the bulk solution, C_b. The driving force behind the movement of solute molecules through the stagnant film is the concentration gradient that exists between the saturation concentration of the solute, Cs, in the stagnant layer at the surface of the solid and its concentration on the farthest side of the stagnant film, C_b.

DISSOLUTION TEST APPARATUS

The study of dissolution process has been developing since the end of nineteenth century by physical chemists. Hence, most of the fundamental research was not related to the drugs, mostly in engineering sciences. The basic laws in pharmaceutical sciences were developed in the early 1950s. Till then, there was only test to be conducted was disintegration test, but not the dissolution test[34]. For orally administered dosage form, mostly the non-solution dosage forms, in vitro performances such as dissolution and disintegration tests are to be tested to:

- guide drug development and select formulation for further in vivo studies,
- evaluate comparability between products before and after changes in the formulation and/ or manufacturing,
- serve as a surrogate for in vivo bioequivalence studies, with suitable in vitro/ in vivo correlations and/ or use of the Biopharmaceutics Classification System approach, and
- ensure batch-to-batch consistency for product performance[35].

In pharmaceutical industries, in vitro dissolution test is performed earlier times to validate initial screening among potential formulation to detect the influence of critical manufacturing variables and to help in the selection of the candidate formulation[36-38]. The use of dissolution test can speed up the formulation development, enabling a prompt identification of potential problems in drug release[39].

The shaft and the components of basket of the stirring element are fabricated of stainless steel, type 316, or other inert material, to the specifications shown in Fig.4.6. A basket having a gold coating of about 0.0001 inch (2.5 μm) thick may be used. A dosage unit is placed in a dry basket at the beginning of each test. The distance between the inside bottom of the vessel and the bottom of the basket is maintained at 25 ± 2 mm during the test.

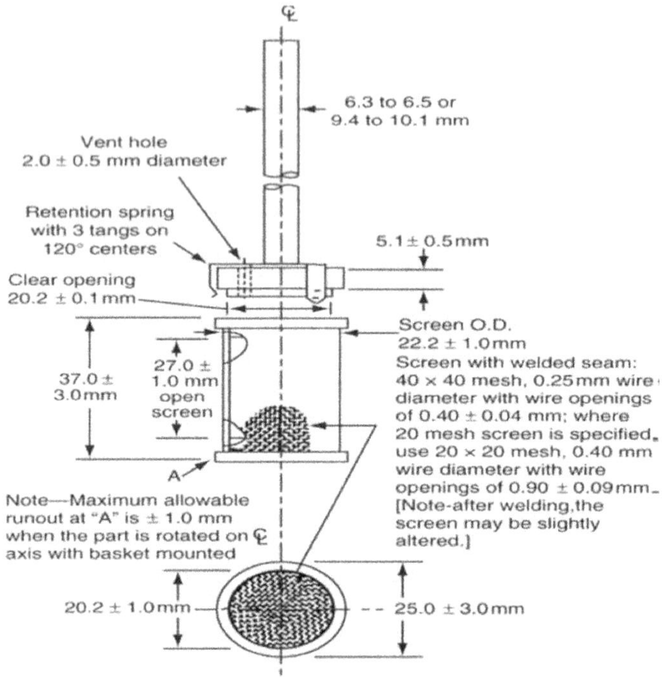

Fig.4.6 Schematic diagram of USP type I (Basket Apparatus).

Apparatus 1 (Basket Apparatus)

The assembly consists of the following: a vessel, which may be covered, made of glass or other inert, transparent material, basket stirring element, controlled thermostatic heating arrangement.

Apparatus type 2 (Paddle Apparatus)

The assembly can be used from Apparatus 1, except that a paddle formed from a blade and a shaft is used as the stirring element. The shaft is positioned so that its axis is not more than 2 mm from the vertical axis of the vessel at any point and rotates smoothly without significant wobble that could and rotates smoothly without significant wobble that could through the axis of the shaft so that the bottom of the blade is flush with the bottom of the shaft. The paddle conforms to the specifications shown in Fig 4.7. The distance of 25 ±2 mm between the bottom of the blade and the inside bottom of the vessel is maintained during the test. The metallic or suitably inert, rigid blade and shaft comprise a single entity. A suitable two-part detachable design may be used provided the assembly remains firmly engaged during the test. The paddle blade and shaft may be coated with a suitable coating so as to make them inert. The dosage unit is allowed to sink to the bottom of the vessel before rotation of the blade is started. A small, loose piece of nonreactive material, such as not more than a few turns of wire helix, may be attached to dosage units that would otherwise float. An alternative sinker device is shown in Fig 4.7. Other validated sinker devices may be used.

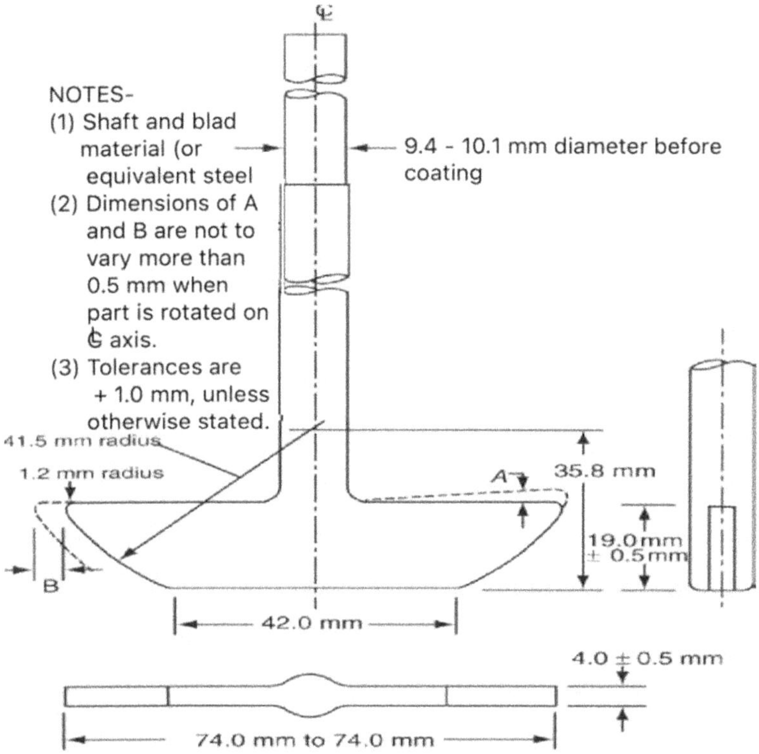

Fig.4.7 Schematic diagram of paddle stirring element.

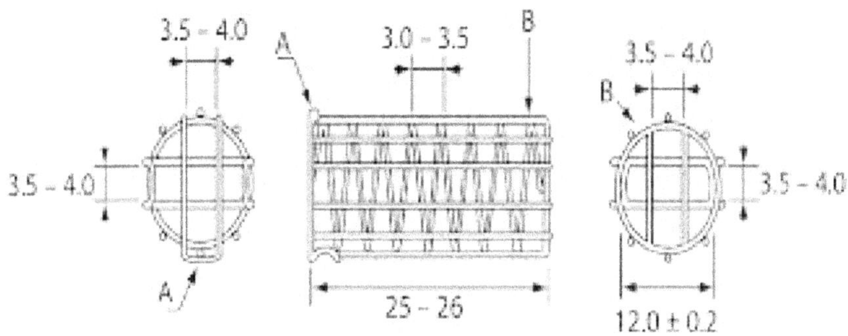

A: Acid-resistant wire clasp B:Acid-resistant wire support

Fig.4.7(a) Alternative sinker. Dimensions are in mm.

Apparatus 3 (Reciprocating Cylinder)

The assembly consists of a set of cylindrical, flat-bottomed glass vessels; a set of glass reciprocating cylinders; inert fittings (stainless steel type 316 or other suitable material), and screens that are made of suitable non-absorbing and non-reactive material and that are designed to fit the tops and bottoms of the reciprocating cylinders; and a motor and drive assembly to reciprocate the cylinders vertically inside the vessels and, if desired, index the reciprocating cylinders horizontally to a different row of vessels. The vessels are partially immersed in a suitable water bath of any convenient size that permits holding the temperature at 37 ±0.5°C during the test. No part of the assembly, including the environment in which the assembly is placed, contributes significant motion, agitation, or vibration beyond that due to the smooth, vertically reciprocating cylinder. A device is used that allows the reciprocation rate to be selected and maintained at the specified dip rate given in the individual monograph within ±5%. An apparatus that permits observation of the specimens and reciprocating cylinders is preferable. The vessels are provided with an evaporation cap that remains in place for the duration of the test. The components conform to the dimensions shown in Figure 3 unless otherwise specified in the individual monograph.

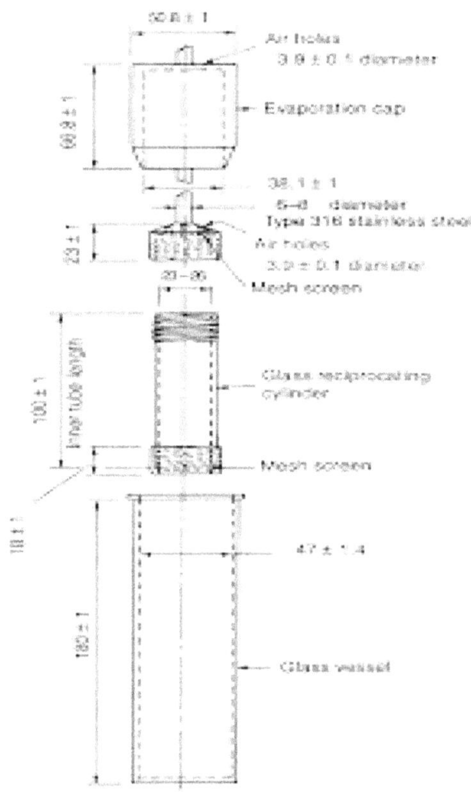

Fig.4.8 Diagram of USP type 3 dissolution test apparatus (Reciprocating Cylinder.

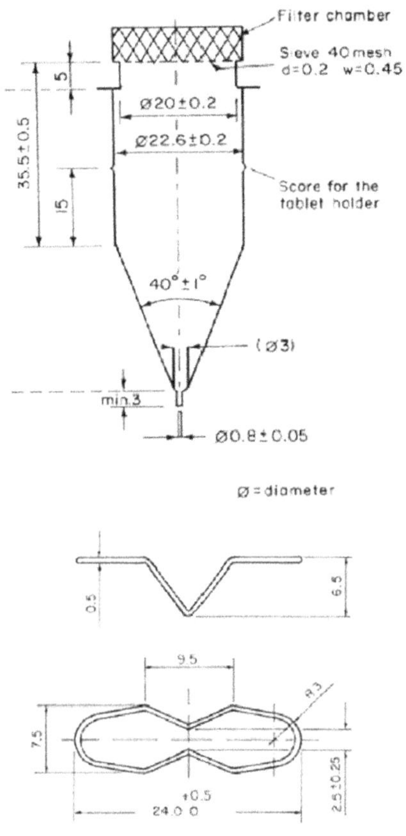

Fig.4.9 Large cell for tablets and capsules (top) Tablet holder for the large cell (bottom) (All measurements are expressed in mm unless noted otherwise.)

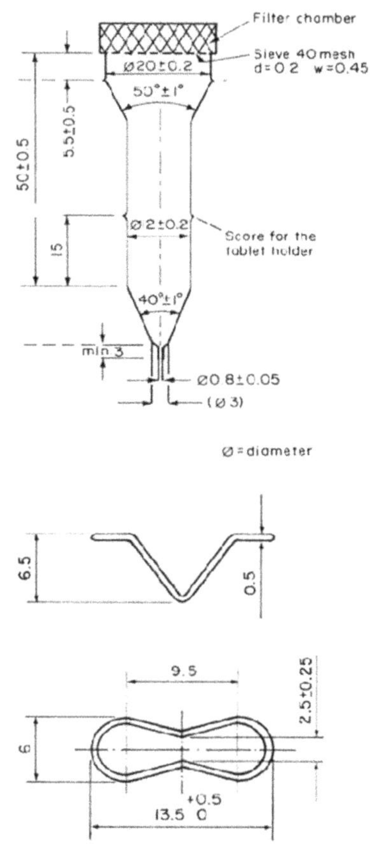

Fig.4.10 Small cell for tablets and capsules (top) Tablet holder for the small cell (bottom) (All measurements are expressed in mm unless noted otherwise).

Apparatus 4 (Flow-Through Cell)

The assembly consists of a reservoir and a pump for the Dissolution Medium; a flow-through cell; and a water bath that maintains the Dissolution Medium at 37 ±0.5°. Use the specified cell size (as given in the individual monograph). The pump forces the Dissolution Medium upwards through the flow-through cell. The pump has a delivery range between 240 and 960 mL per hour, with standard flow rates of 4, 8, and 16 mL per minute. It must deliver a constant flow (± 5% of the nominal flow rate); the flow profile is sinusoidal with a pulsation of 120 ±10 pulses per minute. A pump without pulsation may also be used. Dissolution test procedures using a flow-through cell must be characterised with respect to rate and any pulsation.

The flow-through cell (Figures 4.9 and 4.10), of transparent and inert material, is mounted vertically with a filter system (specified in the individual monograph) that prevents escape of undissolved particles from the top of the cell; standard cell diameters are 12 and 22.6 mm; the bottom cone is usually filled with small glass beads of about 1-mm diameter with one bead of about 5 mm positioned at the apex to protect the fluid entry tube; and a tablet holder is available for positioning of special dosage forms, for example, inlay tablets. The cell is immersed in a water bath, and the temperature is maintained at 37 ±0.5°. The apparatus uses a clamp mechanism and two O-rings to assemble the cell. The pump is separated from the dissolution unit in order to shield the latter against any vibrations originating from the pump. The position of the pump should not be on a level higher than the reservoir flasks. Tube connections are as short as possible. Use suitably inert tubing, such as polytef, with about 1.6-mm inner diameter and chemically inert flanged-end connections.

DESIGNS DISSOLUTION TESTING for CONTROLLED RELEASE PRODUCTS

Prior to the emergence of dissolution tests as being official in the United States Pharmacopeia (USP) in the early 1960s, disintegration tests were the only official in vitro tests used by major pharmacopoeias throughout the world as means of in vivo release predictability and product performance. Although the disintegration test is only indirectly related to drug bioavailability[40], this test has been the number one choice for the pharmaceutical industry in assessing the quality and performance of any conventional oral solid dosage form. This is perhaps due to the fact that this test is inexpensive, quick and does not require skilled personnel. With modernisation of technology, advancement in research in drug delivery and more emphasis on in vivo predictability of therapeutic effect by means of in vitro tests, dissolution tests have been gaining more and more popularity. Initially, dissolution tests were introduced to characterise the release profiles of low solubility (< 1%) drugs in aqueous media. But now the emphasis is to adopt dissolution tests in monographs of all oral solid dosage forms with minor exceptions (e.g. non-absorbed drugs). Not surprisingly, any report in literature on formulation and development of any solid dosage form starts with dissolution testing.

The dissolution tests have been successfully implemented on conventional dosage forms, and generalised monographs described in pharmacopoeias are usually sufficient to test any such new formulation. Unfortunately, this is not the case with sustained or controlled release dosage forms. Formal guidelines to evaluate sustained or controlled release products do not exist. The current trend is to evaluate each and every sustained or controlled release dosage form on individual basis. The formulation scientists and regulatory authorities face an enormous challenge of generalising the test conditions for dissolution testing because most individual drug candidates for sustained or controlled release dosage forms and their delivery design possess diverse physico-chemical and pharmacokinetic properties requiring specific considerations. The difficulties are also in simulating in vivo conditions in in vitro. Since most sustained or controlled release preparations are designed for prolonged release and therapeutic effect, variabilities in in vivo conditions (such as presence and nature of food in the gastrointestinal tract, time of the day the dosage form is administered) which can substantially affect the release profile of the drug are bound to happen. The formulation aspects of sustained or controlled release oral dosage forms for some water-soluble drugs were addressed in a recent review[41]. The overall design aspects of sustained/ controlled release dosage forms were also addressed by other reviewers[42]. But despite significant emphasis given on dissolution testing of sustained or controlled release dosage forms by regulatory authorities[43,44]. The difficulties faced by formulation scientists and regulatory authorities in generalising the test conditions have not been addressed in recent years. Almost a decade ago, it was discussed dissolution testing and bioavailability of various dosage forms covering sustained/controlled release preparations briefly, but ever since, the sustained/controlled release technology has progressed substantially. The main objective of this review is to focus on various factors that deserve consideration during dissolution testing of sustained or controlled release oral dosage forms and to summarise the recent trends and progress in overcoming these difficulties with an emphasis on in vivo predictability.

Performance Verification Test, Apparatus 1 and 2

Test USP Prednisone Tablets RS according to the operating conditions specified. The apparatus is suitable, if the results obtained are within the acceptable range stated in the technical data sheet specific to the lot used and the apparatus used for the test.

Performance Verification Test, Apparatus 3

The USP Performance Verification Test (PVT) assesses the suitable performance of apparatus used in dissolution testing. This assures reliability of dissolution results that reflects the quality of the drug product and not the condition of the test equipment. As such, the PVT in USP General Chapter <711> Dissolution is a core building block for dissolution instrument qualification. The PVT appraises the suitable performance of the entire apparatus. By using standardised materials and procedures, your laboratory can compare results from your instrument with other laboratories worldwide. Results that do not meet the acceptance criteria can indicate the improper operation of the dissolution assembly, deviation from the procedure, or an error in conducting the test. The USP Performance Verification Test (PVT) is an integral part of the General Chapter <711> Dissolution and assesses proper dissolution apparatus performance. PVT is a holistic test and by using the reference standard material and the standard procedure, laboratories can compare results from their instrument with other laboratories worldwide. The PVT acceptance criteria for geometric mean (GM) and coefficient of variation (%CV) are a measure for the accuracy and precision of the results within the context of ISO 5725-6. Based on the studies that have been performed, the new product is more sensitive to operational and mechanical variables of instrument setup, less sensitive to media degassing, and delivers more consistent results.

Qualification and Calibration

Prior to undertaking the task of dissolution procedure development and validation, it is necessary to invest some time and energy up-front to ensure that the dissolution system itself is validated or qualified. Qualification is a subset of the overall validation process that verifies proper module and system performance prior to the instrument being placed on-line in a regulated environment[45]. Analysts for years have used salicylic acid tablets to qualify and "chemically" calibrate dissolution instruments. While UV spectrophotometric methods are commonly used for dissolution sample analysis.

Dissolution Procedure Development

The dissolution procedure has several distinct components. These components include a dissolution medium, an apparatus, the study design (including acceptance criteria) and the mode of assay. All of these components must be properly chosen and developed to provide a method that is reproducible for within laboratory day-to-day operation and robust enough to enable transfer to another laboratory. The Dissolution Medium When selecting the dissolution medium, physical and chemical data for the drug substance and drug product need to be considered, e.g. the solubility and solution state stability of the drug as a function of pH value. Other critical drug product properties include the release mechanism (immediate, delayed or modified) and disintegration rate as affected by formulation hardness, friability, presence of solubility enhancers and other excipients. When selecting the composition of the medium, the influence of buffers, molarity, pH, and surfactants on the solubility and stability of the drug also need to be evaluated. The most common dissolution medium is dilute hydrochloric acid, however other media commonly used includes buffers in the physiologic pH of 1.2 to 7.5, simulated gastric or intestinal fluid (with or without enzymes), water and surfactants (with or without acids or buffers) such as polysorbate 80, sodium lauryl sulphate and bile salts. The use of aqueous-organic solvent mixtures, while generally discouraged, can also be used if justified. Enzymes are also sometimes used in the media when testing gelatine capsule products. Media volumes are typically in the range of 500-1000 ml, with 900 ml the most common volume. Volumes as high as 2-4 L have been used and as low as 100 ml for high potency (low dosage strength) drug formulations. Media deaeration is usually required and can be accomplished by heating the medium or (more commonly) filtering the medium or placing it under vacuum for short period of time. USP chapter 711 contains additional information on deaeration (USP 32-NF 27). During method development, results from dissolution samples run in non-deaerated medium versus a deaerated medium should be compared to determine whether deaeration is necessary. When developing dissolution procedure, one general goal is to have "sink" conditions. Sink conditions are defined as the volume of medium that is at least three times that required in order to form a saturated solution of drug substance. Dissolution results will more accurately reflect the properties of the dosage form when sink conditions are present.

The Dissolution Apparatus

The choice of apparatus is based on the dosage form performance in the in vitro test system. USP dissolution apparatus I and II illustrate the . Somewhat recently, an AAPS committee published recommendations for the type of apparatus recommended for novel or special dosage forms. These recommendations are summarised. While changes to the approved apparatuses are allowed, justification must be provided. For some dosage forms, particularly capsules that might float on the media surface, "sinkers" may be required.

USP chapter 711 (USP 32-NF 27, 2009) and USP chapter 1092 (USP 32-NF 27, 2009) provides additional detail for construction and usage of sinkers. If sinkers are required, steps must be taken in method development to evaluate different types and construction, as sinkers can significantly affect dissolution. Agitation is also an important part of dissolution procedure. Coning or mounding problems can be solved by increasing the paddle speed. If justified, 100 rpm may be used, especially for extended-release products. Decreasing or increasing the apparatus rotation speed may also be justified. Selection of site for placing apparatus is also important; vibrations from doors closing or pumps (mass spectrometry instrument vacuum pumps) can cause significant variability.

Dissolution Study Design

Dissolution is evaluated by measuring rate release profile or the amount dissolved over time. Single or multiple points in time can be measured, depending upon the dosage type or data desired.

For immediate release dosage forms, the procedure duration is usually 30 to 60 minutes and in most cases, a single time point specification is adequate. However, for formulation development comparison purposes, profile comparison is required, and it is common to collect data from numerous time point.

For extended-release dosage forms, at least three test time points are typically chosen to characterise the in vitro drug release profile. Sampling probe can affect the hydrodynamic of the system and so that change in dissolution rate. For position of sampling, USP / NF states that sample should be removed at approximately half the distance from the basket or paddle to the dissolution medium and not closer than 1 cm to the side of the flask. Filter material must be saturated with the drug by repeated passage to avoid losses that might go undetected during the test sampling. Accumulation of the particulate matter on the surface may cause significant error in the dissolution testing. Acceptance criteria must also be considered during test development. The acceptance criteria should be representative of multiple batches from the same nominal composition and manufacturing process, include key batches used in pivotal studies and batches that are representative of the drug product performance in stability studied. Acceptance criteria are derived in the form of "Q-factors" a minimum amount dissolved at a given time as a percentage of the labelled content. Dissolution tests can have a single Q-factor, or may have multiple Q-factors. A Q value in excess of 80% is not generally used, because allowance needs to be made for assay and content uniformity ranges. Finally, the dissolution test procedure should be discriminating enough to be capable of distinguishing significant changes in a composition or manufacturing process that might be expected to affect in vivo performance. In general, a properly designed dissolution test should result in reproducible data. Too much result variability can make it difficult to identify trends, true batch differences or effects of formulation changes. If too much variability is observed, the usual remedies include changing the apparatus type, speed of agitation, or deaeration; consideration and/ or examination of sinker type; and changing the composition of the medium. During routine testing of the product, variability outside the expected range should be investigated from analytical formulation and processing perspectives.

Evaluation

There are two common ways of analysing dissolution test samples, spectrophotometric (UV) determinations and HPLC. Typically, the drug substance UV spectrum is observed to choose the optimum wavelength for analysis. Cells with path lengths ranging from 0.02 to 1 cm are used. HPLC methods, however, have distinct advantages, particularly when there is significant interference from excipients or between multiple active ingredients in the formulation. It also requires less sample volume.

DESIGNS OF DISSOLUTION TESTING for CONVENTIONAL PRODUCTS

Dissolution is the process by which a solid solute enters a solution. In the pharmaceutical industry, it may be defined as the amount of drug substance that goes into solution per unit time under standardised conditions of liquid/solid interface, temperature and solvent composition. Drug dissolution testing plays an important role as a routine quality control test, for characterising the quality of the product and also plays a major role in drug development. Dissolution testing is an official test used by pharmacopeia's for evaluating drug release of solid and semisolid dosage forms dissolution tests were first developed to quantify the amount and extent of drug release from solid oral dosage forms including immediate/sustained release tablets and capsules. More recently, dissolution has become important in testing drug release of dosage forms such as, buccal and sublingual tablets, chewing gums, soft gelatine capsules, suppositories, transdermal patches, aerosols and semisolids the study of the dissolution process has been developing since the end of the 19th century by physical chemists. The goal is to have a fully functional set of USP performance tests for all kinds of dosage forms.

Conditions (for all in general):

1. Temp. - 37±0.5°C
2. pH - ±0.05 unit in specified monograph
3. Capacity – 1000 ml
4. Distance between inside bottom of vessel and paddle/basket is maintained at 25±2 mm
5. For enteric coated dosage form it is first dissolved in 0.1 N HCl and then in buffer of pH 6.8 to measure drug release. (Limit – NMT 10% of drug should dissolve in the acid after 2hr.and about 75% of it should dissolve in the buffer after 45 min.)

The dissolution apparatus has been evolved gradually and considerably from a simple beaker type to a highly versatile and fully automated instrument. Based on absence or presence of sink conditions, there are three principal types of dissolution apparatus[45]:

1. **Apparatus I** – Closed-compartment- Basically a limited volume apparatus operating under non-sink conditions. For example, Apparatus-I and II.
2. **Apparatus II** – Open compartment- One in which dosage form is contained in a column which is brought in continuous contact with fresh, flowing dissolution medium (perfect sink condition) Useful for: Tablets, Capsules, Beads, Delayed release, enteric coated dosage forms, Standard volume: 900/1000 ml.
3. **Apparatus III** – Reciprocating cylinder: The assembly consists of a set of cylindrical, flat-bottomed glass vessels; a set of glass reciprocating cylinders; stainless steel fittings (type 316 or equivalent) and screens that are made of suitable nonasorbing and nonreactive material (polypropelene) and that are designed to fit the tops and bottoms of the

reciprocating cylinders; and a motor and drive assembly to reciprocate the cylinders vertically inside the vessels. The vessels are partially immersed in a suitable water bath of any convenient size that permits holding the temperature at 37 ±0.5 during the test. The dosage unit is placed in reciprocating cylinder and the cylinder is allowed to move in upward and downward direction constantly. Release of drug into solvent within the cylinder measured.

- Useful for: Tablets, Beads, controlled release formulations.
- Standard volume: 200-250 ml/station.

4. **Apparatus IV** – flow through cell: The assembly consists of a reservoir and a pump for the Dissolution Medium; a flow through cell; a water bath that maintains the Dissolution Medium at 37 ±0.5. The cell size is specified in the individual monograph. The pump forces the Dissolution Medium upwards through the flow-through cell. Place the glass beads into the cell specified in the monograph, Place 1 dosage unit on top of the beads or, if specified in the monograph, on a wire carrier and then assemble the filter head, and fix the parts together by means of a suitable clamping device. By introducing the pump the Dissolution Medium warmed to 37 ±0.5 through the bottom of the cell to obtain the flow rate specified in the individual monograph. Collect the elute by fractions at each of the times stated, Perform the analysis as directed in the individual monograph.

   - Useful for: Low solubility drugs, Micro particulates, Implants, Suppositories, Controlled release formulations.
   - Variations : (A) Open system and (B) Closed system.

5. **Apparatus V**–Paddle over disk: Use the paddle and vessel assembly from Apparatus 2 with the addition of a stainless-steel disk assembly designed for holding the transdermal system at the bottom of the vessel. Other appropriate devices may be used, provided they do not sorb, react with, or interfere with the specimen being tested. The disk assembly for holding the transdermal system is designed to minimise any "dead" volume between the disk assembly and the bottom of the vessel, the disk assembly holds the system flat and is positioned such that the release surface is parallel with the bottom of the paddle blade, the vessel may be covered during the test to minimize evaporation.

   - Useful for: Transdermal patches
   - Standard volume: 900 ml.

6. **Apparatus VI**–cylinder: Use the vessel assembly from Apparatus 1 except to replace the basket and shaft with a stainless-steel cylinder stirring element and to maintain the temperature at 32°C± 0.5 during the test. The dosage unit is placed on the cylinder at the beginning of each

test, to the exterior of the cylinder such that the long axis of the system fits around the circumference of the cylinder and removes trapped air bubbles. Place the cylinder in the apparatus, and immediately rotate at the rate specified in the individual monograph.

7. **Apparatus VII** – Reciprocating Holder: The assembly consists of a set of volumetrically calibrated solution containers made of glass or other suitable inert material, a motor and drive assembly to reciprocate the system vertically and a set of suitable sample holders. The solution containers are partially immersed in a suitable water bath of any convenient size that permits maintaining the temperature, inside the containers at 32 ±0.5. For Coated tablet drug delivery system attach each system to be tested to a suitable sample holder (e.g., by gluing system edge with 2- cyano-acrylate glue onto the end of a plastic rod or by placing the system into a small nylon net bag at the end of a plastic rod or within a metal coil attached to a metal rod).

For Transdermal drug delivery system attach the system to a suitable sized sample holder with a suitable O-ring such that the back of the system is adjacent to and centered on the bottom of the disk-shaped sample holder or centered around the circumference of the cylindrical shaped sample holder, trim the excess substrate with a sharp blade for Other drug delivery systems attach each system to be tested to a suitable holder as described in the individual monograph. Suspend each sample holder from a vertically reciprocating shaker such that each system is continuously immersed in an accurately measured volume of Dissolution Medium within a calibrated container reciprocate at a frequency of about 30 cycles per minute with amplitude of about 2 cm, or as specified in the individual monograph, for the specified time in the medium specified for each time point. Perform the analysis as directed in the individual monograph.

DATA HANDLING

Drug regulatory systems worldwide have always depended upon the knowledge of organisations that develop, manufacture and package, test, distribute and monitor pharmaceutical products. Implicit in the assessment and review process is trust between the regulator and the regulated that the information submitted in dossiers and used in day-to-day decision making is comprehensive, complete and reliable. The data on which these decisions are based should therefore be complete as well as being attributable, legible, contemporaneous, original and accurate, commonly referred to as "ALCOA"

These basic ALCOA principles and the related good practice expectations that assure data reliability are not new and much high- and mid-level normative guidance already exists. However, in recent years, the number of observations made regarding good data and record management practices

(GDRP) during inspections of good manufacturing practice (GMP)[46,] good clinical practice (GCP) and good laboratory practice (GLP) has been increasing. The reasons for the increasing concern of health authorities regarding data reliability are undoubtedly multifactorial and include increased regulatory awareness and concern regarding gaps between industry choices and appropriate and modern control strategies.

Contributing factors include failures by organisations to apply robust systems that inhibit data risks, to improve the detection of situations where data reliability may be compromised, and/or to investigate and address root causes when failures do arise. For example, organisations subject to medical product good practice requirements have been using validated computerised systems for many decades but many fail to adequately review and manage original electronic records and instead often only review and manage incomplete and/or inappropriate printouts. These observations highlight the need for industry to modernise control strategies and apply modern quality risk management (QRM) and sound scientific principles to current business models (such as outsourcing and globalisation) as well as technologies currently in use (such as computerised systems).

Examples of controls that may require development and strengthening to ensure good data management strategies include, but are not limited to:

- A QRM (Quantitative Risk Management) approach that can effectively assures the patient safety and product quality and validity of data by ensuring that management aligns expectations with actual process capabilities. Management should take responsibility for good data management by first setting realistic and achievable expectations for the true and current capabilities of a process, a method, an environment, personnel, or technologies, among others;

  Monitoring of processes and allocation of the necessary resources by management to ensure and enhance infrastructure, as required (for example, to continuously improve processes and methods, to ensure adequate design and maintenance of buildings, facilities, equipment and systems; to ensure adequate reliable power and water supplies; to provide necessary training for personnel; and to allocate the necessary resources to the oversight of contract sites and suppliers to ensure adequate quality standards are met). Active engagement of management in this manner remediates and reduces pressures and possible sources of error that may increase data integrity risks;

- Adoption of a quality culture within the company that encourages personnel to be transparent about failures so that management has an accurate understanding of risks and can then provide the necessary resources to achieve expectations and meet data quality standards: a reporting mechanism independent of management hierarchy should be provided for;

- Mapping of data processes and application of modern QRM and sound scientific principles throughout the data life cycle;
- Ensuring that all site personnel are kept up to date about the application of good documentation practices (GDoCP) to ensure that the GXP principles of ALCOA are understood and applied to electronic data in the same manner that has historically been applied to paper records;
- Implementation and confirmation during validation of computerised systems and subsequent change control, that all necessary controls for GDoCP for electronic data are in place and that the probability of the occurrence of errors in the data is minimised;
- Training of personnel who use computerised systems and review electronic data in basic understanding of how computerised systems work and how to efficiently review the electronic data, which includes metadata and audit trails;
- Definition and management of appropriate roles and responsibilities for quality agreements and contracts entered into by contract givers and contract acceptors, including the need for risk-based monitoring of data generated and managed by the contract acceptor on behalf of the contract giver;
- Modernisation of quality assurance inspection techniques and gathering of quality metrics to efficiently and effectively identify risks and opportunities to improve data processes.

Principle

- GDRP are critical elements of the pharmaceutical quality system and a systematic approach should be implemented to provide a high level of assurance that throughout the product life cycle, all GXP records and data are complete and reliable.
- The data governance programme should include policies and governance procedures that address the general principles listed below for a good data management programme. These principles are clarified with additional detail in the sections below.
- Applicability to both paper and electronic data. The requirements for GDRP that assure robust control of data validity apply equally to paper and electronic data. Organisations subject to GXP should be fully aware that reverting from automated or computerised to manual or paper-based systems does not in itself remove the need for robust management controls.

- Applicability to contract givers and contract acceptors. The principles of these guidelines apply to contract givers and contract acceptors. Contract givers are ultimately responsible for the robustness of all decisions made on the basis of GXP data, including those made on the basis of data provided to them by contract acceptors. Contract givers should therefore perform risk-based, due diligence to assure themselves that contract acceptors have in place appropriate programmes to ensure the veracity, completeness and reliability of the data provided.
- Good documentation practices. To achieve robust decisions, the supporting data set needs to be reliable and complete. GDoCP should be followed in order to ensure all records, both paper and electronic, allow the full reconstruction and traceability of GXP activities.
- Management governance. To establish a robust and sustainable good data management system it is important that senior management ensure that appropriate data management governance programmes are in place. Elements of effective management governance should include:
  - application of modern QRM principles and good data management principles that assure the validity, completeness and reliability of data;
  - application of appropriate quality metrics;
  - assurance that personnel are not subject to commercial, political, financial and other
  - allocation of adequate human and technical resources such that the workload, work organisational pressures or incentives that may adversely affect the quality and hours integrity of their work; and pressures on those responsible for data generation and record keeping do not increase errors;
  - ensure staff are aware of the importance of their role in ensuring data integrity and the relationship of these activities to assuring product quality and protecting patient safety.

Quality Culture

Management with the support of the quality unit, should establish and maintain a working environment that minimises the risk of non-compliant records and erroneous records and data. An essential element of the quality culture is the transparent and open reporting of deviations, errors, omissions and aberrant results at all levels of the organisation, irrespective of hierarchy. Steps should be taken to prevent, and to detect and correct weaknesses in systems and procedures that may lead to data errors so as to continually improve the robustness of scientific decision-making within the organisation. Senior management should actively discourage any management practices that might reasonably be expected to inhibit the active and complete reporting of such issues, for example, hierarchical constraints and blame cultures.

Quality Risk Management and Sound Scientific Principles

Robust decision making requires appropriate quality and risk management systems, and adherence to sound scientific and statistical principles, which must be based upon reliable data. For example, the scientific principle of being an objective, unbiased observer regarding the outcome of a sample analysis requires that suspect results be investigated and rejected from the reported results only if they are clearly attributable to an identified cause. Adhering to good data and record-keeping principles requires that any rejected results be recorded, together with a documented justification for their rejection, and that this documentation is subject to review and rejection.

Data Life Cycle Management

Continual improvement of products to ensure and enhance their safety, efficacy and quality requires a data governance approach to ensure management of data integrity risks throughout all phases of the process by which data are created, recorded, processed, transmitted, reviewed, reported, archived and retrieved and this management process is subject to regular review. To ensure that the organisation, assimilation and analysis of data into information facilitates evidence-based and reliable decision-making, data governance should address data ownership and accountability for data process(es) and risk management of the data life cycle. To ensure that the organisation, assimilation and analysis of data into a format or structure that facilitates evidence-based and reliable decision making, data governance should address data ownership and accountability for data process(es) and risk management of the data life cycle.

Design Of Record-Keeping Methodologies and Systems

Record-keeping methodologies and systems, whether paper or electronic, should be designed in a way that encourages compliance with the principles of data integrity.

Examples include, but are not restricted to:

- restricting the ability to change any clock used for recording timed events, for example, system clocks in electronic systems and process instrumentation.
- ensuring controlled forms used for recording GXP data (e.g. paper batch records, paper case report forms and laboratory worksheets) are accessible at the locations where an activity is taking place, at the time that the activity is taking place, so that ad hoc data recording and later transcription is not necessary;
- controlling the issuance of blank paper templates for data recording of GXP activities so that all printed forms can be reconciled and accounted for;

- restricting user access rights to automated systems to prevent (or audit trail) data amendments;
- ensuring automated data capture or printers are attached and connected to equipment, such as balances, to ensure independent and timely recording of the data;
- ensuring proximity of printers to sites of relevant activities;
- ensuring ease of access to locations of sampling points (e.g. sampling points for water systems) to allow easy and efficient performance of sampling by the operators and therefore minimising the temptation to take shortcuts or falsify samples; ensuring access to original electronic data for staff performing data checking activities.

Data and record media should be durable. For paper records, the ink should be indelible. Temperature-sensitive or photosensitive inks and other erasable inks should not be used. Paper should also not be temperature-sensitive, photosensitive or easily oxidisable. If this is not feasible or limited (as may be the case in printouts from legacy printers of balance and other instruments in quality control laboratories), then true or certified copies should be available until this equipment is retired or replaced.

Maintenance of Record-Keeping Systems

The systems implemented and maintained for both paper and electronic record-keeping should take account of scientific and technical progress. Systems, procedures and methodology used to record and store data should be periodically reviewed for effectiveness and updated as necessary.

CORRECTION FACTOR

In recent years, the concept and application of the in vitro-in vivo correlation (IVIVC) for pharmaceutical dosage forms have been a main focus of attention of pharmaceutical industry, academia, and regulatory sectors. Development and optimization of formulation is an integral part of manufacturing and marketing of any therapeutic agent which is indeed a time consuming and costly process. Optimization process may require alteration in formulation composition, manufacturing process, equipment and batch sizes. If these types of changes are applied to a formulation, studies in human healthy volunteers may be required to prove that the new formulation is bioequivalent with the old one. Certainly, implementation of these requirements not only halts the marketing of the new formulation but also increases the cost of the optimization processes. It would be, desirable, therefore, to develop in vitro tests that reflect bioavailability data. A regulatory guidance for both immediate- and modified-release dosage forms has been, therefore, developed by the FDA to minimize the need for bioavailability studies as part of the formulation design and optimization. IVIVC procedures are specific to certain countries but could be adopted or used as the background for regulatory recommendations by other countries. IVIVC can be used in the development of new pharmaceuticals to reduce the number of human studies during the formulation development. The main objective of an IVIVC is to serve as a surrogate for in vivo bioavailability and to support bio-waivers. IVIVCs could also be employed to establish dissolution specifications and to support and/or validate the use of dissolution methods.

This is because the IVIVC includes in vivo relevance to in vitro dissolution specifications. It can also assist in quality control for certain scale up and post-approval changes, for instance, to improve formulations or to change production processes. There must be some in vitro means of assuring that each batch of the same product will perform identically in vivo. With the proliferation of modified-release products, it is essential to examine the concept of IVIVC in greater depth. Therefore, a more detailed article covering various aspects of an IVIVC study including complete process of developing the correlation with high quality, accurate and precise predictability, and identifying specific applications for such correlations might be of importance. Although the focus of discussion, in this review, will primarily be centered on modified-release formulations for which IVIVC is believed to be more defined, various aspects of the IVIVC of immediate-release dosage forms are also discussed.

The term correlation is frequently employed within the pharmaceutical and related sciences to describe the relationship that exists between variables. Mathematically, the term correlation means interdependence between quantitative or qualitative data or relationship between measurable variables and ranks. From biopharmaceutical standpoint, correlation could be referred to as the relationship between appropriate in vitro release characteristics and in vivo bioavailability parameters. Two definitions of IVIVC have been proposed by the USP and by the FDA. United State Pharmacopoeia (USP) definition The establishment of a rational relationship between a biological property, or a parameter derived from a biological property produced by a dosage form, and a physicochemical property or characteristic of the same dosage form. Food and Drug Administration (FDA) definition IVIVC is a predictive mathematical model describing the relationship between an in vitro property of a dosage form and a relevant in vivo response. Generally, the in vitro property is the rate or extent of drug dissolution or release while the in vivo response is the plasma drug concentration or amount of drug absorbed.

CORRELATION LEVELS

Five correlation levels have been defined in the IVIVC FDA guidance. The concept of correlation level is based upon the ability of the correlation to reflect the complete plasma drug level-time profile which will result from administration of the given dosage form. Level A Correlation This level of correlation is the highest category of correlation and represents a point-to-point relationship between in vitro dissolution rate and in vivo input rate of the drug from the dosage form. Generally, percent of drug absorbed may be calculated by means of model dependent techniques such as Wagner-Nelson procedure or Loo-Riegelman method or by model-independent numerical deconvolution. These techniques represent a major advance over the single-point approach in that these methodologies utilise all of the dissolution and plasma level data available to develop the correlations and will be discussed more in detail later in this article. The purpose of Level A correlation is to define a direct relationship between in vivo data such that measurement of in vitro dissolution rate alone is sufficient to determine the biopharmaceutical rate of the dosage form. In the case of a level A correlation, an in vitro dissolution curve can serve as a surrogate for in vivo performance. Therefore, a change in manufacturing site, method of manufacture, raw material supplies, minor formulation modification, and even product strength using the same formulation can be justified without the need for additional human studies. It is an excellent quality control procedure since it is predictive of the dosage form's in vivo performance. Level B Correlation A level B IVIVC utilises the principles of statistical moment analysis. In this level of correlation, the mean in vitro dissolution time (MDTvitro) of the product is compared to either mean in vivo residence time (MRT) or the mean in vivo dissolution time (MDTvivo). MRT, MDTvitro and MDTvivo will be defined throughout the manuscript where appropriate. Although a level B correlation uses all of the in vitro and in vivo data, it is not considered to be a point-to-point correlation, since there are a number of different in vivo curves that will produce similar mean residence time values. A level B correlation does not uniquely reflect the actual in vivo plasma level curves. Therefore, one can not rely upon a level B correlation alone to justify formulation modification, manufacturing site change, excipient source change, etc. In addition, in vitro data from such a correlation could not be used to justify the extremes of quality control standards. Level C Correlation In this level of correlation, one dissolution time point ($t_{50\%}$, $t_{90\%}$, etc.) is compared to one mean pharmacokinetic parameter such as AUC_{tmax} or C_{max}. Therefore, it represents a single point correlation and doses do not reflect the entire shape of the plasma drug concentration curve, which is indeed a crucial factor that is a good indicative of the performance of modified-release products. This is the weakest level of correlation as partial relationship between absorption and dissolution is established. Due to its obvious limitations, the usefulness of a Level C correlation is limited in predicting in vivo drug performance. The usefulness of this correlation level is subject to the same caveats as a Level B correlation in its ability to support product and site changes as well as justification of quality control standard extremes. Level C correlations can be useful in the early stages of formulation development when pilot formulations are being selected. While the information may be useful in formulation development, waiver of an in vivo bioequivalence study (biowaiver) is generally not possible. Multiple-level C correlation A multiple level C correlation relates one or several pharmacokinetic parameters of interest (Cmax, AUC, or any other suitable parameters) to the amount of drug dissolved at several time points of the dissolution profile. A multiple point level C correlation may be used to justify a biowaiver, provided that the correlation has been established over the entire dissolution profile with one or more pharmacokinetic parameters of interest. A relationship should be demonstrated at each time point at the same parameter such that the effect on the in vivo performance of any change in dissolution can be assessed. If such a multiple level C correlation is achievable, then the development of a level A correlation is also likely. A multiple Level C correlation should be based on at least three dissolution time points covering the early, middle, and late stages of the dissolution profile. Level D correlation Level D correlation is a rank order and qualitative analysis and is not considered useful for regulatory purposes. It is not a formal correlation but serves as an aid in the development of a formulation or processing procedure[47].

SYSTEMATIC DEVELOPMENT OF A CORRELATION

Any well designed and scientifically sound approach would be acceptable for establishment of an IVIV correlation. As the development of an IVIVC is a dynamic process starting from the very early stages of development program through the final step, the following practical and detailed approach with industrial application is summarised from reference number 5 without modifications. "To understand how an IVIVR is used throughout the product development cycle, it is useful to become familiar with the following terms as they relate to a typical product development cycle for oral extended-release product. An assumed IVIVR is essentially one that provides the initial guidance and direction for the early formulation development activity. Thus, during stage 1 and with a particular product concept in mind, appropriate in vitro targets are established to meet the desired in vivo profile specification. This assumed model can be the subject of revision as prototype formulations are developed and characterized in vivo, with the results often leading to a further cycle of prototype formulation and in vivo characterisation. Out of this cycle and in vivo characterisation and, of course, extensive in vitro testing is often developed what can be referred to as retrospective IVIVR. With a defined formulation that meets the in vivo specification, stage 2 starts. At this stage based on a greater understanding and appreciation of defined formulation and its characteristics, a prospective IVIVR is established through a well-defined prospective IVIVR study. Once the IVIVR is established and defined it can be then used to guide the final cycle of formulation and process optimization leading into Stage 3 activities of scale-up, pivotal batch manufacture, and process validation culminating in registration, approval and subsequent post-approval scale-up and other changes. Thus rather than viewing the IVIVR as a single exercise at a given point in a development program, one should view it as a parallel development in itself starting at the initial assumed level and being built on and modified through experience and leading ultimately to a prospective IVIVR"

Absorption Number (A_n)

The Absorption Number (A_n) is the ratio of the Mean Residence Time (T_{res}) to the Mean Absorption Time (T_{abs}) and is calculated by equation 1.

$$A_n = T_{res} / T_{abs} = (\pi R^2 L/Q) / (R/P_{eff}) \quad .....(4.1)$$

Dissolution Number (D_n)

The Dissolution Number (D_n) is the ratio of T_{res} to Mean Dissolution Time (T_{diss}) and could be estimated using equation 2.

$$D_n = T_{res} / T_{diss} = (\pi R^2 L/ Q)/(\rho r_o^2 / 3DC_s^{min}) \quad .....(4.2)$$

Dose Number (D_o)

The Dose Number (D_o) is calculated using equation 3:

$$D_o = Dose / (V_o \times C_s^{min}) \quad .....(4.3)$$

Where, L is tube length, R is tube radius, $\pi = 3.14$, Q is fluid flow rate, r_o is initial particle radius, D is particle acceleration, ρ is particle density, P_{eff} is effective permeability, V_o is the initial gastric volume equal to 250 ml which is derived from typical bioequivalence study protocols that prescribe administration of a drug product to fasting human volunteers with a glass of water at the time of drug administration and C_s^{min} is minimum aqueous solubility in the physiological pH range of 1-8.

The dose, dose number, solubility, and estimated dissolution number for a number of drugs. The fraction dose absorbed could be estimated using these three major dimensionless parameters. However, the extent of solubilization and potential particle aggregation in the small intestine is unknown and therefore, the solubility, dose and dissolution number of a drug in vivo is difficult to estimate precisely. As the drug dissolution and intestinal permeability are the fundamental parameters governing rate and extent of drug absorption, drugs could be categorized into high/low solubility and permeability classes. Thus, the expectations regarding IVIVC could be stated more clearly[48].

Comparison between dissolution profiles could be achieved using a difference factor (f_1) and a similarity factor (f_2) which originates from simple model independent approach. The difference factor calculates the percent difference between the two curves at each time point and is a measurement of the relative error between the two curves:

equation

Where, n is the number of time points, R_t is the dissolution value of the reference batch at time t, and T_t is the dissolution value of the test batch at time t.

The similarity factor is a logarithmic reciprocal square root transformation of the sum squared error and is a measurement of the similarity in the percent dissolution between the two curves.

Generally, f_1 values up to 15 (0 -15) and f_2 values greater than 50 (50 -100) ensure sameness or equivalence of the two curves.

The mean in vitro dissolution time (MDT_{vitro}) is the mean time for the drug to dissolve under in vitro dissolution conditions. This is calculated using the following equation (3):

$$MDT_{vitro} = \int_0^{\infty} (M_{\infty} - M(t))dt / M_{\infty} \qquad .....(4.6)$$

BIO-RELEVANT MEDIA

Dissolution of drugs from solid dosage forms is a key parameter in assessing the product quality and uniformity at the formulation stage as well as throughout the shelf-life of the product. In case of lipophilic drugs dissolution rate can be the rate-limiting step in the in vivo absorption process and hence the dissolution medium is a critical component of the test that can cause problems[49,50]. Therefore, dissolution method should be discriminative, reproducible, scientifically justifiable and more importantly biorelevant[51]. This clinical relevance of dissolution testing can be achieved in the context of Quality by Design derived from a specific case study for a BCS II compound. Approaches usually used in the design of a dissolution media for poorly water-soluble drugs include:

1) Bringing about drug solubility by increasing the volume of the aqueous sink or removing the dissolved drug.
2) Solubilisation of drug by cosolvents up to 40% by addition of anionic or non-anionic surfactants to dissolution medium in post micellar concentration.
3) Alteration of pH to enhance the solubility of insoluble drug molecule.

Surfactant solutions are often proposed as dissolution media for drugs characterised by low water solubility. Generally, aqueous solutions of such surfactants may simulate the physiological environment more accurately rather than using adsorbents or hydroalcoholic and aliphatic media. However, Tang and coworkers showed that for a low solubility drug, increase in solubility by addition of surfactants to meet sink conditions (based on bulk drug solubility data) may not always produce biorelevant results[48]. Aqueous buffers can be used to reflect typical pH conditions in the stomach or small intestine, but do not represent other key aspects of the composition of the GI contents (Osmolality, ionic strength, viscosity, surface tension) that can be relevant to drug release from the dosage form to be tested. In particular, they cannot be used to simulate the influence of food ingestion on drug release. Normal adult diet contains about 150gm of lipids, 95% of which are long-chain triglycerides and 4 - 8gm of phospholipids mainly composed of lecithin. In fed state bioavailability of drug can be increased when there will be change in GIT environment, such as

1) Prolonged gastric emptying and decrease in intestinal motility increasing the time available for Solubilisation.
2) Increased dissolution rate and Solubilisation of drug substances in mixed micelles due to simulation of pancreatic secretion of bile salts and lipase
3) Protection from gastric/luminal degradation, due to protection in lipids.
4) Increased lymphatic transport, thus avoiding first pass metabolism.

Specifically in the case of poorly soluble compounds, it is often observed that the in vivo fraction absorbed increases when the drug is given with a meal. Thus, in order to simulate the effects of food on dissolution in the GI tract, it is equally important to develop representative dissolution tests for both the fasted and fed states[52]. This article mainly focuses on composition of Biorelevant dissolution medium for poorly water-soluble drug with the necessary steps that need to be considered for development of Biorelevant Dissolution Medium.

Bio-relevant Dissolution Media

Compendial dissolution media often fail to yield IVIVC's for class II drugs because relevant physiological parameters are not taken into account. A suitable *in vitro* model should include a medium that mimics as much as possible the GIT contents after food intake. Biorelevant in vitro dissolution testing is useful for qualitative forecasting of formulation and food effects on the dissolution and availability of orally administered drugs. These biorelevant media can be used to assess the performance of different formulations for poorly water-soluble compounds. Biorelevant media have been successfully applied over the past decade to obtain IVIVCs. Two bio-relevant dissolution media simulating conditions in the proximal small intestine FaSSIF and FeSSIF were proposed in 1998. Bio-relevant dissolution methods, combined with permeability measurements and computational simulations, were used to predict the oral absorption of drug[53]. Due to their complex composition, these media are expensive and need to be prepared on the day of the experiment. Before the development of biorelevant dissolution medium the following steps should be considered

1) Fluid composition in the GIT
2) Hydrodynamics in the GIT
3) API/formulation properties
4) Prediction of plasma profile
5) Development of IV-IVCs (*in vitro in vivo* correlation)

1) Fluid composition of GIT

The features of GI fluid are altered in fasted and fed condition and they affect the dissolution. Several physiochemical and physiological properties of GI fluids such as pH, buffer capacity, bile component concentration and state of aggregation and enzyme activity can greatly influence the drug dissolution process. For simulation of GI fluid the composition of GI fluid plays important role because upon simulating biological environment after a convenient alternative could facilitate routine and experimental in vitro dissolution work. Several physiologically based models for GI transit and absorption have been developed recently[54].

Motility in the stomach and small bowel is organised into two basic motor patterns fasting and fed. Fasting motor pattern is characterised by cyclic repetition of periods of quiescence altering with periods of contractile activity. Fed motor pattern is characterized by irregular but persistant phasic contractile activity. It develops almost immediately after ingestion of food and replaces the fasting pattern at whatever point in the interdigestive cycle the meal is eaten. Under fasting condition pH of healthy human stomach is acidic, ranging between 1 and 3. Fluid volume in the stomach would initially be around 300ml in fasted state and 500ml or more in the fed state. The problem while carrying out the dissolution test in FeSSGF is that the medium contains milk, which cannot be filtered using filters with a pore size in the range of 20-500 nm.

- **Stomach**

  Motility in the stomach and small bowel is organised into two basic motor patterns fasting and fed. Fasting motor pattern is characterized by cyclic repetition of periods of quiescence altering with periods of contractile activity. Fed motor pattern is characterized by irregular but persistant phasic contractile activity. It develops almost immediately after ingestion of food and replaces the fasting pattern at whatever point in the interdigestive cycle the meal is eaten[55]. Under fasting condition pH of healthy human stomach is acidic, ranging between 1 and 3. Fluid volume in the stomach would initially be around 300ml in fasted state and 500ml or more in the fed state. The problem while carrying out the dissolution test in FeSSGF is that the medium contains milk, which cannot be filtered using filters with a pore size in the range of 20-500 nm.

Table 4.1 Composition of human bile salt.

Conjugated bile acids	Percentage in bile salt
Sulfolithocholylglycine	3
Sulfolithocholytaurine	1
Lithocholyglycine	0.7
Lithocholyltaurine	0.3
Cholyglycine	24
Chenglycine	24
Deoxycholyglycine	16
Cholyltaurine	12
Chenyltaurine	12
Deoxycholytaurine	8

- **Intestine**

Motility of intestine comprises of intraluminal flow, motion of the wall that induce the flow and systems that regulate the wall motions. Fluid volume in small intestine is of 200 ml in fasted state and 1L in the fed state[56]. It has been found that the bioavailability of poorly soluble drug can be markedly enhanced by meal intake and its related changes in GI tract physiology such as secretions, digestion processes and motility. The human intestinal fluid contains bile salts, phospholipids, monoglycerides, free fatty acids and cholesterol. The increased solubility in FeSSIF-V2 can be explained by the formation of solubilising micelles from bile salts, lecithin, GMO and sodium oleate. Vertzoni et al have proposed that the surface tension could be lowered appropriately with combination of pepsin and very low concentration of bile salt. Bile salts and lecithin can increase the wetting process for the lipophilic drugs and solubilise the drug into the micelles formed by bile salts and lecithin. Composition of bile salts in human.

- **Colon**

  Unlike the motility of the stomach and small intestine which is characterized by the cyclic appearance of the migrating motor complex under fasted conditions, colonic motility is rather limited and in progress due to its inaccessibility and regional differences in structure and function.

The composition of biorelevant media which are proposed by dissolution scientist in fasted and fed state. for stomach, intestine and colon are shown in table from 2-6 pH decreases with increase in temperature and decreases when the temperature is lowered to 24°C. The pH changes at elevated temperature necessitated addition of different amounts of NaOH for maintaining the medium within the physiological range. This could in turn have an influence on osmolality changes. Osmolality is determined by freezing-point depression using an osmometer, buffer capacity is determined by titration with 1 M hydrochloric acid and surface tension is measured using stalagmo meter. The dissolved gases can cause changes in the performance of the dissolution medium by changing pH, forming bubbles on the dosage form or altering the interaction of the medium and the API. Extensive studies have been performed examining appropriate technique for the removal of dissolved gases from aqueous media which include a combination of heating and vaccum filtration followed by stirring under vaccum , vaccum filtration, heating, Sonication, helium sparing and membrane filtration[56]. For stability reason all media were used within 24 hrs after preparation. Taupitz et al suggested that these biorelevant media can be simplified by using SLS and Tween 80 to replace bile compounds. In some cases of poorly water-soluble drugs, existing media such as FaSSIF and FeSSIF were not enough to predict the absorption behaviour of drug so that MREVID 1 and 2 was proposed as a new in-vitro dissolution medium to describe the in-vivo dissolution behavior. The composition of MERVID dissolution medium. Diakidou et al performed simulation of gastric lipolysis and predicted the Felodipine release from a matrix tablet in the fed stomach and concluded that modeling intragastric lipolysis is necessary in order to simulate felodipine release from extended release tablet in fed stomach.

Table 4.2 Composition of the gastric fluid in fasted condition.

Gastric Contents	SGF_{SLS}	SGF_{Triton}	FaSSGF
Sodium lauryl sulfate(%w/v)	0.25/0.05	-	-
Triton X 100 (%w/v)	-	0.1	-
Pepsin (mg/ml)	-	-	0.1
NaTc (μm)	-	-	80
Lecithin (μm)	-	-	20
NaCl	34.2	34.2	34.2
pH	1.2	1.2	1.6
Surface Tension (mN/m)	33.7	32.0	42.6
Osmolality (mOsml/Kg)	180 ± 3.6	157.7 ± 2.9	120.7 ± 2.5

Table 4.3 Composition of the gastric fluid in fed condition.

Gastric contents	Early	Middle	Late
Sodium chloride (mM)	148	237.02	122.6
Acetic acid (mM)	–	17.12	–
Sodium acetate(mM)	–	29.75	–
Ortho-phosphoric acid (mM)	–	–	5.5
Sodium dihydrogen phosphate (mM)	–	–	32
Milk: buffer	1:0	1:1	1:3
Hydrochloric acid/sodium hydroxide	qs pH 6.4	qs pH 5	qs pH 3
pH	6.4	5	3
Osmolality (mOsmol/Kg)	559± 10	400±10	300±10
Buffer capacity (mml/pH)	21.33	25	25

Table 4.4 Composition of the Media to Simulate the Small Intestine in fasting state.

Contents of the Small Intestine	FaSSIF	FaSSIF-V2
Sodium Taurocholate (mM)	3	3
Lecithin (mM)	0.75	0.2
Dibasic sodium phosphate (mM)	28.65	–
Maleic acid (mM)	–	19.12
Sodium hydroxide (mM)	8.7	34.8
Sodium chloride (mM)	105.85	68.62
pH	6.5	6.5
Osmolality (mOsmol/Kg)	270± 10	180± 10
Buffer capacity (mmol/l/pH)	12	10

2) Hydrodynamics in the GIT

The dissolution fluid flow characteristics should consist of a predictable pattern that is free of irregularities or variable turbulence. Hydrodynamics is predominant for the overall dissolution rate if the mass transfer process is mainly controlled by convection/diffusion as is usually the case for poorly soluble substances. A thorough knowledge of hydrodynamics is useful in the course of dissolution method development and formulation development for pharmaceutical industries quality needs. The dissolution apparatus used for different formulation. Muscular contraction in the wall of the small intestine achieves two objectives one is stirring of the contents to increase exposure to enzymes and to bring the luminally digested products close to the wall and second propulsion of indigestible material towards the distal gut. Abrahamsson demonstrated that human intestinal hydrodynamics were reflected in vitro using the paddle method at stirring rates of about 140rpm.

Table 4.5 Composition of the media to stimulate the contents of the Small Intestine in the fed state.

Contents of the Small Intestine	FeSSIF	Early	Middle	Late	FeSSIF-V2
Sodium Taurocholate (mM)	15	10	7.5	4.5	10
Lecithin (mM)	3.75	3	2	0.5	2
Glyceryl monooleate (mM)	-	6.5	5	1	5
Sodium oleate (mM)	-	40	30	0.8	0.8
Acetic acid	140	–	–	–	–
Maleic acid	-	28.6	44	58.09	55.02
Sodium hydroxide (mM)	101	52.5	65.3	72	81.65
Sodium chloride (mM)	173	145.2	122.8	51	125.5
pH	5.0	6.5	5.8	5.4	5.8
Osmolality (mOsmol/Kg)	635± 10	400± 10	390± 10	240± 10	390± 10
10 Buffer capacity (mmol/L/pH)	76	25	25	15	25

However, human studies to establish such correlation are expensive and time consuming. He had used, Labradors as the anatomy and physiology of GI tract of Labradors resembles those of the human GI tract. This canine breed can serve as a model to simulate human intestinal hydrodynamics. The pharmacokinetic of felodipine matrix tablet (poorly soluble, neutral and lipophilic) in Labrador was studied. On the other hand micronised and coarse felodipine dissolution was carried out in biorelevant medium at various speeds (slower, medium, fast). In vitro AUC ratio of this particular experimental set up showed best agreement with the pharmacokinetic parameters. Cammarn et al have established a model for the dissolution of non-disintegrating salicylic acid tablets as a function of hydrodynamic conditions in the Flow Through Cell system (USP Apparatus 4). The approach was to model the dissolution rate of the material as a function of the Reynolds's number. Reynolds number is commonly described as the ratio of momentum forces to viscous forces in a moving fluid. D'Arcy et al, simulated hydrodynamics in the Levy beaker dissolution apparatus and explored the hydrodynamic characteristics of the apparatus. They also determined the hydrodynamics relevance to *in vivo* data used in IVIVCs through comparison of the magnitudes of velocities in the regions of the paddle, basket and Levy apparatuses where a dosage form would be located, with functions of *in vitro* dissolution rate data used in IVIVC studies. Gao Zongming compared dissolution testing under finite and infinite sink conditions, this study applied both paddle and flow-through methods for dissolution testing with disintegrating prednisone and nondisintegrating salicylic acid tablets. The closed- and open-loop configurations of the flow-through method were used to provide comparisons with the paddle method and the dissolution rates obtained using the two configurations were similar if the sink condition maintained. Mirza et al evaluated the dissolution Hydrodynamics in the USP, Peak and Flat-Bottom Vessels Using Different Solubility Drugs. The existence of the 'dead zone' at the bottom of the USP vessel was confirmed by performing perturbation (vessel tilt) studies using the USP Prednisone calibrator tablets, and two Novartis Development tablet formulations containing a low and a high solubility drug. All formulations formed a 'cone‘ of disintegrated mass at the bottom of the vessels. The hydrodynamic environment in the Peak and in flatbottom vessels was also evaluated using the low and high solubility drug formulations. There was no significant difference between the dissolution rates obtained by using the USP and flat-bottom vessels. The Peak vessel provided the highest release rates that were significantly different from those obtained by using USP and flatbottomed vessels. Finally, at higher paddle speeds of 60 and 75 rpm, the results obtained from USP vessels were comparable to results from the Peak vessel operated at 50 rpm. The NJIT group under Prof. Armenante studied the hydrodynamics of dissolution testing using LaserDoppler Velocimetry (LDV) and Computational Fluid Dynamics (CFD), respectively, to experimentally map and computationally predict the velocity distribution and the turbulent intensity inside a standard USP Apparatus II under the typical operating conditions mandated by the dissolution test procedure and concluded that the velocity in the region below the paddle is very low in magnitude.

3) API/Formulation characteristics

Knowledge of the physiochemical nature of a compound in biorelevant media is useful for formulation development, which follows API phase selection. Based on this information the pKa profile of compound could be improved by modifying the surfactants or excipients in the formulation. Many new chemical entities possess physiochemical characteristics unfavourable for oral absorption[56]. The following properties of the API/Formulation are also considered to influence effectively:

i) The solubility and permeability of a drug depends on in which group of the Biopharmaceutical Classification System drug belongs. Accordingly, the characteristics of the formulation will vary.

ii) Solubility of the drug

iii) Particle size of the drug/dosage form

iv) pKa of the drug and pH of the gastrointestinal fluid

4) Prediction of plasma profile

In vitro drug dissolution/release tests are conducted to estimate or predict in vivo drug release characteristics of a product. Direct estimation of in vivo drug dissolution is usually not possible and therefore blood drug concentration-time profiles are used for this purpose. The prediction of plasma profile can be done by using model dependent or model independent approaches. Wagner-Nelson, Loo-Riegelman and numerical deconvolution are such methods. Wagner-Nelson and Loo-Riegelman are both model dependent methods in which former is used for a one-compartment model and the latter for multi-compartment system[57]. The prediction method using convolution analysis consists of following processes-

1) The drug amount–time profile in each segment is calculated by the convolution method.
2) The absorption rate–time profile in each segment is calculated by using the drug amount–time profile in each segment, calculated in step 2.
3) The absorption rate–time profile in the whole GI tract is calculated as the sum of the absorption rate–time profiles of four segments obtained in step 2.
4) Prediction of the plasma concentration–time curve of orally administered drug is performed by means of the convolution method.
5) **Development of IV-IVCs (*in vitro in vivo* correlation):** The total absorption rate– time data obtained in step 3 and pharmacokinetic parameters after intravenous administration correspond to the input function and the weight function, respectively. The inverse Laplace transformation of the obtained equation by the convolution program gives the predicted plasma concentration profile after oral administration without the first-pass metabolism in intestinal epithelium and/or liver.

The pharmacokinetic parameters determined by taking following consideration as study design, population study, study conditions, characteristics investigated during bioavailability study, bioanalytical methodology and statistical evaluation. Rahman et al derived absorption profiles of Theophylline by using Wagner-Nelson equation. Fujioka et al tried to predict the in-vivo absorption kinetics of griseofulvin orally administered as a powder into rats, based on gastrointestinal transit absorption model (GITA), consisting of absorption, dissolution and GI- transit processes[58].

5) Development of IV-IVCs (*in vitro in vivo* correlation)

From biopharmaceutical point of view, in vitro - in vivo correlation (IV-IVC) is a predictive mathematical treatment describing the relationship between an in vitro property of a dosage form (usually the rate or extent of drug release) and a relevant in vivo response, (e.g., plasma or urine drug concentrations or amount of drug absorbed). It is recommended by various regulatory bodies and mostly applicable to drug dosage forms for oral routes and sustained release products. It is a useful tool for drug dosage form development, because a successful correlation can assist in the selection of drug formulation with appropriate and acceptable dissolution criteria, and depending on its predictiveness, it can be used as a forecast or surrogate for further bioequivalence studies. There are different categories of IVIVC; A, B, C and D. In the rapidly emerging field of novel drug delivery systems, the need to establish correlation between in vitro drug release (dissolution) data and in vivo drug profiles is ever growing. Such correlations would not only allow more efficient drug and product development but also economise resources and lead to improved product quality. The bioavailability implications of dissolution should never be accepted on faith; rather it has to be proved through carefully designed in vitro-in vivo correlation studies. Long back, Wagner had stated that, "*Future research in dissolution rate should be directed mainly towards establishing correlation of in vitro data with in vivo data.*"

Objectives of *in vitro - in vivo* Correlation

In vitro dissolution is one of the vital tools for characterisation of biopharmaceutical quality of a dosage form at different stages of drug development. In vitro dissolution data helps in the evaluation and interpretation of possible risks especially in the modified release dosage form and the food effects on bioavailability that influence the gastrointestinal conditions. It also plays a great role while assessing changes in the manufacturing process. However, none of these purposes will be fulfilled by in vitro dissolution testing without sufficient knowledge of its in vivo relevance. IVIVC have been defined in many ways and have been a subject to much controversy. A meaningful correlation must be quantitative5 so as to allow interpolation between data thus making the in vitro model predictive. IVIVC also ensures batch to batch consistency in the physiologic performance of a drug product.

Parameters to be considered while developing IVIVC

1. **Metabolic factors**

   A drug must pass sequentially from the gastrointestinal lumen, through the gut wall, and the liver, before entering in the systemic circulation. This sequence is an anatomic requirement because blood perfusion virtually all gastro- intestinal tissues drain into the liver via the hepatic portal vein. Drug loss may occur in the GIT due to the instability of the drug in the GIT and/or due to complexation of drug with the components of the GI fluids, food, formulation excipients or other co-administered drugs. In addition, the drug may undergo destruction within the walls of the GIT and/or liver.

2. **Drug loss in GIT**

   Any reaction that completes with the absorption of a drug may reduce oral bioavailability of a drug. Reaction can be both enzymatic and non-enzymatic. Acid hydrolysis is a common non-enzymatic reaction. Enzymes in the intestinal epithelium and within the intestinal microflora, which normally reside in the large bowel, metabolise some drug. The reaction products are often inactive or less potent than the large molecule.

3. **Stereochemistry**

   When one enantiomer has higher affinity towards receptors than other, the phenomenon is termed as stereo selectivity which results in pharmacokinetics or pharmacodynamics. If such stereoisomers in the form of racemate are administered orally, one form may have higher bioavailability than the other. Obviously, use of in vitro dissolution data of racemate will not be useful in the development of IVIVC and hence prediction of in vivo availability of active enantiomer. So, consideration of stereoisomerism in the development of IVIVC may provide more meaningful relationship.

Physicochemical properties play a major role in predicting the *in vivo* absorption of drug candidates. For almost all drugs administered orally, dissolution is a prerequisite to drug absorption and clinical efficacy. Dissolution is dependent on several physicochemical properties, including solubility, pH dependency, salt forms, and particle size. A classical mechanistic equation that attempts to model dissolution is the Noyes-Whitney dissolution equation given by equation 1, which incorporates several of the physicochemical factors.

$$dM/dt = [DS(Cs - Cb)]/h \qquad \text{.....(4.1)}$$

Where, M is the amount of the drug dissolved,

t is time,

D is the diffusion coefficient of the drug in the liquid, unstirred boundary layer surrounding the dissolving drug particle,

S is the surface area of drug particle,

h is the diffusion layer thickness, and

C_s and C_b represent drug solubility and drug concentration in the bulk medium at time t, respectively.

The Noyes-Whitney equation describes dissolution rate as a function of the change in drug concentration over time. If the sink condition is assumed, equation 1 can be transformed into the following form:

$$dM/dt = (D.S.Cs)/h \qquad .....(4.2)$$

Where, Cs is approximated by the solubility of the drug substance. This agrees with our previous statement that the rate of dissolution is dependent on solubility. Although the Noyes-Whitney equation is a useful approach to model dissolution, it cannot be utilised to describe all types of dissolution data and may not apply in clinical settings[58].. Another relatively simple model developed, presents the concept of maximum absorbable dose (MAD) as an initial guide to determine dissolution characteristics. In this approach, the MAD is calculated by:

$$\text{MAD} = \text{S. K}_{\text{A}}\text{. SIWV. SITT} \qquad .....(4.3)$$

where S is the solubility at pH 6.5, Ka is the intestinal absorption rate constant, SIWV is the small intestinal water volume, and SITT is the residence time of the drug in the small intestines. In general, the SIWV is considered to be 250 mL and the SITT is assumed to be 3h. This rather simplistic approach has many limitations and can only be utilised as an initial assessment of drug dissolution. To develop a more comprehensive model, all relevant physicochemical properties must be considered. In addition to solubility, another important factor is the compound's ionisation constant or its logarithmic equivalent, the pKa value. The pKa values determine the stability, solubility and absorption of compounds under different environmental pH conditions. This is highly relevant because the human body contains inherent pH gradients, especially in the gastrointestinal (GI) tract, which give rise to pH-dependent absorption profiles in vivo. The salt form of the drug compound is yet another important factor to be considered. In general, a salt form has a higher dissolution rate than that of its free acid or base form. However, under certain pH conditions in the GI tract, the reverse may also be true. Perhaps a more obvious source of effect on dissolution is the particle size. It is commonly recognised that a reduction in particle size would increase surface area and enhance rate of dissolution. It is, however, less well established how particle size reduction affects the dissolution rate. In the study conducted by Johnson and Swindell, it was found that the effect of particle size on absorption is dependent on the drug dose and drug solubility. All these factors add to the complexity of the model building process.

Biopharmaceutical Properties

Drug permeability plays a major role in drug absorption, particularly in orally administered dosage forms. The transcellular permeability (P_m) of a compound is defined as:

$$P_m = (K_p X D_m)/ L_m$$

where Kp is the membrane-water partition coefficient, D_m is the membrane diffusivity, and L_m is the membrane thickness[59]. Various models have been developed to estimate membrane permeability. One such model is based on the pH-partition theory, which states that the membrane uptake of unionised solutes is favoured over the ionised solutes. For weakly acidic compounds, ionisation is suppressed at low pH values, resulting in relatively high absorption rate. At high pH values, equilibrium is shifted towards the ionisation of the compound, resulting in decreased membrane permeability. The opposite conclusions can be deduced for weakly basic compounds. It is also predicted that the pH value at which the half maximal absorption occurs is approximately equal to the compound's p*K*a value. This particular model is not without limitations and deviations have been observed, possibly due to factors such as microenvironmental pH and solubility issues. Another parameter that may be useful in model development is the oil-water partition coefficient. In particular, octanol-water partition coefficient (P or logP) of neutral or unionised species is often used to provide insight into the ability of compounds to pass through membranes for absorption. Using computer and multiple linear regression, Hansch and Fujita were able to quantitate the structure activity relationships based on lipophilicity. They discovered that in general, a bell-shaped distribution exists between absorption and logP values. Kramer was able to further establish that compounds with logP between 0 and 3 generally had high permeability, and those with logP values less than −1.5 or greater than 4.5 had lower membrane permeability.

It is important to note that although the n-octanol-water partition coefficient is a good indicator of membrane permeability, by itself it is not a sufficient parameter to predict *in vivo* absorption. Other measures of membrane permeability have been developed, such as absorption potential (AP) and polar surface area (PSA). The concept of absorption potential was developed by Dressman and is defined as:

$$AP = \log (P. F_{un} /D_o)$$

Where P is the partition coefficient

F_{un} is the fraction of unionised drug at pH6.5, and

D_0 is the dose number equal to the ratio of dose concentration to solubility.

Studies indicate that AP correlates well with the fraction of drug absorbed. PSA is the surface area of a drug molecule occupied by polar atoms. The PSA value has demonstrated good correlation with the passive transport of molecules through membranes, making it a candidate parameter to include in an *in vivo* absorption model[59].

LEVELS OF CORRELATIONS

Although the concepts of correlation and regression are intimately related, they are nevertheless different. Correlation may be described as the degree of association between two variables, whereas regression expresses the form of the relationship between specified values of one (the independent, exogenous, explanatory, regressor, carrier or predictor) variable and the means of all corresponding values of the second (the dependent, outcome, response variable, the variable being explained) variable. In general, we can say that the study of interdependence leads to the investigation of correlations, while the study of dependence leads to the theory of regression. When the x variable is a random covariate to the y variable, that is, x and y vary together (continuous variables), we are more interested in determining the strength of the linear relationship than in prediction, and the sample correlation coefficient, rxy (r), is the statistics employed for this purpose. The Pearson (Product–Moment) correlation r was developed by Pearson (1896) and was based on the work of others, including Galton (1888), who first introduced the concept of correlation. As a matter of fact, correlation charts, also known as scatter diagrams, is one of the seven basic tools of statistical quality control. Empirical relationships can be used, i.e., to determine yield vs. conditions, so process optimization can be achieved, or in linear free-energy relationships (LFR), quantitative structure-activity relationships (QASR) and quantitative structure property (QSPR) relationships[60]. The correlation, however, is a concept of much wider applicability than just 2D scatterplots. There is also "multiple correlation," which is the correlation of multiple independent variables with a single dependent. Also, there is "partial correlation," which is the correlation of one variable with another, controlling for a third or additional variables. If the parameter estimates associated with any one factor in a multi-factor design are uncorrelated with those of another, the experiment design is said to be orthogonal. This is the basic principle of the orthogonal design, which often permits simple formulas to be used to calculate effects, thus avoiding on this way tedious manual calculations. Correlation and covariance play a central role in clustering; correlation is used as such to measure similarity between objects. Factor analysis, behavioural genetic models, structural equations models and other related methodologies use the correlation coefficient as the basic unit of data. Canonical correlation analysis is a way of measuring the linear relationship between two multidimensional variables. There are a number of different correlation coefficients to handle the special characteristics of such types of variables as dichotomies, and there are other measurements of association for nominal and ordinal variables (and for time-series analysis as well). The literature provides a variety of measures of dependence (i.e., Spearman's ρ, the point biserial correlation and the φ coefficient), which are either improved versions of the correlation coefficient or based on complementary different concepts.

In vitro dissolution is one of the vital tools for characterisation of biopharmaceutical quality of a dosage form at different stages of drug development. In vitro dissolution data helps in the evaluation and interpretation of possible risks, especially in the modified release dosage form and the food effects on bioavailability that influence the gastrointestinal conditions. It also plays a great role while assessing changes in the manufacturing process. However, none of these purposes will be fulfilled by *in vitro* dissolution testing without sufficient knowledge of its in vivo relevance. IVIVC have been defined in many ways and have been a subject to much controversy. A meaningful correlation must be quantitative so as to allow interpolation between data, thus making the in vitro model predictive. IVIVC also ensures batch to batch consistency in the physiologic performance of a drug product.

Fundamentals of Correlation

The purpose of establishing the *in vitro in vivo* correlation is to know or to get the vast knowledge about the drug release study from a drug delivery system by oral route. This is important to study the in vitro availability to produce the correlation *in vitro/ in vivo* for suitable drugs. The purpose of identifying the various parameters like pharmacokinetics and pharmacodynamics and various biopharmaceutical parameters also in presence of the food is to prepare the efficacious and validate[61]

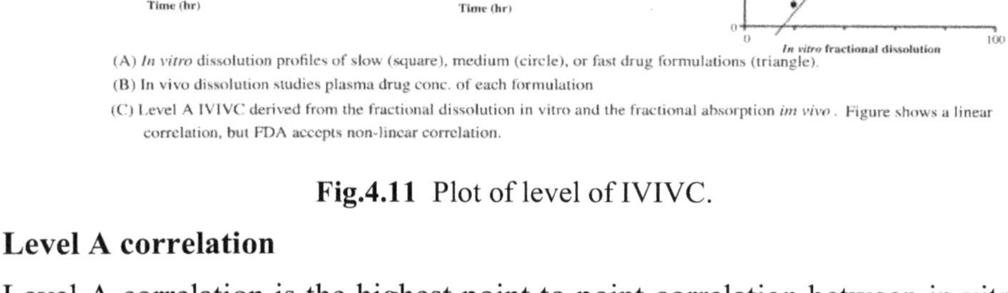

(A) *In vitro* dissolution profiles of slow (square), medium (circle), or fast drug formulations (triangle).

(B) In vivo dissolution studies plasma drug conc. of each formulation

(C) Level A IVIVC derived from the fractional dissolution in vitro and the fractional absorption *im vivo*. Figure shows a linear correlation, but FDA accepts non-linear correlation.

Fig.4.11 Plot of level of IVIVC.

Level A correlation

Level A correlation is the highest point to point correlation between in vitro dissolution profile and in vivo input rate concentration time of drug release. The percent of absorbed drug can be calculated by the model independent techniques such as model dependent numerical deconvolution. These are the mostly use all data obtain from dissolution profile and plasma level to develop a correlation. The purpose of this correlation is to define the in vivo direct relationship such as in vitro dissolution rate single is enough to determine the biopharmaceutical rate of the dosage form.in the level A correlation dissolution curve show surrogate for in vivo performance. Therefore, changing in raw material, method of manufacture, change in manufacture site, minor modification in formulation, and strength of product can b use without additional justification of human studies. It's an excellent quality control which predicts the dosage form in vivo performance[62].

Level B Correlation

A level B by using the principle of statically moment analysis we correlate it here we compare the in vitro dissolution time (MDT) of the product with the mean in vivo dissolution time or means residence time. Although level B can be used for all in vivo and in vitro data, it is not considered to be the point to point of correlation but there are different curves which produce the similar means of residence time. It does not justify the exact plasma curve so that is why a person can't rely upon it, because it's not enough to justify the quality control of standard.

Level C correlation

It also establishes the single point relationship. It is done between dissolution like percent half of drug dissolve in 4 hours and its pharmacokinetics parameters such as AUC, C_{max}, T_{max}[63].

Multiple Level C Correlation

It relates on several pharmacokinetics time points like amount of drug dissolve at several time points of the dissolution profile cover the 3 dissolution time points early, middle and last stage of the dissolution profile.

Exercise

Multiple Choice Questions

1. Fill in the blank with an appropriate word from the words given below.

   The term, dissolution can be defined as the process by which a known amount of solid substance goes into solution per unit of time under .... conditions.

   a) Standardised
   b) Any
   c) The specific pressure
   d) Specific Temperature

2. Which of the following can influence the dissolution of a drug substance?
   a) Crystalline property
   b) Wettability of the dosage form,
   c) Amorphous structure
   d) None of the above
3. Fill in the blank with an appropriate word from the words given below.

   In dissolution test of solid dosage form the solid must ……….. first, and the drug in solution state must then pass through the gastrointestinal membrane.

   a) Disintegrate b) Deaggreate
   c) Dissolve d) None of the above
4. Fill in the blank with an appropriate word from the words given below.

   Due to ,,,,,,,,,,,,,,,,,,,,,, surface area of insoluble solid or compound, the rate of dissolution will increase and hence, absorption through oral route would increase.

   a) Decreased b) Unchanged
   c) Changed d) Increased
5. Which of the following statements stand for PVT?
   a) Private Veterinary Test
   b) Performance Verification Test
   c) Private Limited Company
   d) None
6. Fill in the blank with an appropriate statement from the statements given below.

   A Q value ………………….. is not generally used, because allowance needs to be made for assay and content uniformity ranges.

   a) Less than 60% b) Less than 80%
   c) More than 80% d) Less than 95%
7. The data on which these decisions are based should therefore be complete as well as being attributable, legible, contemporaneous, original and accurate, commonly referred to as ……?

   a) ALCOHOL b) COHA
   c) COHAL d) ALCOHA

8. What for QRM stands?
   a) Quantitative Risk Management
   b) Qualitative Risk Management
   c) Quality Risks and Management
   d) None of these

9. Which of the following is the Noyes-Whitney dissolution equation?
   a) =
   b) =
   c) =
   d) None of the above

10. Which of the following statements is correct?
    a) Particle size affects the dissolution rate.
    b) Particle size reduction affects the dissolution rate.
    c) Particle size reduction does not affect the dissolution rate.
    d) Particle size reduction increases the dissolution rate.

11. Which of the following statements is correct?
    a) For weakly basic compounds, ionisation is suppressed at low pH values, resulting in relatively high absorption rate.
    b) For weakly acidic compounds, ionisation is suppressed at high pH values, resulting in relatively high absorption rate.
    c) For weakly acidic compounds, ionisation is suppressed at low pH values, resulting in relatively high absorption rate.
    d) For strongly acidic compounds, ionisation is suppressed at low pH values, resulting in relatively low absorption rate.

12. Which of the following statements is correct?
    a) The iso-octanol-water partition coefficient is a good indicator of membrane absorption.
    b) The iso-octanol-water permeability is a good indicator of distribution of drug in the membranes.
    c) The benzene-water partition coefficient is a good indicator of membrane permeability.
    d) The n-octanol-water partition coefficient is a good indicator of membrane permeability.

13. Fill in the blank with an appropriate word from the words given below.

    Correlation may be described as the degree of .... between two variables,

    a) Dissociation
    b) Association
    c) All the above
    d) None of the above

14. Fill in the blank with an appropriate statement from the statements given below.

    The correlation is a concept of much wider applicability than just .... scatterplots.

    a) 2D b) 3D
    c) Scatter plots d) Normal plots

15. Fill in the blank with an appropriate word given below.

    .... also ensures batch to batch consistency in the physiologic performance of a drug product.

    a) VIVIC b) IVIVIC
    c) IVIVC d) IVIVIC

16. Fill in the blank with an appropriate word given below.

    The purpose of establishing the in vitro in vivo correlation is to know or to get the vast knowledge about the drug .... study from a drug delivery system by oral route.

    a) absorption b) distribution
    c) metabolism d) release

17. Fill in the blank with an appropriate word given below.

    Level A correlation is the .... point to point correlation between in vitro dissolution profile and in vivo input rate concentration time of drug release.

    a) lowest b) highest
    c) middle d) None of the above

18. Fill in the blank with an appropriate word given below.

    Leve B .... considered to be the point to point of correlation.

    a) is b) is not.
    c) can be d) None of the above

19. Fill in the blank with an appropriate word given below.

    Multiple Level C correlation .... on several pharmacokinetics time points.

    a) does not relate.
    b) does not mean.
    c) does not indicate.
    d) relates

20. Fill in the blank with an appropriate word given below.

    Spearman's ρ, the point biserial correlation and the φ coefficient are either improved versions of the .... coefficient or based on complementary different concepts.

    a) correlation b) coordinating
    c) dissolution d) none of the above

Short Questions

1. Define the term, dissolution. Write down the factors that influence the dissolution characteristics of drugs.
2. Explain how the complexes are formed that favor the dissolution of a dosage form.
3. What is meant by the sink condition and non-sink condition with respect to the dissolution of dosage form? Write down how the sink method for dissolution testing are generally performed.
4. Write down how the solubility, particle size of the drug, and salt formation can influence the dissolution of the drug.
5. Write down how the parameters of dissolution apparatus can affect the dissolution rate of a drug substance.
6. What are the inherent problems of intrinsic dissolution testing? What is saturation concentration of a drug in the dissolution medium?
7. Explain mathematically, the process of dissolution testing. What are different types of apparatuses used for dissolution testing?
8. When the apparatus I and II, and III to VII are used for dissolution testing? Describe how can the 'flow through cell 'be used?
9. Explain 'dissolution number,' 'absorption number', and 'dose number ' with the help of appropriate equation. What is bio-relevant media?
10. What is meant by 'Prediction of plasma profile'. Write about the objective of *in vitro- in vivo* correlation.

Long Questions

1. Pictorially mention the process of dissolution. Explain the Carstensen proposal on a scheme incorporating some sequences.
2. 'The mechanism by which the improvement of dissolution rate can be made- is not fully understood. – 'explain the statement.
3. Describe in short how the interaction between the drug molecule and functional group of carrier molecule can influence the dissolution rate of the drug. Is there any correlation between the solubility of a drug and its dissolution rate.

4. Explain the surface activity and micellar solubilisation, and how do the carrier molecule swell to produce the capillaries.
5. Explain the effect of processing factors on the dissolution of a drug substance.
6. Define intrinsic dissolution rate. 'By use of the intrinsic dissolution testing, the data on the chemical purity and bioequivalence of the available APIs can be obtained'. – justify the statement.
7. Discuss why the management of a pharmaceutical company should take responsibility for good data management by first setting realistic and achievable expectations for the true and current capabilities of a process, a method, an environment, personnel, or technologies, among others.
8. What is meant by 'Quality culture 'in a manufacturing company? Explain 'Quality risk management and sound scientific principle 'and 'Data life cycle management'.
9. Explain correlation levels in dissolution testing. What are MDT and MRT?
10. Explain the levels of correlation.

Answers

1	2	3	4	5	6	7	8	9	10	11	12	13	14	15	16	17	18	19	20
a	b	c	d	b	c	d	a	a	b	c	d	b	a	c	d	b	c	d	a

References

1. Leuner C, Dressman J., Improving drug solubility for oral delivery using solid dispersions, Eur J Pharm and Biopharm., 2000, 50, 47-60.
2. Duncan Q.M. Craig., The mechanisms of drug release from solid dispersions in water-soluble polymers, Int J Pharm., 2002, 231, 131–144.
3. Sekiguchi K. and Obi N., Studies on Absorption of Eutectic Mixture II. Absorption of Fused Conglomerates of Chloramphenicol and Urea in Rabbits, Chem. Pharm. Bull, Tokyo, 1964, 12, 134–144.
4. Sekiguchi K. and Obi N., Studies on absorption of eutectic mixtures I. A comparison of the behavior of eutectic mixtures of sulphathiazole and that of ordinary sulphathiazole in man, Chem. Pharm. Bull., 1961, 9, 866–872.
5. Levy G., Effect of particle size on dissolution and gastrointestinal absorption rates of pharmaceuticals, Am. J. Pharm. Sci. Support Public Health., 1963, 135, 78–92.

6. Kanig J.L., Properties of Fused Mannitol in Compressed Tablets, J. Pharm. Sci., 1964, 53, 188–192.
7. Goldberg A.H. et al., Increasing dissolution rates and gastrointestinal absorption of drugs via solid solutions and eutectic mixtures. IV . Chloramphenicol-urea system, J. Pharm. Sci., 1966, 55, 581–583.
8. Yu L., Amorphous pharmaceutical solids: preparation, characterization and stabilization, Adv Drug Del Rev., 2001, 48, 27-42.
9. Hancock BC., Zograf G., Characteristics and significance of the amorphous state in pharmaceutical systems, J Pharm Sci., 1997, 86, 1-12.
10. Zahedi P, Lee PI., Solid molecular dispersions of poorly water-soluble drugs in poly (2- hydroxyethyl methacrylate) hydrogels, Eur J Pharm Biopharm., 2007,65,320-328.
11. Goldberg A.H., Gibaldi M., Kanig J.L., Mayersohn M., Increasing dissolution rates and gastrointestinal absorption of drugs via solid solutions and eutectic mixtures IV : chloramphenicol-urea system, J Pharm Sci., 1966, 55, 581-583.
12. Verheyen S., Blaton N., Kinget R., Van den Mooter G., Mechanism of increased dissolution of diazepam and temazepam from polyethylene glycol 6000 solid dispersions, Int J Pharm., 2002, 249, 45-58.
13. Konno H., Taylor L.S., Influence of different polymers on the crystallization tendency of molecularly dispersed amorphous felodipine, J Pharm Sci., 2006, 95, 2692-2705.
14. Guillory JK., Generation of polymorphs, hydrates, solvates, and amorphous solids in: Brittain HG (Ed.), Polymorphism in pharmaceutical solids, Marcel Dekker, New York, 1999, 95, 209-210.
15. Martınez-Oharriz M.C., Martın C., Rodrıguez- Espinosa C., Tros-Ilarduya M.C., Zornoza A., Influence of polyethylene glycol 4000 on the polymorphic forms of Diflunisal, Eur J Pharm Sci., 1999, 8,127–132.
16. Perissutti B., Rubessa F., Mariarosa V oinovich D., Formulation design carbamazepine fast- release tablets prepared by melt granulation technique, Int J Pharm., 2003, 256,53-63.
17. Davis, M.E., Brewster, M.E., Cyclodextrin- based pharmaceutics: past, present and future, Nat. Rev. Drug Dis., 2004, 3, 1023–1035.
18. Amin A.F., Shah T.J., Dua R., Mishra R., Superdisintegrants an economical alternative, Pharma Focus Asia., 2006, 47-48.
19. Marderosian A. H. D. et al., editors. Remington: The science and practice of pharmacy, Lippincott Williams and Wilkins, Philadelphia, 2000, 20, 862.

20. Ghaderi R. et al., Preparation of biodegradable microparticles using solution enhanced dispersion by supercritical fluids (SEDS), Pharm. Res., 1999, 16, 676–681.
21. Vasconcelos T. and Costa P., Development of a rapid dissolving ibuprofen Solid dispersion, In PSWC-Pharmaceutical Sciences World Conference, 2007.
22. The United States Pharmacopeia and National Formulary USP38–NF-33. United States Pharmacopeial Convention, Inc.: Rockville, MD, 2015
23. Zakeri-Milani, P.; Barzegar-Jalali, M.; Azimi, M.; Valizadeh, H. Biopharmaceutical classification of drugs using intrinsic dissolution rate (IDR) and rat intestinal permeability. Eur. J. Pharm. Biopharm. 2009, 73 (1), 102–106.
24. Sehić, S.; Betz, G.; Hadžidedić, S.; El-Arini, S. K.; Leuenberger, H. Investigation of intrinsic dissolution behavior of different carbamazepine samples. Int. J. Pharm. 2010, 386 (1–2), 77–90.
25. Lehto, P.; Aaltonen, J.; Niemelä, P.; Rantanen, J.; Hirvonen, J.; Tanninen, V. P.; Peltonen, L. Simultaneous measurement of liquidphase and solid-phase transformation kinetics in rotating disc and channel flow cell dissolution devices. Int. J. Pharm. 2008, 363 (1), 66–72.
26. Steele, G. Preformulation Predictions from Small Amounts of Compound as an Aid to Candidate Drug Selection. In Pharmaceutical Preformulation and Formulation: A Practical Guide from Candidate Drug Selection to Commercial Dosage Form; Gibson, M., Ed. Interpharm/CRC Press: Boca Raton, FL, 2004, 21–88.
27. Azarmi, S.; Roa, W.; Löbenberg, R. Current perspectives in dissolution testing of conventional and novel dosage forms. Int. J. Pharm. 2007, 328 (1), 12–21.
28. Kulinowski, P.; Woyna-Orlewicz, K.; Rappen, G-M.; HaznarGarbacz, D.; Węglarz, W.P.; Dorożyńskib, P.P. An understanding of modified release matrix tablets behavior during drug dissolution as the key for prediction of pharmaceutical product performance – case study of multimodal characterization of quetiapine fumarate tablets, Int. J. Pharm. 2015, 484 (1–2), 235–245,
29. Sehić, S.; Betz, G.; Hadzidedić, S.; El-Arini, S.K.; Leuenberger, H. Investigation of intrinsic dissolution behavior of different carbamazepine samples. Int. J. Pharm. 2010, 386 (1–2), 77–90.
30. Horkovics-Kovats, S. Disintegration rate and properties of active pharmaceutical ingredient particles as determined from the dissolution time profile of a pharmaceutical formulation: An inverse problem. J. Pharm. Sci. 2014, 103 (2), 456–464.

31. Dokoumetzidis, A., Macheras, P.A.; Century of dissolution research: From Noyes and Whitney to the Biopharmaceutics Classification System.; Int. J Phar.; 321, 1 – 11, 2006.

32. Hauck, W.W., Foster, T., Sheinin, E., Cecil, T., BBrown, W., Marques, M., Williams, R.L.; Oral Dosage Form Tests: New Dissolution Approaches.; Pharm Res.; 22, 2, 182 – 187, 2005.

33. Chevalier, E., Viana, M., Artaud, A., Chomette, L., Haddouchi, S., Devidts, G., Chulia, D.; Comparison of Three Dissolution Apparatuses for Testing Calcium Phosphate Pellets used as Ibuprofen Delivery Systems.; AAPS Pharm Sci Tech.; 10, 2, 597 – 605, 2009.

34. Pillay, V., Fassihi, R.; Evaluation and comparison of dissolution data derived from different modified release dosage forms: an alternative method.; J Control Rel.; 55, 45 – 55, 1998.

35. Missaghi, S., Fassihi, R.; Release characterization of dimehydrinate from aneroding and swelling matrix: selection of appropriate dissolution apparatus.; Int J Pharm.; 293, 35 – 42, 2005.

36. Joshi, A., Pund, S., Nivsarkar, M., Vasu, K., Shishoo, C.; Dissolution test for site-specific release isomiazid pellets in USP apparatus 3 (reciprocating cylinder): optization using response surface methodology.; Eur J Pharm Biopharm.; 69, 769 – 775, 2008.

37. Cohen, J.L., Hubert, B.B., Leeson, L.J., Rhodes, C.T., Robinson, J.R., Roseman, T.J. and Shefter, E., The development of USP dissolution and drug release standards. Pharm. Res..7 (1990) 983 987.

38. 38. Khan, M.Z.I., Recent trends and progress in sustained or controlled oral delivery of some water soluble drugs: morphine salts, diltiazem and captopril. Drug Dev. Ind. Pharm., 21 (1995) 1037-1070.

39. Skelley, J.P., Amidon, G.L., Barr, W.H., Benet, L.Z., Carter, J.E., Robinson, J.R., Shah, V.P. and Yacobi, A., Report of the workshop on in vitro and in vivo testing and correlation for oral controlled/modified-release dosage forms. J. Pharm. Sci., 79 (1990) 849-854.

40. AAPS/FDA Workshop Committee, Scale-up of oral extendedrelease dosage forms. 37.

41. Pharm. Teehnol., 19(5) (1995) 46, 48, 50, 52, 54.

42. Lezoray, O., Cardot, H.; A neural network architecture for data classification; International Journal of Neural Systems, Vol. 11, No. 1 (2001) 33-42

43. Dor PJM, Fix JA. In vitro determination of disintegration time of quick-dissolve tablets using a new method. Pharm Dev Tech.; 2000; 5(4):575–577.

44. United States Pharmacopoeia. In vitro and In vivo Evaluations of Dosage Forms, 27th edition, Revision, Mack Publishing Co., Easton, PA., 2004.

45. Guidance for industry, extended release oral dosage forms: development, evaluation and application of an in vitro/in vivo correlation. FDA, CDER, 1997 Bolton, S. Correlation in Pharmaceutical Statistics: Practical and Clinical Applications, 2nd ed., Marcel Dekker Inc., New York, 1991; 211- 245.

46. Gander B, Ventouras K, Gurny R, Doelkar E. In vitro dissolution medium with supramicellar surfactant concentration and its relevance for in vivo absorption. Int J of Pharma. 1985; 27: 117-124.

47. Lehto P. Academic Dissertation; Division of Pharmaceutical Technology Faculty of Pharmacy University of Helsinki Mechanistic Studies of Drug Dissolution Testing

48. Implications of solid phase properties and in vivo prognostic media; Academic Dissertation 2010; 1-49

49. Jamzad S, Fassihi R. Role of Surfactant and pH on Dissolution Properties of Fenofibrate and Glipizide-A Technical Note. AAPS PharmSciTech. 2006; 7 (2): E1-E6.

50. Marques M. Dissolution Media Simulating Fasted and Fed States; Dissolution Technol. 2004; 11(2):16.

51. Juenemann D, Jantratid E, Wagner C, Reppas C, Vertzoni M, Dressman J. B. Biorelevant in vitro dissolution testing of products containing micronized or nanosized fenofibrate with a view to predicting plasma profiles. Eur J of Pharma and Biopharmaceutics; 2011; 77: 257-264.

52. Willmann S, Thelen K, Becker C, Dressman J, Lippert J. Mechanism-based prediction of particle size-dependent dissolution and absorption: Cilostazol pharmacokinetics in dogs Eur J of Pharm and Biopharmaceutics. 2010; 76: 83-94

53. Jantratid E, Janssen N, Chokshi H, Tang K, Dressman J. Designing biorelevant dissolution tests for lipid formulations: case example--lipid suspension of RZ-50. Eur J Pharm Biopharm. 2008; 69:776-785.

54. Yasir M, Asif M. Ammeduzafar, Chauhan I, Singh A. In Vitro - In Vivo Correlation: A Review.; Drug Invention Today; 2010; 2(6): 282-286.

55. Rahman N, Tulain U. Comparative bioavailability and in vitro in vivo correlation of two sustained release brands of theophylline: tablets and pellets. Pak J Pharm Sci. 2008; 21(2): 131-138.

56. J. M. Vergnaud, I. D. Rosca. Assessing Bioavailability of Drug Delivery Systems – Mathematical Model. Taylor & Francis Group., 2005, 81-89.

57. T. J. Sullivan, R. G. Stoll, E. Sakmar, D. C. Blair, J. G. Wagner. J. Pharmakinet. Biopharm. 1974, 2: 29.

58. R. Dietrich, R. Brausse, G. Benedikt, V. W. Steinijans. Arzneim. Forsch. 1988, 38: 1229.
59. Dokoumetzidis A, Papadopoulou V, Macheras P. Analysis of dissolution data using modified versions of Noyes-Whitney equation and the Weibull function. *Pharm. Res.* 2006;23:256–261.
60. Li SF, He HD, Parthiban LJ, Yin HQ, Serajuddin ATM. IVIVC considerations in the development of immediate-release oral dosage form. *J. Pharm. Sci.* 2005;94:1396–1417.
61. A. R. Leach and V. J. Gillet, An Introduction to Chemoinformatics (Dordrecht: Kluwer, 2003), 79.
62. Sirisuth N, Eddington, ND. In-vitro-in-vivo correlation definitions and regulatory guidance. Int J. Generic Drug. 2002;1-11.
63. Lu, Ying, Sungwon Kim, and Kinam Park. "In vitro–in vivo correlation: Perspectives on model development." Int J Pharm. 2011; 418.1:142-148.
64. Nainar, Sundaramoorthi, et al. Biopharmaceutical Classification System in Invitro/In-vivo Correlation: Concept and Development Strategies in Drug Delivery. Tropical J Pharm. Res.2012;11(2): 319-329.

CHAPTER - 5

Product Stability

Degradation Kinetics, Mechanisms, Stability Testing of Drugs and Pharmaceuticals, Factors Influencing-Media Effects and Ph Effects, Accelerated Stability Studies, Interpretation of Kinetic Data (API & Tablets). Solid State Stability and Shelf-Life Assignment. Stability Protocols, Reports and ICH Guidelines

DEGRADATION KINETICS

Stability of pharmaceuticals is a critical quality attribute (CQA) and thus, it is an integral part of the pharmaceutical drug development program. The term stability primarily refers to a drug's ability to maintain its chemical nature, strength, and efficacy within pharmacopoeial limits. Stability also includes considerations regarding shape and size, palatability, uniformity of content, dissolution rate, suspendability, resistance to microbial growth, and, most importantly, therapeutic effect without significant increase in toxicity during its shelf life[1,2]. Stability of pharmaceutical products can be determined by assessing their quality with -in a variety of environmental factors such as relative humidity, light, and temperature. Stability testing of pharmaceuticals is important to describe product's safety, quality, and efficacy, as well as to determine its shelf life. Degradation of a pharmaceutical product includes various chemical reactions initiated by different factors including pH, temperature, and light. Therefore, it is necessary to study the kinetic behaviour of these reactions to get predictive data for the calculation of shelf life of pharmaceutical products[3,4]. The term degradation kinetic refers to the study of the rate at which a drug degrades. Data obtained from the degradation kinetic study can be used to generate a better understanding of the mechanism of drug degradation. Moreover, it also helps to suggest better packaging and storage conditions for pharmaceuticals to improve their shelf life[5].

Stability testing can be carried out under accelerated conditions of increased temperature and humidity to increase the rate of pharmaceutical degradation for obtaining stability data in a short period. There are various degradation kinetics models and many of them have already been applied to basic systems such as drug crystals or API. Study of drug degradation kinetic in its solid form is significantly more complex due to the overlapping of one or more degradation reactions at a time. However, the initial decrease in potency is mainly due to pharmaceutical stability issues which depends on order of their degradation kinetics. Sometimes, residual moisture present in drug substances and drug products can lead to a large number of solid-state reactions[6]. Degradation kinetics commonly refers to the degradation of a drug under various stress conditions. Different kinetic variables can be subsequently used to evaluate the order of drug degradation through the best-fitted line model based on regression coefficient. Thereafter, various kinetic parameters such as rate constant, half-life ($t_{1/2}$), time taken for 10% degradation (t_{90}), and activation energy (E_a) required to initiate the degradation reaction are determined. The t_{90} data are used to interpret shelf life of the pharmaceuticals and to calculate their expiration date[7].

Therefore, it is necessary to study the degradation kinetics of pharmaceuticals to ascertain their shelf life under different environmental conditions. Evaluation of degradation rate under different stress conditions reveals the critical quality attributes (CQAs) of drug stability. The details of kinetic deviations have been described later.

Stability of Pharmaceuticals

Physicochemical properties of drug substances and drug products can be changed during their use, storage, and transport. The significance of instabilities that occur in drug products are primarily described by stability of drug products. Pharmaceuticals may produce toxic substances because of unfavourable environmental factors like moisture, temperature, pH, light, and air. This affects the quality, efficacy, and other properties of drugs. For example, Fanconi syndrome is caused due to the toxicity of epianhydrotetra-cycline, a degraded product of tetracycline. Pharmaceutical stability can be defined as *the potential of a drug substance or drug product to resist any change in its physical, chemical, biopharmaceutical, and microbiological property with respect to change in environmental factors (temperature, light, humidity, etc.).* Pharmacological stability can be defined *as the ability of a pharmaceutical product to preserve its original pharmacological effect to the same extent throughout its shelf life.* Toxicological stability can be defined *as the ability of a drug product to resist any increase in its toxicity during shelf life.* Physical stability means that the physical characteristics of the pharmaceutical product, such as size, shape, hardness, appearance, brittleness, and particle size, remain unchanged during its shelf life. Abrasion, vibrations, and temperature variations are the main causes of physical shape change. These characteristics must be maintained throughout the development of formulation and shelf-life processes. The drug efficacy and safety are ensured by stability and to be maintained throughout the production, formulation, packing, and storage stages[8]. Table 5.1 presents different types of pharmaceutical stability and their requirements. Precipitation, sorption, and leaching are examples of physical instability. Chemical stability includes the absence of any change in the chemical constituent of the drug product. Drug products can undergo chemical degradation reactions, such as, oxidation, hydrolysis, and photolysis. Such chemical reactions can decrease in the concentration of the active ingredient present in a formulation. Moreover, it may cause formation of unwanted degradation products. Microbial stability is related to the sterility of drug substances or products and the absence of contamination with any microorganism in them. Microbial growth in drug products can decrease the safety of products and may lead to serious unwanted effects. Toxicological studies are performed to check the development of any toxic compounds because of the degradation of pharmaceuticals[9].

Kinetics of Drug Degradation

From the previous discussion, it is known that degradation kinetic study is very much important because it affects the stability of pharmaceuticals throughout the stages of product development and testing. With the help of proper storage conditions, reduction in the rate of their degradation reaction can be possible. This ensures the stability of pharmaceuticals throughout their shelf life.

Order of Drug Degradation Reaction

Order of degradation reactions of pharmaceuticals is generally categorised as zero, first, and second order. Knowledge of the order of drug degradation can help pharmaceutical scientists to establish shelf life and optimise storage conditions for drug substances and drug products. Table 5.2 expresses different orders of degradation reaction and formulas for calculating kinetic parameters.

Parameters for Degradation Kinetics

Rate constant, activation energy, half-life, shelf life, and mean kinetic temperature are the primary parameters measured in degradation kinetics. Rate constant can be defined as a proportionality constant that is seen in the rate law. Rate constants are mostly independent of concentration and sometimes depend on other factors, mainly temperature. Activation energy can be defined as *the lowest amount of energy needed to start any kind of chemical reaction.* It is the energy gradient between reactants and state of activation. The lower the activation energy, the faster is the reaction rate. Arrhenius equation can be used for calculation of the activation energy. Half-life of a reaction is *the time taken by the reactant to reach 50% of its initial concentration.* It is used in pharmaceuticals to predict the concentration of drugs over a specific time. It plays an important role in degradation of the drug during stability study. Formula for the calculation of half-life for different orders of reactions is mentioned in Table 5.2. Shelf life is *the time during which the pharmaceutical product is predicted to be stable and remains fit for its intended use under specified storage conditions.* Shelf life of pharmaceuticals can be estimated by using mean kinetic temperature. The idea of mean kinetic temperature is utilised to ensure that real-time storage conditions do not have a direct impact on the drug's stability and shelf life. This happens mostly because degradation rate constants are temperature sensitive. It may be evaluated following the procedures described in USP and FDA. The USP method can be used to calculate the mean kinetic temperature by averaging the temperatures measured over one year. Hayne's equation, which is a modified form of the Arrhenius equation. This equation is used to calculate 52 data points[10].. Arrhenius equation is,

$$k = Ae^{-Ea/RT}$$

Arrhenius regression equation is the most commonly used mathematical model for the assessment of stability of the drug during different types of stability studies. It helps to establish a relationship between temperature and rate constant, to measure the shelf life of a drug substance and drug product during developmental phase. With the help of this method, the effect of temperature and catalyst on chemical stability and decomposition can be established. In the above equation, A represents frequency factor, T represents the temperature (kelvin), E_a is the activation energy require to start degradation reaction in J mol^{-1}, k is a rate constant of any order reaction as a function of absolute temperature, and R is the Gas constant (R = 1.987 Cal mol^{-1} K^{-1}).

Arrhenius equation is the most important equation that predicts the stability of drug at room temperature, at temperature, higher than or lower than the room temperature.

Table 5.1 Different types of pharmaceutical stability and its requirement.

Sl. nos.	Types of stability	Stability problems	Stability requirements
1.	Physical	Precipitation, sorption, leaching, color change	Physical appearance, palatability, uniformity
2.	Chemical	Reduction in active concentration of API	Chemical integrity and labeled strength
3.	Microbiological	Microbial growth	Sterility, no microbial contamination
4.	Toxicological	Toxicity	No increase in toxicity
5.	Therapeutic	No therapeutic activity	Drug action does not change on storage

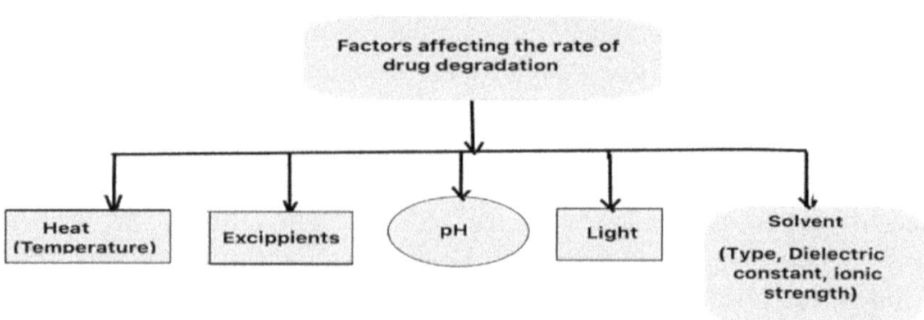

Fig.5.1 Factors affecting the drug degradation process.

Factors affecting the quality of degradation kinetic data of pharmaceuticals

Degradation kinetics of pharmaceuticals can be affected by several factors including pH, temperature, medium used for degradation kinetic study (solvent, dielectric constant, and ionic strength), intensity of light, duration of exposure, and excipients. These factors individually and/or synergistically can affect the quality of data obtained from the degradation kinetic study of pharmaceuticals. For generation of good quality kinetic study data, it is important to study the individual effect of each variable on the rate of degradation. An overlapping effect of variables can make the interpretation of kinetic data more complicated. Simultaneous effect of variables can change the rate as well as the order of the degradation reaction which can further lead to false positive data. Among all these factors, temperature used for degradation kinetic study is one of the most important factors which can directly affect the rate of degradation. It is necessary to control and carry out degradation kinetic at an appropriate temperature to provide optimum degradation of the drug. If the temperature is increased the order of degradation reactions also increases. *A 10°C increase in temperature can double the reaction rate with the same activation energy*. This increase in reaction rate is mainly due to an increase in numbers of useful collision of molecules with right orientation above activation energy level. Degradation kinetics can also be affected by the type of solvent used for performing degradation kinetic study of pharmaceuticals. Iqbal et al. had reported the linear increase in the degradation of riboflavin (vitamin B2) to form two major degradation products formyl methyl flavin and lumichrome with an increase in polarity of solvent under photolytic conditions[11]. Dielectric constant and ionic strength of the medium can also sometimes affect the rate of drug degradation. T pH is another important variable for degradation kinetic study. The rate of hydrolysis of ester and amide-containing drugs is greatly affected by pH of the medium in which degradation is supposed to happen. Barbosa et al. had reported in a study the effect of pH on the rate of hydrolysis of nitazoxanide (NZN), a broad-spectrum antiparasitic and antiviral drug[12].They found an increase in the rate of hydrolysis of NZN at neutral and slightly alkaline pH. Excipients present in the drug formulation can also influence the rate of degradation of drug substances. Natasa et al. studied the impact of different excipients on the degradation of olanzapine an antipsychotic drug in its solid-state. Olanzapine is reported to be sensitive to light and moisture[13]. They found an increase in the formation of hydrolytic degradation product in the presence of lactose monohydrate when used as a filler in tablet formulation. Their study concluded that hydrolysis of olanzapine was excipient mediated. Degradation kinetics of pharmaceuticals can be studied by considering individual factors based on their impact to generate good quality kinetic data for a better understanding of drug stability which can help to develop a stable formulation and to improve the shelf life of the drug.

Systematic Strategies to Perform Degradation Kinetics

Degradation kinetics require the selection of different kinetic variables including pH, temperature, stressor concentration, excipient type and quantity, ionic strength, and radiation intensity. This study is performed to evaluate the rate of drug degradation under different environmental conditions such as hydrolytic (acid, base, and neutral), oxidative, photolytic, and thermolytic stress conditions. Figure 5.1 shows the factors generally affect the rate of degradation of a drug. Selection of variables for degradation kinetic study is an important step, since it can provide information regarding rate-limiting factors for each degradation reaction. To study the degradation kinetics of a drug under hydrolytic conditions, different variables such as temperature, light, and pH of the reaction mixture can be used. It is important to consider one variable at a time to evaluate the effect of an individual variable on the kinetics of drug degradation reaction. Multiple variables when used simultaneously to study degradation kinetics can provide false positive or false negative data because the effects of multiple variables can overlap at a time. The degradation kinetic study is carried out by using different selected variables. The data are plotted as a percentage of drug remaining vs time. From this graph, the best-fitted line can be obtained to determine the order of reaction based on the regression coefficient value of each graph with an individual variable. The data obtained from this graph can be used to calculate different kinetic parameters such as degradation rate constant (k), $t_{1/2}$, and t_{90}. The Arrhenius equation is used to calculate the activation energy for the reaction. Vasantakumar et. al. have studied the degradation kinetics of butacaine sulfate by sodium chlorobenzene sulfonamide (CAB) in the presence of perchloric acid at 303 K. This reaction shows first-order kinetics, since the substrate showed fractional order dependence. It did not depend on perchloric acid. Measure of elements of the reaction was found to be 1:3 and the oxidation product formed was recognised. The degradation kinetics by oxidation was studied at different temperatures, and activation parameters have been assessed. Shubha et al., have reported a study on oxidation of a local anesthetic benzocaine hydrochloride with the help of sodium n-halo-p-toluene sulphonamide in the perchloric acid medium at 303K. As per the study, oxidative degradation of benzocaine hydrochloride was found to follow first-order degradation kinetics. When the dielectric constant of the medium decreased by the addition of methanol, the rate of reaction was increased. The rate of reaction was not affected much with the variation in ionic strength and the addition of p-toluene sulphonamide. The reaction has been studied at various temperatures, and activation parameters were calculated. The elements of the reaction were measured which was found to be 1:1 and the degradation product formed by oxidation was identified by using spectral analysis[14]. Oliviera et al., investigated the mechanism of atorvastatin degradation in acidic and basic environments. In acidic environments it was found to be the first-order kinetics and in basic environment it was found to follow zero-order kinetics, which were less stable when examined in acidic medium. The rate constant for degradation in acidic medium was found to be 1.88×10^{-2} $s^{-1.}$ This suggests first-order kinetics. On the other hand, the rate constant for degradation in the basic medium was found to be 2.35×10^{-4} mol L^{-1}, indicating zero-order reaction and the drug was less stable in acid media. Berge et al. studied the kinetics and degradation mechanism of cefotaxime sodium in a pH 0 – 10 solution at 25°C. HPLC was used for analysis of the samples to find out the rate of degradation reaction, which revealed pseudo-first order with the drug concentration. According to the research, hydrogen ion, solvolysis, and hydroxide ion catalysis improved the rate of degradation kinetics substantially. The pH rate profile at 25°C showed that cefotaxime had the best stability between 4.5 and 6.5. In an aqueous solution, cefotaxime degraded by two concurrent reactions, namely C-3 position de-esterification and β-lactam cleavage. Vaucher et al. employed a UV lamp at a wavelength of 254 nm and a power of 15 watts to study the photodegradation of telithromycin in a chamber with internal mirrors. Zhao et al., studied amoxicillin degradation kinetic in an aqueous medium. Amoxicillin was found to be degraded by active persulfate under oxidative conditions. Each time, the drug was found to obey pseudo-first-order degradation kinetics. When the energy of activation was 126.9 kJ mol^{-1} and the temperature of the reaction was changed from 35 to 60°C, the reaction was matched with the Arrhenius equation. When the initial concentration of persulfate, reaction temperature, concentration of chlorine, and concentration of humic acid were high, the degradation efficiency was improved[15]. Moreno et al. studied thermal and photodegradation kinetics of ceftazidime and the dependability of microbiological assay for it. During stress process, the degradation of the antibiotic was found to follow first-order reaction kinetics. In an aqueous solution, ceftazidime showed extensive degradation when it was compared with solid state. Paczkowska et al. studied the degradation process of Cefozopran with the help of HPLC by using a DAD detector. Total two DPs were calculated when analysed with Q-TOF mass spectrometer. They investigated the effect of relative humidity and temperature on stability of cefozopran. The degradation kinetic profile of solid-state cefozopran hydrochloride was found to obey the first-order reaction where the rate of drug degradation reaction depends on the concentration of the drug.

Degradation Kinetic Study of Pharmaceuticals Employing Advanced Models

Many advanced degradation models have been developed to perform forced degradation studies by using mixed effects of different stressors. This advancement in degradation study requires the study of degradation kinetic data to evaluate deviation from normal degradation kinetics of drug substance and drug product.

Autocatalytic Kinetic of Hydrolysis

Autocatalytic process generally involves modification in the reaction kinetic of many chemical reactions including degradation of pharmaceuticals. The change in chemical kinetics includes the formation of a product that can further increase or decrease the rate of drug degradation reaction. Antheunis et al. have developed a mathematical kinetic model to describe and predict the rate and extent of degradation of different polyester molecules. The polyester molecule includes polycaprolactone (PCL), poly (4-methyl caprolactone), polylactide, and the copolymer poly (D, L-lactide-co-glycolide) by autocatalytic hydrolysis in an aqueous medium. This model helps to calculate the degradation rate of polyesters by plotting a decrease in molecular weight as a function of time. The model considers autocatalytic effect of carboxylic acid on the hydrolysis of polyesters to predict the degradation rate. It describes the formation of carboxylic acid as a product of hydrolysis of polyesters which further catalyse this hydrolysis process by decreasing pH of the media up to 2. Sudden decrease in pH leads to more degradation and faster decrease in molecular weight which further affect the kinetic of this hydrolytic reaction and increase the rate of degradation.

Oxidation/Reduction Models

Advanced oxidative degradation uses oxidising agents with UV exposure for degradation of the system followed by generation of highly reactive radicals which increases the rate of oxidative degradation of the drug. Rosenfeldt et al. studied the effect of UV radiation on oxidative degradation kinetics of endocrine-disrupting compounds such as ethynyl estradiol, bisphenol, and estradiol by exposing hydrogen peroxide stressed compound to ultraviolet radiation. They have reported that by adding hydrogen peroxide to UV exposed samples accelerates oxidative degradation of compounds. The change in drug degradation was caused by addition of hydrogen peroxide. When hydrogen peroxide was added, the primary mechanism of endocrine-disrupting chemical destruction changed to hydroxyl radical-mediated accelerated oxidation. This mechanism results in the creation of highly reactive species, such as OH• radicals, which appear to react rapidly with endocrine-disrupting compounds. Several endocrine-disrupting compounds are destroyed by chemical oxidation using different oxidative metal stressors such as TiO_2, chlorine, potassium permanganate, and ozone-based photocatalysis. The UV absorption spectrum of chemical pollutants and contaminating agents denoted a higher degradation rate after the addition of hydrogen peroxide to generate a harsh oxidative system which led to an increased rate of degradation.

Oxidation by using Fe(II) Activated Bisulphate

Wang et al. used advanced oxidation techniques such as Fe (II)-activated bisulphate (BS) to degrade diclofenac from waste-water. Degradation mechanisms were studied concerning Fe(II) dose, bisulfite concentration, initial pH, reaction temperature, and dissolved oxygen. Fe(II)/bisulfite had a better removal rate of diclofenac than Fe (II)/persulphate, and its degradation followed a pseudo-first-order kinetic model. The best pH for diclofenac decomposition was 4 due to the morphology of Fe(II) and bisulfte. Excess Fe (II) or bisulfite inhibited diclofenac degradation as an SO_4 scavenger, but with higher initial Fe (II) or bisulfte concentration, the diclofenac degradation increased. Although dissolved oxygen did not influence the elimination of diclofenac in the pH range of 4.6–8.3 mg L^{-1}, it was found to be an important factor in promoting the conversion of SO_3 to SO_4. Based on the increased diclofenac degradation with rising temperature, the activation energy of this process was found to be 120.75 3.43 kJ mol^{-1}. As per the radical scavenging studies, SO_4 –, HO•, and other reactive species contributed 71.1%, 24.6%, and 4.3% to diclofenac degradation in the Fe(II)/bisulphate system, respectively. UPLC-Q-TOF–MS was used to detect nine transformation products. The degradation pathways of diclofenac were hydroxylation, dehydration, decarboxylation, dichlorination, and formylation[16].

UV-activated Persulphate Model

Xian Lu et al. demonstrated the effect of different degradation processes that were evaluated using three different approaches, namely direct UV radiation, persulfate (PS) oxidation alone, and UV/PS combination. It was found that there was a considerable increase in the degradation of diclofenac under the impact of UV/PS. After 60 min of irradiation, direct UV photolysis was removed 75% of the material. With a rate constant of 3.9104 s^{-1}, the degradation was found to follow a pseudo-first order[17].

Oxidation by UV-activated Sulfate Radical

Lou et. al investigated the removal efficiency of trimethoprim in the UV-activated persulphate system. By using a pseudo-first-order reaction kinetic model, degradation behaviour of trimethoprim in UV-activated persulphate was studied. Because of the poor molar absorptivity and quantum yield of trimethoprim at 254 nm, direct photolysis was slower. The degradation rate increased dramatically with the addition of H_2O_2 and persulphate. In the UV-activated persulphate model, the SO_4 radical plays a major role in the degradation reaction. In the presence of a UV-activated persulphate system, the model built by them can assess and elaborate the effect of natural organic matter, persulphate concentration, and chloride ion on trimethoprim degradation. The pseudo-first-order rate constant for trimethoprim was increased with an increase in persulfate concentration. On the other hand, rate constant was decreased in the presence of chloride.

Mixed Oxidation Catalysis

Wols et al., investigated UV/H_2O_2-based mixed oxidation catalysis, which is a well-known method for degrading organic micro-pollutants[18]. The degradation of organic micro-pollutants in UV/H_2O_2 reactors was predicted using a computational fluid dynamics model combined with an advanced kinetic model. It takes into account the influence rate, hydraulics complex photochemical reactions in the water matrix, and interactions between these processes. The compound was degraded with the help of UV photolysis, carbonate radicals, and HO• radicals. The scale of UV/H_2O_2 reactors in the plot, the pharmaceutical degradations were monitored and shown under various operating settings. The study concluded that temperature affects the decomposition of organic micropollutants during mixed oxidation catalysis.

Photo-assisted Fenton Reagent-Based Model

Kusic, H. et al. Used Fenton-type (Fe^{3+}/H_2O_2, Fe/ H_2O_2 Fe^{2+}/H_2O_2) and photo-assisted processes (UV/ Fe/H_2O_2, UV/Fe^{3+}/H_2O_2, and UV/Fe^{2+}/H_2O_2) for the degradation of phenol as a model organic pollutant in wastewater. They described the entire kinetic model as phenol degradation. The analytical models anticipated the degradation of phenol and the generation of main oxidation by-products such as catechol, hydroquinone, and benzoquinone. In this study, the mineralization kinetics of the phenol solution was predicted using advanced oxidation. Additional reactions that describe the removal of Fe from the catalytic cycle through the creation of ferric complexes and their regeneration triggered by UV light are included. HPLC analysis and total organic carbon content measurements were used to examine the phenol breakdown kinetics. The procedures used were successful in removing all phenols by degradation[19].

Table 5.2 Different orders of degradation reaction and formulas for calculating kinetic parameters.

Order of degradation reaction	Kinetic parameters			Example
	Rate equation	Half-life	Shelf life	
Zero-order	$R = -d[A]/dt = k_0$	$t_{1/2} = [A]_0/2k$	$t_{0.9} = 0.1[A]_0/k_0$	Hydrolysis of atorvastatin Electrochemical degradation ceftriaxone
First-order	$R = -d[A]dt = kA$	$t_{1/2} = \ln(2)/k$	$t_{0.9} = 0.105/k$	Oxidation of butacaine Oxidation of benzocaine hydrochloride Hydrolysis of atorvastatin Thermal and photodegradation of ceftazidime
Second-order	$d[A] = -k[A]^2/dt^2$	$t_{1/2} = 1/k[A]_0$	$t_{0.9} = (0.11/k)[A]_0$	Photodegradation of formamethylfavin in acidic solution Thermolysis of formamethylfavin, hydrolysis of esters in alkaline solution

Thermal Degradation

Vieira et al. studied thermal degradation kinetics of ascorbic acid by using two mathematical models in replication to regenerate experimental conditions and data. With the help of linear regression, all kinetic parameters were identified on the logarithmic curve of experimental data. The mathematical model has been used to calculate the loss of ascorbic acid and to study the degradation kinetics of ascorbic acid. Quantification of ascorbic acid has been determined with UHPLC-MS/MS. The degradation parameter was determined using data after fitting in 243 inearized equations, and the final result showed fast degradation with a low activation energy value. Since, the average error achieved is low, both of the generated kinetic models may be used to represent the deterioration rate. To achieve isothermal heating and to prevent air oxidation, the samples were put in screw cap tubes with a diameter of 1 cm.

Acid hydrolysis and photolysis under near-UV light in the presence of TiO2

Kwiecien et al. Studied two mechanisms of roxithromycin degradation under near-UV irradiation to perform acidic hydrolysis and photocatalytic degradation of drug by TiO_2 photosensitizer. This was used for analysis of acidic degradation samples. Dense spots of drug and its degradation products were observed. HPLC can be used to track photocatalytic degradation experiments by using TiO_2 as a stressor. The results revealed that both ways of roxithromycin degradation are quite effective. The Langmuir–Hinshelwood theory for photocatalytic microheterogeneous systems govern the kinetics of first-order photocatalytic degradation reactions. For elucidating the structure of degradation product under photocatalytic and acidic conditions. The UPLC-MS/MS technique was used for this purpose. The structure proposed was based on its fragmentation pattern[20].

Accelerated degradation by Ferrous/Chloride Ions

Mao et al. determined the mechanism and degradation kinetics of ibuprofen and sulfamethoxazole. The study showed that reactive chlorine species had a major role in the degradation of ibuprofen at pH 3. Fe(IV) was not found to be the main contributor in degradation reaction because of the low reaction rate between Fe and the targeted compound. In the acidic conditions, degradation of the pharmaceuticals was facilitated. Chlorine showed significant degradation of sulfamethoxazole but showed negligible effect on the degradation of ibuprofen. The reactive species like OH•, Fe(IV), and reactive chlorine species showed a major contribution to the degradation of the drug[s21].

Boron-Doped Diamond Electrode Mediated Electrochemical Oxidation

In a study Loos et al., assessed the degradation kinetics using a boron-doped diamond electrode for electrochemical oxidation. In this research, electrochemical oxidation was carried out for selected drugs, such as iopromide, sulfamethoxazole, 17-ethinylestradiol, and diclofenac, in simulated wastewater and hospital effluent wastewater. The degradation kinetics follows pseudo-first-order reaction kinetics in all experimental conditions. The result showed that sulfamethoxazole, 17-ethinylestradiol, and diclofenac degraded rapidly. The degradation of iopromide was significantly slower in simulated wastewater and real wastewater. The activation energy was determined on the basis of reaction rate constant at different temperatures[22].

Computation-Based Kinetic Models

On the basis of computation, kinetic modeling is gaining more attention to predict the degradation behaviour of pharmaceutical products under defined stress conditions. This can help to understand the effect of individual variables on degradation rate kinetics. The study of degradation kinetics using a computation-based model helps to predict different kinetic parameters such as rate constants, activation energy (Ea), and mean kinetic temperature. These provide a better understanding of the degradation kinetic behaviour of the drug. While using computation-based models to study drug degradation kinetics, initial experimental data are required to predict the effect of the individual variable on the rate of drug degradation. The success of computation-based prediction of kinetic parameters mainly depends on the quality of initial data generated from different experiments. Blaž et al. reported a study on computation-based kinetic model to assess the degradation kinetic behaviour of complex solid dosage form using saxagliptin as a model drug[23].

MECHANISMS

Kinetics of Drug Degradation

Degradation kinetic study is important. It affects the stability of pharmaceuticals throughout the stages of product development and testing. With the help of proper storage conditions, reduction in the rate of their degradation reaction can be possible. This ensures the stability of pharmaceuticals throughout their shelf life[24].

Order of Drug Degradation Reaction

Order of degradation reactions of pharmaceuticals is generally categorised as zero, first, and second order. Knowledge of the order of drug degradation can help pharmaceutical scientists to establish shelf life and optimum storage conditions for drug substances and drug products. Table 5.3 shows different orders of degradation reaction and formulas for calculating the kinetic parameters.

First-order Degradation Reaction

Most pharmaceutical products are found to degrade through first-order reactions. The reaction rate of first-order degradation of drugs under different environmental conditions can be determined through a decrease in the initial concentration of the drug with time. The degradation reaction rate is proportional to a decrease in the initial concentration of the drug as a function of time. Equation 1 denotes the formula for the rate of drug degradation through a first-order reaction. A negative sign denotes a decrease in the initial concentration of the drug as a function of time.

$$r = -d[A]/dt = k_1[A] \qquad .....(5.1)$$

Where, A is the concentration of a drug,

k_1 is the first-order rate constant, and

t is the time.

It has been established that the degradation of imidapril hydrochloride under hydrolytic (acid/base catalysed) conditions follows first-order degradation kinetics[25]. Another example of describing first-order degradation such as the thermal decomposition of meropenem a beta-lactam antibiotic when exposed to a higher temperature (70, 80, and 90°C) for 335, 295, and 95 days, respectively. The degradations were found to follow first-order degradation kinetics[26].

Second-order Reaction

Rate of second-order drug degradation reaction mainly depends on the concentration of the drug substance and stressor. Equation 2 indicates the rate of drug degradation through a second-order reaction.

$$dA/dt = -k_2[A]^2 \qquad .....(5.2)$$

Where, k_2 represents second-order rate constant and

A represents concentration of the drug.

Photodegradation of formamethylflavin in acidic solution, thermolysis of formamethylflavin, hydrolysis of esters in alkaline solution reported to follow second-order degradation reaction[27]. Degradation of trans-lutein (carotenoids) via isomerization into cis-lutein under ultrasonic waves was reported to follow second-order degradation kinetic at 30–50°C temperature.

Zero-order Reaction

In zero-order kinetics, the degradation reactions do not depend on the concentration of the drug and stressor. Equation 3 expresses the rate of zero-order drug degradation reactions. Zero-order reactions mainly include rearrangement or radical-mediated cleavage of chemical bonds under photolytic and oxidative stress conditions.

$$r = -d[A]/dt = k_o \quad .....(5.3)$$

where, A is the concentration of the drug and

k_0 represents rate constant for zero-order degradation reaction and

t is the time.

Table 5.3 Degradation mechanism and order or degradation of different drugs.

Sr. nos	Name of drug	Reaction type	Variables	Order of degradation
1.	Bedaquilline	Hydrolysis	pH	First-order reaction
2.	Tenofovir	Hydrolysis Oxidation	pH, H_2O_2	First-order reaction
3.	Cefotaxime	Hydrolysis of the lactam ring	UV, pH, temperature	Pseudo-frst order
4.	Ceftriaxone	Electrochemical oxidation of thiazole side chain (R1-CONH-)	Electrolysis, temperature	First-order reaction Zero order reaction
5.	Amoxicillin	Hydroxylation of β lactam ring	pH, temperature	Pseudo-frst-order reaction
6.	Moxalactam	Hydroxylation of β lactam ring	pH, temperature	Pseudo-frst order reaction
7.	Telithromycin	Oxidation, Photolysis	UV light, H_2O_2	First-order reaction
8.	Azithromycin	Ester hydrolysis	pH, temperature	Pseudo-frst order
9.	Erythromycin	Ester hydrolysis	Concentration, ionic strength, bufer concentration, pH, temperature	Pseudo-frst order
10.	Cefozopran	Amide hydrolysis	Temperature, humidity	First-order reaction
11.	Ciprofbrate	Acid hydrolysis	pH, temperature	First-order reaction
12.	Ceftazidime	Amide hydrolysis	pH, temperature	First-order reaction

For example, ultrasonic degradation of diclofenac under acidic (pH = 3) oxidative condition at higher concentration (40–80 mg/L) occurs through zero-order degradation kinetics. The degradation of atorvastatin an antilipemic drug under basic hydrolytic conditions follows a zero-order rate of degradation[28].

Pseudo-zero-Order Reaction

The principle of pseudo-zero-order kinetics is that the drug concentration is kept constant throughout the reaction. Thus, the degradation rate does not depend on the concentration of the drug at saturation. Pseudo-zero-order reactions are mainly observed in solid dose-age forms and suspensions. Degradation kinetic study of pharmaceutical formulation such as tablet or capsule containing API sometimes represents mixed order of degradation due to overlapping effect of more than one degradation mechanism. During the degradation phase, overall degradation kinetic of the drug follows a zero-order rate. However, the first-order degradation kinetics can also be observed. Equation 4 shows the formula for the calculation of rate of pseudo-zero-order reaction, where A is the concentration of reactant and k_1 is the pseudo-zero-order rate constant.

$$d[A]/dt = -k_1[A] \quad .....(5.4)$$

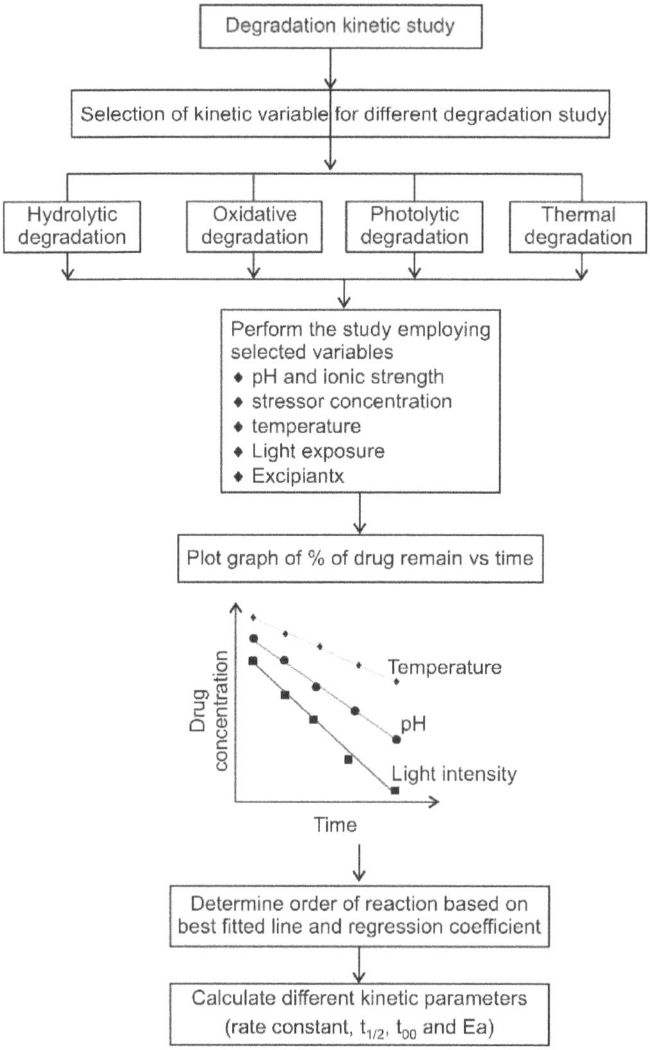

Fig.5.2 General strategy to perform degradation kinetic study of pharmaceutic.

Interaction between the drug and moisture present in the drug product can cause degradation of drug through pseudo-zero order. The presence of moisture forces the system to function as a suspension, and the increased concentration of solid drug makes it pseudo-zero order, and drug degradation to be linear with time. Equation 5 describes the mixed order behaviour of pseudo-zero-order reaction, where $[A]_S$ denotes solubility of drug due to moisture present in the system, $[A]$ denotes concentration of the drug, k_0 denotes zero-order rate constant, and k_1 is the first-order rate constant.

$$k_1[A] = k_1[A]_S = k_0 \qquad \text{.....(5.5)}$$

It has been reported from a study on the degradation of dacarbazine (antineoplastic agent) in an aqueous solution. As per the study, photolytic degradation of dacarbazine was found to be accelerated in light even at lower concentration (0.05 mg/ml) and there was a reduction in the over-all degradation rate above 0.05 mg/ml concentration. This was caused due to the absorption of light by the degradation product at higher concentrations. Therefore, photolysis of dacarbazine was shown to follow pseudo- zero-order kinetics[29].

Pseudo-First-Order Reaction

It only occurs when one of the reactants is in a higher concentration or remains constant in comparison with another substance. Thus, the rate of reaction is determined by only one reactant although both the reactants are present. In such a case, no significant effect of the second reactant on the change in concentration during the period of degradation reaction is observed. Degradation of ascorbic acid and hydrolysis of aspirin follows pseudo-first-order reaction. As per the study, hydrolytic degradation of oxytocin at lower pH (~2) follows pseudo-first-order degradation kinetics[30].

STABILITY TESTING OF DRUGS AND PHARMACEUTICALS

Stability testing of pharmaceutical products is a complex set of procedures. This includes considerable cost, time consumption and scientific expertise to achieve quality, efficacy and safety in a drug formulation. Scientific and commercial success of a pharmaceutical product can only be achieved with the understanding of the drug development process and the myriad tasks and milestones that are important to a comprehensive development plan. The most important steps during the developmental stages are the pharmaceutical analysis and stability studies. These are necessary to determine and ensure the identity, potency and purity of ingredients, as well as those of the formulated products. Stability of a pharmaceutical product may be defined as *the capability of a particular formulation in a specific container/closure system to remain within its physical, chemical, microbiological, toxicological, protective and informational specifications.* In other words, it is the extent to which a product retains the same properties and characteristics possessed at the time of its packaging within the specified limits, throughout its period of storage and use. Thus, stability testing evaluates the effect of environmental factors on the quality of the drug substance or a formulated product which is utilised for prediction of its shelf life, and to determine proper storage conditions and suggest labelling instructions. Moreover, the data generated during the stability testing is an important requirement for regulatory approval of any drug or formulation[31].

Stability testing is considered as a complex process because of involvement of a variety of factors influencing the stability of a pharmaceutical product. These factors include stability of the active ingredient(s); interaction between active ingredients and excipients, and the manufacturing process followed. For the type of dosage form, container/closure system used for packaging and light, heat and moisture conditions encountered during shipment, storage and handling. Moreover, the degradation reactions such as oxidation, reduction, hydrolysis or racemizatoon, can play important role in stability of a pharmaceutical product. The stability also depends on the conditions such as concentration of reactants, pH, radiation, catalysts etc., as well as on the raw materials used and the length of time between manufacture and usage of the product. A pharmaceutical product may undergo change in appearance, consistency, content uniformity, clarity (solution), moisture contents, particle size and shape, pH, package integrity affecting its stability. Such physical changes may occur because of the impact, vibration, abrasion, and temperature fluctuations such as freezing, thawing or shearing etc. The chemical reactions, such as solvolysis, oxidation, reduction, racemizatoon etc. may occur in the pharmaceutical products leading to the formation of degradation product, loss of potency of active pharmaceutical ingredient (API), loss of excipient activity like antimicrobial preservative action and antioxidants etc. Stability of a pharmaceutical product can also be affected due to the microbiological changes such as growth of microorganisms in non-sterile products and changes in preservative efficacy.

Importance of Stability Testing

The primary reason for stability testing is the concern for the well-being of the patient suffering from the disease for which the products is designed. Apart from degradation of the unstable product into toxic decomposition products, loss of activity up to a level of 85% of that claimed on the label may result in failure of the therapy resulting in death, for example, nitroglycerine tablets for angina and cardiac arrest. As a result, it has become a legal requirement to provide data for certain types of stability tests for the regulatory agencies before approval of a new product. Second important point is to protect the reputation of the manufacturer by assuring that the product will retain fitness for use with respect to all functionally relevant attributes for till they are on the market. Other benefits of stability studies at the developmental stage or of the marketed products are to provide a database. These may be of useful in selecting the adequate formulations, excipients and container closure systems for development of a new product, to determine shelf life and storage conditions for development of a new product, preparation of registration dossier, to prove the claimed shelf life for the registration dossier and to verify that no changes have been introduced in the formulation or manufacturing process that can adversely affect the stability of the product[32].

FACTORS INFLUENCING-pH EFFECTS

Stability studies correspond to a set of tests are designed to assess changes in the quality of a given drug over time and under the influence of a number of factors. Among these factors, pH plays an important role, due to the catalytic effect that hydronium and hydroxide ions can play in several reactions. For example, (1) the study on the degradation kinetics of nitazoxanide has been measured over a wide pH range, the major degradation product produced has been identified by LC-MS/MS. Nitazoxanide showed the first-order degradation kinetics in the pH range of 0.01 to 10.0 and showed the greater stability within the pH ranging from1.0 to 4.0. The degradation rate constant calculated for these pH was 0.0885×10^{-2} min^{-1} and 0.0689×10^{-2} min^{-1}, respectively. The highest degradation rate constant value was observed at pH 10.0 (0.7418×10^{-2} min^{-1}) followed by at pH 0.01 (0.5882×10^{-2} min^{-1}). (2) The major degradation product (DP-1) was observed in all conditions tested. Through LC-MS/MS analysis, DP-1 was identified as a product of nitazoxanide deacetylation. The effect of pH on the stability of nitazoxanide and the kinetic data obtained contribute to a better understanding of the intrinsic stability characteristics of nitazoxanide. The *in vivo* tests were time consuming and were difficult to measure directly the drug release amount in the body fluid or target tissue. Many studies were carried out *in vitro* using the fluids that can mimic the body environment. These studies demonstrates that how the release condition such as pH, osmotic pressure and ionic strength can affect polymer degradation and thus, affect the drug release kinetics[33-35]. Among these factors, pH is predominant one, it has been under concentrated investigation. But little knowledge is available for the importance of the pH conditions on elucidating the correlation between degradation and drug release kinetics. On the other hand, the most of degradation studies were performed with strings, sutures, or matrix cylinders. The microparticles were rarely related. Besides, the degradation of block copolymer PLGA-mPEG showed different mechanism as compared with PELA or PLGA, has been rarely investigated. It has been pointed out that morphology and polymer composition could be responsible for the polymer matrix degradation behaviour[36].

The impact of pH triggered polymer degradation on drug release kinetics is helpful for developing new products prepared on the basis of polyester block copolymers for different incubating-condition application. The degradation patterns under acid or basic catalysis, compared with those under pH 7.4 conditions, were investigated from polymer composition profile by measuring degradation products, weight loss, and molecular weight (Mw) change of the polymer matrix and etc. High performance liquid chromatography (HPLC), gel permeation chromatography (GPC), differential scanning calorimetry (DSC), scanning electron microscopy (SEM), and Fourier transform infrared (FTIR) spectrum were applied as analysing tools. The model drug, methotrexate (MTX) is one of the most frequently used antirheumatic drugs in the treatment of rheumatoid arthritis (RA). Methotrexate was employed to evaluate the release kinetics of small molecule drugs.

pH effects on the Polymer Degradation

In degradation studies, the molecular weight (Mw) and dry weight of the microparticles were monitored during 6 weeks incubation under different pH conditions. Degradation products released into the incubation media were detected as further evidence. SEM and FTIR were also used for monitoring morphological changes of microparticles.

- *Change of molecular weight (Mw) and weight loss*

The decrease of molecular weight was followed pseudofirstorder kinetics[41,42] The decrease of polymer molecular weight can be calculated as follows:

$$M_w(t) = M_{w0}e^{-k_{deg}{}^{2}}$$

where $M_w(t)$ is the polymer molecular weight before exposure to the release medium and k_{deg} is the pseudo-first-order degradation rate constant of the polymer. The weight loss (WL) is the percent of microparticles during degradation, this is calculated as:

$$WL(\%) = W(t)/\ W(t{=}0) \times 100$$

where, W(t) is the dry weight of microparticles at time t. From the calculated k_{deg} data, the decrease of Mw was the fastest in acidic condition, but almost same at pH 10.08 and pH 7.4.

On the other hand, the weight loss rate increased with the growth of pH value of the release medium. A pronounced weight loss occurred in the basic medium at the first 2 weeks and then the loss of water-soluble degradation of oligomers continued at a reduced rate. At the end of incubation, only trace of degradation residues remained in contrast to the degradation at pH 1.2 and 7.4. At pH 7.4, the erosion onset was observed at the end of the third week but no more than 10% in total. Whereas, the microparticles hardly lost any weight under acidic condition.

The introduction of mPEG chain caused some local interference in the PLGA crystalline region, and the hydrophilic nature made the end units of polymer very susceptible to water molecule attacks. Consequently, the ester linkage between PLGA and mPEG was more at risk to hydrolysis than that between LA and GA. This can be concluded from the liberation data: In all pH conditions, mPEG was first detected from the liberation media, and the liberation rate was faster than that of LA. In addition, the higher pH led to the faster mPEG fragments liberated into the medium. The release of LA monomer also shows the same pattern as that of mPEG. This provides another evidence for analysing matrix erosion mechanism besides the weight loss data, as the LA is made up of the most part of the polymer. At pH 10.08, LA release is fastest at the beginning and shows an inflection point on the 15th day. At pH 7.4, an onset of LA release is also observed in the third week compared with the onset of weight loss. However, at pH 1.2, there is hardly any LA detected in the releasing medium[37].

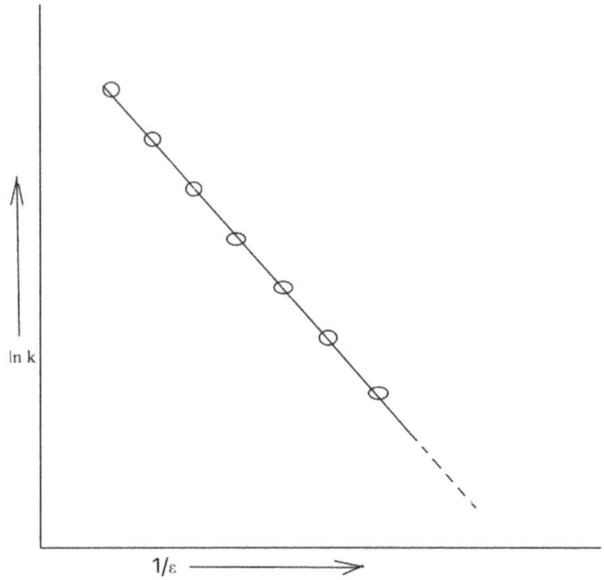

Fig.5.3 Schematic diagram of the plot of ln k vs. 1/ε

FACTORS INFLUENCING-MEDIA EFFECTS

The rate of reaction in the case ionic reaction depends strongly on the nature of the solvent used and ionic strength. The single and double sphere treatment of these reactions can make us studying their detail effect. The application and validity of the influence of solvent and ionic strength on the rate of this type of reaction are:

Effect of Solvent

To study the influence of solvent on the rate of ionic reactions, and the rate equation can be derived using double sphere model, i.e,

$$\text{In } k = \text{In } ko - NZ_AZ_Be^2 / RT4\pi\varepsilon_o\ \varepsilon r \qquad \text{.....(5.1)}$$

where, ε and ε_o are the permitives of the vacuum ($8.854 \times 10^{-12} C^2N^{-1}m^{-1}$) and dielectric constant of the solvent used,

e is the elementary charge having a value of 1.6×10^{-19} C,

k_o is the magnitude of rate constant for the ionic reaction carried out in a solvent of infinite dielectric constant so that the electrostatic interactions become zero,

Z_A and Z_B are the charge numbers of the participating ions,

N and R are the constants, Avogadro's number and gas constant respectively.

Rearranging the above equation we get,

$$\ln k = -(N Z_A Z_B e^2 / RT4\pi\varepsilon_o r.\ 1/\varepsilon) + \ln k_o. \quad ....(5.2)$$

The above equation clearly shows the equation of a straight line, $y = mx + c$ with a negative slope and positive intercept. Thus, the logarithm of the rate constant will vary with the reciprocal of the dielectric constant of the solvent.

It is clear that the equation 2 holds good for a wide range of dielectric constant. However, large deviation is observed with lower values of dielectric constant. From the plot (Fig 5.3) we can derive the value of the slope (m),

$$m = -(NZ_A Z_B e^2/RT\varepsilon_o r) \quad .....(5.3)$$

In the equation 3 the values of every symbol is known, excepting the value of r. Thus, from the equation 3, we can calculate the value of r. The value of r obtained from the equation 3 is quite comparable to other method[38].

By knowing the values of dielectric constant of the solvent, the values of entropy of activation can be known. The entropy of activation is negative and decreases with increase in Z_A and Z_B.

Influence of Ionic Strength

The influence of ionic strength (I) on the rate of tractions can be studied with the help of the following equation.

$$I = \frac{1}{2}\sum_{i=0}^{i=n} m_i z_i^2$$

Where, m_i is the molarity of the ${}_i$th species, z_i is the charge number of the ${}_i$th species,

The value of z for Ca^{2+} and Cl^{-1} in $CaCl_2$ are +2 and -1 respectively. It has been observed that increase in ionic strength increases the rate of reaction, if the charges on the reacting species are of the same sign. On the other hand, the rate of reaction has been found to follow declining trend with increasing ionic strength, if the ions of the reaction are of opposite sign.

To rationalise the effect of ionic strength of the solution on the rate of reaction in case of ionic reactions, let us the imagine

$$A^{Z_A} + B^{Z_B} \longrightarrow X^{Z_A+Z_B} \longrightarrow P$$

The rate equation relating the rate of reaction (R) and activity coefficient is as

$$R = k_o[A][B](Y_A Y_B/Y_X \quad .....(5.5)$$

Where Y_A, Y_B, and Y_X are the activity coefficient for the reactants A, B and activated complex, X, respectively. Bronsted collectively labeled the term, $Y_A Y_B/ Y_X$ as the "kinetic activity factor" and it has been found to be more accurate with experimental data. Now, the equation 5 can be rearranged as follows:

$$R/ [A][B] = k_o(Y_A Y_B/Y_X) \quad ....6$$

Since, the left-hand side of the equation 6 is equals to a second-order rate constant, the equation may bc writtcn as;

$$k = k_o(Y_A Y_{B//} Y_X)$$

Taking logarithm of both the sides, we get

$$\log k = \log ko + \log (Y_A Y_B/ Y_X)$$

or, $$\log k = \log ko + \log Y_A + \log Y_B - \log Y_X$$

The correlation of mean ionic activity coefficient with ionic strength is given by Deye-Huckel theory, that is,

$$\log y_i = - Bz_i^2\sqrt{l}$$

ACCELERATED STABILITY STUDIES

The primary reason for stability testing is the concern for the well-being of the patient suffering from the disease for which the products are designed. Apart from degradation of the unstable product into toxic decomposition products, the loss of activity up to a level of 85% of that claimed on the label may lead to failure of the therapy resulting in death, for example, nitroglycerine tablets for angina and cardiac arrest. As a result, it has become a legal requirement to provide data for certain types of stability tests for the regulatory agencies before the approval of a new product. Second important concern is to protect the reputation of the manufacturer by assuring that the product will retain fitness for use with respect to all functionally relevant attributes for as long as they are on the market. The stability studies are conducted at the developmental stage or of the marketed products[39].

(1) to provide a database that may be of value in selection of adequate formulations, excipients and container closure systems for development of a new product,

(2) to determine shelf life and storage conditions for development of a new product, preparation of registration dossier,

(3) to substantiate the claimed shelf life for the registration dossier and

(4) to verify that no changes have been introduced in the formulation or manufacturing process that can adversely affect the stability of the product.

Real-Time Stability Testing

Real-time stability testing is normally performed for longer duration of the test period to allow significant product degradation under recommended storage conditions. The period of the test depends upon the stability of the product. The testing period is long enough to indicate clearly that no measurable degradation occurs. It must permit one to distinguish degradation from inter-assay variation. During the testing, data is collected at an appropriate frequency such that a trend analysis is able to distinguish instability from day-to-day ambiguity. The reliability of interpretation of data can be increased by including a single batch of reference material for which stability characteristics have already been established. Stability of the reference material also includes the stability of reagents as well as consistency of the performance of the instrument to be used throughout the period of stability testing. However, the system performance and control for drift and discontinuity resulting from changes in both reagents and instrumentation must be monitored[40].

Retained Sample Stability Testing

This is a usual practice for every marketed product for which stability data are required. In this study, stability of samples, for retained storage for at least one batch a year are selected. If the number of batches marketed exceeds 50, stability samples from two batches are recommended to be taken. At the time of first introduction of the product in the market, the stability samples of every batch must be taken, which must not decrease to only not more than 2% to 5% of marketed batches at a later stage. In this study, the stability samples are tested at predetermined intervals, that is, if a product has shelf life of 5 years, it is conventional to test the samples at 3, 6, 9, 12, 18, 24, 36, 48, and 60 months. This conventional method of obtaining stability data on retained storage samples is known as *constant interval method*[41]. Stability testing by evaluation of market samples is a modified method which involves testing the samples already in the marketplace and evaluating stability attributes. This type of testing is inherently more realistic since it challenges the product not just in the idealised retained sample storage conditions, but also in the actual marketplace.

Cyclic Temperature Stress Testing

This is not a routine testing method for marketed products. In this method, cyclic temperature stress tests are designed on knowledge of the product so as to mimic likely conditions in marketplace storage. The period of cycle mostly considered is 24 hours since the diurnal rhythm on earth is 24 hour which the marketed pharmaceuticals are most likely to experience during storage. The minimum and maximum temperatures for the cyclic stress testing is recommended to be selected on a product-by-product basis and considering factors like recommended storage temperatures for the product and specific chemical and physical degradation properties of the products. It is also recommended that the test should normally have 20 cycles[41].

Stability Testing Methods

Stability testing is a routine procedure performed on drug substances and drug products and is used at various stages of the product development. In early stages, accelerated stability testing (at relatively high temperatures and/or humidity) is used to determine the type of degradation products which may be found after long-term storage. Testing under less rigorous conditions i.e. those recommended for long-term shelf storage, at slightly elevated temperatures is used to determine a product's shelf life and expiration dates. Thus, the aim of pharmaceutical stability testing is to provide reasonable assurance that the products will remain at an acceptable level of fitness/quality during they are in market place and available for supply to the patients and will be fit for their consumption until the patient uses the last unit of the product[42]. Depending upon the aim and steps followed, stability testing procedures have been categorised into the following four types.

Accelerated Stability Testing

In accelerated stability testing, a product is stressed at several high (warmer than ambient) temperatures. The amount of heat input required to cause failure of the product is determined. This is done on the product to a condition that accelerates degradation. This information is then used to predict the shelf life of the product or used to compare the relative stability of alternative formulations. This provides an early indication of shelf life of the product and thus, shorten the development schedule. The stress conditions applied during accelerated stability testing are temperature, moisture, light, agitation, gravity, pH and package. In accelerated stability testing the samples are put into a refrigerator, after stressing, assayed simultaneously. Since, the duration of the analysis is short, the possibility of instability in the measurement system is reduced in comparison to the real-time stability testing. Moreover, in accelerated stability testing, comparison of the unstressed product with stressed material is made within the same assay and the stressed sample recovery is expressed as percent of unstressed sample recovery. For statistical reasons, the treatment in accelerated stability projections is recommended to be conducted at four different stress temperatures. For thermolabile and proteinaceous components, relatively accurate stability projections are obtained when denaturing stress temperatures are avoided.

The concept of accelerated stability testing is based upon the Arrhenius equation (1) and modified Arrhenius equation:

$$\ln K = \ln A + \Delta E/RT \quad .....(5.1)$$

Where, K = degradation rate/s,

A = frequency factor/s,

ΔE = activation energy (kJ/mol),

R = universal gas constant (0.00831 kJ/mol), and

T = absolute temperature (K)

The equation describes the relationship between storage temperatures and degradation rate. Using Arrhenius equation, projection of stability from the degradation rates observed at high temperatures for some degradation processes can be determined. If the activation energy is known, the rate of degradation at low temperatures may be projected from those observed at "stress" temperatures[42] The stress tests used in the current International Conference on Harmonization (ICH) guideline (40% for products to be stored at controlled room temperature) were developed from a model that assumes energy of activation of about 83 kJ per mole.

A common practice of manufacturers in pharmaceutical industries was to utilise various shortcuts such as Q rule and bracket tables for prediction of shelf life of the products but these methods are not official either in ICH or FDA. The Q rule states that a product degrades at a rate that decreases by a constant factor Q10 when the storage temperature is decreased by 10°C. Typically, the value of Q10 is set at 2, 3 or 4 because these correspond to reasonable activation energies. This model falsely assumes that the value of Q does not vary with temperature. The bracket table technique assumes that, for a given analyte, the activation energy is between two limits (between 10 and 20 kcal). As a result, a table may be constructed showing days of stress at various stress temperatures. The use of a 10 to 20 kcal bracket table is reasonable because broad experience indicates that most analytes and reagents of interest in pharmaceutical and clinical laboratories have activation energies in this range.

Guidelines for Stability Testing

To assure that optimally stable molecules and products are manufactured, distributed and given to the patients, the regulatory authorities in several countries have made provisions in the drug regulations for the submission of stability data by the manufacturers. The basic purpose was to bring in uniformity in testing from manufacturer to manufacturer. These guidelines provide basic issues related to stability, the stability data requirements for application dossier and the steps for their execution. Such guidelines have been initially issued in 1980s. These were later harmonised (made uniform) in the International Conference on Harmonization (ICH) to overcome the bottleneck to market and register the products in other countries. The ICH was a consortium formed with inputs from both regulatory and industry from European commission, Japan and USA. The World Health Organisation (WHO), in 1996, modified the guidelines because the ICH guidelines did not address the extreme climatic conditions found in many countries and it only covered new drug substances and products and not the already established products that were in circulation in the WHO umbrella countries. In June 1997, US FDA also issued a guidance document entitled 'Expiration dating of solid oral dosage form containing Iron. WHO, in 2004, also released guidelines for stability studies in global environment[39]. ICH guidelines were also extended later for veterinary products. A technical monograph on stability testing of drug substances and products existing in India has also been released by Indian Drug Manufacturers Association. Different test condition and requirements have been given in the guidance documents for active pharmaceutical ingredients, drug products or formulations and excipients. ICH Code Guideline title Q1A Stability testing of New Drug Substances and Products (Second Revision)

Q1B Stability testing indicates the photostability testing of New Drug Substances and Products, Q1C Stability testing of New Dosage Forms, Q1D Bracketing and Martyring Designs for stability testing of Drug Substances and Products Q1E Evaluation of stability data Q1F Stability data package for Registration Applications in Climatic Zones III and IV Q5C Stability testing of Biotechnological/Biological Products. Series of guidelines related to stability testing have also been issued by the Committee for Proprietary Medicinal Products (CPMP) under the European Agency for the Evaluation of Medicinal Products (EMEA) to assist those seeking marketing authorisation for medicinal products in European Union.

Climatic Zones for Stability Testing

For the purpose of stability testing, the whole world has been divided into four zones (I - IV) depending upon the environmental conditions the pharmaceutical products are likely to be subjected to during their storage. These conditions have been derived on the basis of the mean annual temperature and relative humidity data in these regions. On basis of this data, long-term or real-time stability testing conditions and accelerated stability testing conditions have been derived. The standard climatic zones for use in pharmaceutical product stability studies have been presented. The break-up of the environmental conditions in each zone and also the derived long-term stability test storage conditions, as given by WHO have also been presented. The stability conditions have also been harmonised and adjusted to make them more practical for industry application and rugged for generalised application[43].

Protocol for Stability Testing

The protocol for stability testing is a pre-requisite for starting stability testing and is a written document that describes the key components of a regulated and well-controlled stability study. Because the testing condition is based on inherent stability of the compound, the type of dosage form and the proposed container-closure system, the protocol depends on the type of drug substance or the product. Moreover, the protocol can depend on whether the drug is new or is already in the market[41]. The protocol should also reflect the regions where the product is proposed to be marketed, for example, if the product is planned to be used in climatic zones I - III, IVa and IVb, the stability program must include all these zones. A well-designed stability protocol should contain the following information.

Batches

Stability studies at developmental stages are generally carried out on a single batch. The studies pre-decided for registration of new product or unstable established product are done on first three production batches. For stable and well-established batches, even two are allowed. If the initial data is not on a full-scale production batch, first three batches of drug product manufactured, the post-approval should be placed on long-term studies using the same protocol as in approved drug application. Data on laboratory scale batches obtained during development of pharmaceutical products are not accepted as primary stability data but constitute supportive information. In general, the selection of batches should constitute a random sample from the population of pilot or production batches.

Containers and Closures

The testing is done on the product in immediate containers and closures proposed for marketing. The packaging materials include aluminium strip packs, blister packs, Alu-Alu packs, HDPE bottles etc. This may also include secondary packs, but not shippers. Products in all different types of containers/closures, whether meant for distribution or for physician and promotional samples, are to be tested separately. However, for bulk containers, testing in prototype containers is allowed, if it simulates the actual packaging[44].

Orientation of Storage of Containers

Samples of the solutions, dispersed systems and semi solid drug products for stability studies must be kept upright and positioned either inverted or on the side allows full interaction of the product with the container-closure. This orientation helps to determine whether the contact between the drug product or solvent and the closure results in the extraction of chemical substances from the closure components or adsorption of product components into the container-closure.

Sampling Time Points

Frequency of testing should be such that it is sufficient to establish the stability profile of the new drug substance. For products with a proposed shelf life of at least 12 months, the testing frequency at the long-term storage condition should be every 3 months over the first year, every 6 months over the second year and annually thereafter throughout the proposed shelf-life expiration date. In case of accelerated storage conditions, a minimum of three time points, including the initial and end points, for example, 0, 3, and 6 months is recommended. When testing at the intermediate storage condition is necessary as a result of significant change during accelerated storage condition, a minimum of four test points, including the initial and final time points, is recommended, for example, 0, 6, 9 and 12 months.

In case the same product of different strengths, multiple sizes, etc is required to be tested, reduced stability testing plans can be worked out, which involves a smaller number of test points. The reduced testing plans are based on bracketing and matrixing the statistical designs. Bracketing is the design of a stability schedule such that only samples on the extremes of certain design factors, for example, strength, package size, are tested at all time points as in a full design. On the other hand, matrixing involves testing of a subset of the total number of possible samples for all combinations at a specific time point. Subsequently, another subset of samples for all factor combinations is tested. The factors that can be matrixed include batches, strengths with identical formulation, container sizes, fill sizes, and intermediate time points[45].

Sampling Plan

Sampling plan for stability testing involves, planning for the number of samples to be charged to the stability chambers and sampling out of the charged batch so as to cover the entire study. The first step should be the development of the sampling time points. Then the number of samples required, are drawn at each pull point for complete evaluation of all test parameters and finally adding up to get the total number of samples. For example, there would be a requirement of about 100 tablets per pull out in a long term or accelerated stability studies including 10 tabs each for assay, hardness and moisture determination, 6 tabs each for dissolution and disintegration and 50 tabs for friability. This is multiplied by the total number of pull outs will give the total number of tablets required for a study. This is followed by the development of a sampling plan, which includes the selection of the containers representing the batch as a whole but in an unbiased manner. A stratification plan has been suggested whereby from a random starting point every nth container is taken from the filling or packaging line (n is chosen such that the sample is spread over the whole batch).

Test Parameters

The stability test protocol should define the test parameters that would be used for evaluation of the stability samples. The tests that monitor the quality, purity, potency, and identity which could be expected to change upon storage are chosen as stability tests. Therefore appearance, assay, degradation products, microbiological testing, dissolution, and moisture are standard tests performed on stability test samples. Microbiological tests include sterility, preservative efficacy and microbial count as applicable, for example, for liquid injectable preparations. The batches used for stability study must meet all the testing requirements including heavy metals, residue on ignition, residual solvents etc. Some of these are required at the time of product release but not required to be repeated during stability testing. Other tests like enantiomeric purity, particle size and polymorphic form etc have also been discussed in ICH guidance Q6A.

Test Methodology

It is always recommended to follow the procedures given in the official compendia, as the results obtained using the official tests, in general find better acceptance. If alternate methods are used, they are required to be duly validated. The assay of the drug should be carried out using a stability-indicating method, established by carrying out stress tests on the drug under forced decomposition conditions. This method should be validated for specificity, accuracy, precision and linearity, in the range to which the drug is expected to fall during stability studies. For the assay of degradation products, the validated method should also include the limits of detection/quantification. The methods reported in literature should be used after confirming reproducibility and carrying out minimal validation, say of linearity, range, etc. It is always recommended to prepare a standard test protocol (STP) for each test.

Acceptance Criteria

The acceptance criteria for the analytical results and for the presence of degradation products should also be fixed beforehand. The acceptance criteria for each test in the stability study is fixed in the form of numerical limits for the results expressed in quantitative terms, for example, moisture pick-up, viscosity, particle size, assay, degradation products, etc. and pass or fail for qualitative tests, for example, odour, colour, appearance, cracking, microbial growth, etc. These acceptance criteria should also include individual and total upper limits for degradation products. ICH guideline Q3B(R2) related to impurities in new drug products addresses degradation products in new drug formulations. The degradation products of the active or interaction products from the active ingredients and excipients and/or active and container component should be reported, identified, and/or qualified when the proposed thresholds are exceeded. The reporting threshold of impurities is based upon the intended dose. If the maximum daily dose is less than or equal to 1gm, the limit is 0.1% and if greater than 1, the limit is 0.05%. The identification threshold of impurities is between 1.0 - 0.1% for the maximum daily dose ranging between 1mg and 2gm[46].

Conduct of Stability Studies

The stability study is conducted by keeping the drug substance or the product in their proposed final packs (e.g. Aluminium strip, blister pack, HDPE container etc.), or prototype containers in the case of bulk drugs, in sufficient numbers in the stability chambers set at appropriate storage conditions as per the protocol. The samples are then withdrawn, as per the stability protocol, at the prescribed sampling intervals and are then analyzed by a suitable method. The sampling should preferably be from unopened container. The samples are placed for testing, they have been prepared and analysed without delay after they have been withdrawn. Delay in placing the samples and analysis of withdrawn samples is known to affect the results. If there is an unavoidable delay, then the samples are frozen until they are subjected to analysis. To minimize the effect of day-to-day variability on the results, the following two approaches are followed. Samples are drawn in replicate. One of the samples is tested and others are kept at temperatures sufficiently low to prevent further drug loss and then all the samples are subjected to analysis on the same day at the end of study (after withdrawal of the last sample). Second approach is to freeze the initial samples till the expiration period and test them at appropriate times by using them as internal standards in the assays.

Presentation and Recording of Stability Data

Stability data is recorded in an organised, comprehensive and cumulative format. The stability data table is the means for reporting the results of the stability study in a concise format for ease of review and interpretation. The data is recorded in a proper tabular format and encompassing information on a batch is recorded at one place. Similar sheets are prepared for each batch. When it is not possible to collect a sample exactly at the designed time (3, 6, 9, 12 months, etc.), the sample may be withdrawn conveniently, and the actual time of collection should be indicated in the format sheet. The data can be grouped by storage condition and time interval to present the stability as a function of time for each environmental condition studied. Data can be presented in multiple tables taking care, so that it can be easily interpretable. In addition, a graphical presentation of stability data versus time for the test data can be used to illustrate the trends in data and may be helpful for data evaluation. A graphical presentation of the data cannot replace the tabular presentation for a regulatory filing. The results of the statistical analysis, wherever appropriate and analysis of impurities should also be discussed. Details on the above are available in ICH Q3A and Q3B.

Mean Kinetic Temperature

The Mean kinetic temperature is the single calculated temperature at which the total amount of degradation over a particular period is equal to the sum of the individual degradations that would occur at various cycles of higher and lower temperature. It is an isothermal storage temperature that simulates the non-isothermal effects of storage temperature variation. The MKT takes into account seasonal and daily temperature variations during a year. The assurance that the actual storage conditions will not affect adversely the stability and shelf life of the product. This is based upon the fact that the degradation rate constants are temperature dependent. A controlled room temperature maintained thermostatically to the usual working environment of 20°C to 25°C results in a mean kinetic temperature calculated to be not more than 25°C. This concept is applied to pharmacies, hospitals, distribution and storage areas and vehicles and warehouses. Articles may be labeled for storage at "controlled room temperature" or at "up to 25°C", or any other relevant word/phrase based on the same mean kinetic temperature, (USP 1995). The distribution of the countries and regions of the world into four different climatic zones has been on the basis of the mean kinetic temperature. Mean kinetic temperature is calculated by two methods i.e. USP method and FDA method. In the USP method, MKT is calculated from the average storage temperatures recorded over a 1-year period and the running average calculated from the average of weekly high and low temperatures recorded over the preceding 52 weeks. This results in entering 52 data points and calculation is done by Hayne's equation, which is derived from Arrhenius equation and relates degradation rate constants at different temperatures to the activation energy.

The FDA recommends the method of entering both the individual highest and the lowest temperatures (rather than averages) in the equation for the calculation of MKT. This results in entering 104 data points, in contrast to USP's 52 points. If temperatures are electronically recorded at many times during a day and all the values are used in the calculation of MKT, then there is no difference between the USP and FDA method.

Expiration Date/ Shelf Life

An expiration date is defined as the time up to which the product will remain stable when stored under recommended storage conditions. Thus, an expiration date is the date beyond which it is predicted that the product may no longer retain fitness for use. If the product is not stored in accordance with the manufacturer's instructions, then the product may be expected to degrade more rapidly. Shelf life is the time during which the product, if stored appropriately as per the manufacturer's instructions, will retain fitness for use (>90% of label claim of potency). The expiration date is also defined as the date placed on the container/labels of a drug product designating the time during which a batch of the product is expected to remain within the approved shelf-life specifications, if stored under defined conditions and after which it should not be used.

Estimation of Shelf Life

The shelf life is determined from the data obtained from the long-term storage studies. The data is first linearised and test for goodness of fit is applied. The linearised data is then analyzed to see that the slope and the intercepts are matching. The data is pooled accordingly and used for estimation of the common slope.

For determination of significance of difference in case of slope or intercept, statistical tests like t-test should be applied. The data is available in the form of only five data points (0, 3, 6, 9 and 12 months), either pooled from the three batches or from the three individual batches if they are not fit for pooling. In case data is not fit for pooling, stability estimates are to be made on the worst batch. The shelf life/expiry date is determined from the regression line of this five-point data based on calculation of 95% one-sided confidence limit. For reading the expiry date, 90% drug concentration is considered as the lowest specification limit and the point where the extension line cuts the 95% confidence limit line is taken as an expiry date. The shelf life derived from the intersection of the 90% confidence bound and 90% potency value has a 95% confidence level, therefore there is only a 5% chance that our estimate of the shelf life will be too high. For new drugs, it is a general practice to grant only two-year expiry initially, which is based on satisfactory one year long-term and 6 months accelerated stability data. The expiry date for third and later years is allowed only on production of real-time data for the subsequent years. Most pharmaceutical products are characterized by only one shelf life. However, in some cases a product may have two, for example, a freeze-dried (lyophilised) protein product may have only 1 shelf life, say 2 years, for the product stored in the dry condition and a 2nd shelf life, say 2 days, for the product when it has been reconstituted with the appropriate vehicle and is ready for injection[47].

Photostability Testing

USA FDA in 1996 issued ICH guidelines for industry and stated that "the intrinsic photostability characteristics of new drug substances and products should be evaluated to demonstrate that, as appropriate, light exposure does not result in unacceptable change". In this photostability testing is recommended to be carried out on a single batch of material, these studies should be repeated if certain variations and changes are made to the product (e.g., formulation, packaging). While D65 is the internationally recognized standard for outdoor daylight as defined in ISO 10977 (1993), ID65 is the equivalent indoor indirect daylight standard. After this, testing of drugs in photostability chamber is increasingly followed as a standard procedure, especially for the products intended to be marketed in Asian countries.

Stability Test Equipment

The equipment used for stability testing is called stability chamber. These are specialised environmental chambers that can simulate the storage condition and enable evaluation of product stability based on real-time, accelerated and long-term protocols. Smaller chambers are preferred for accelerated testing, as the retention time of products is much less in these cabinets, while the walk-in chambers are preferred for long-term testing. Such chambers or rooms are engineered and qualified to ensure uniform exposure of the set conditions to all the samples in the chamber. These chambers are expected to be dependable and rugged because of the requirement of uninterrupted use for years. They are fitted with appropriate recording, safety and alarm devices. In addition, photostability chambers are also available and utilized both with and without temperature and humidity control. Two types of light sources are usually employed in photostability chambers, one is the combination of cool white and near UV fluorescent tubes, while second are the artificial daylight lamps, for example, xenon or metal halide. It is obtained a total exposure of 1.2 millions lux hours. The visible light intensity is estimated using a lux meter. The calculation is made on how many hours of exposure is needed.

Out-of-Trend Results

According to the ICH Q1A and WHO guidance results are considered out-of-trend (OOT) if the assay data is 5% different from the initial data for the previous batch, because the results are significantly different. If OOT results are generated, a formal mechanism for investigating these results is rigorously followed, as defined by Barr decision. This procedure must have the ability to evaluate the data collection procedures and, in the case of an error, identify the root cause of the error, which might have caused the difference in results. The possible reasons for the same could be a) storage of different batches of products at different locations within the chamber, b) the batches are manufactured at different times and are charged to the chamber at whatever place available. It has been reported that despite that the temperature and humidity having been same at all the points within a chamber, the air velocity still varied at different locations, and this resulted in differential moisture pick up by a hygroscopic drug. Hence it has been advised that stability testing chambers should be designed in a manner that air velocity also remains constant to the best possible within the test chambers[48].

Current Trends in Stability Testing

Current trend, especially amongst the multinational pharmaceutical companies, is to define conditions for stability testing for global marketing. For this the companies are orienting their protocols to single set of conditions that covers extreme environmental conditions. The specific changes for global testing include increase in duration of accelerated testing period from 6 to 12 months and conduct of additional tests at 50°C/ 75% RH for 3 months. The concept behind this change is to avoid repetition of stability testing for other regions and efficient and optimum use of resources as all tests are done in one laboratory. Moreover, testing under combination of three environmental factors, viz., temperature, humidity and light, has been reported to result in stronger deleterious effect on drug substances and products, than under temperature and humidity conditions only.

INTERPRETATION OF KINETIC DATA (API & TABLETS)

The design and execution of formal stability studies should follow the principles outlined in the parent guideline. The purpose of a stability study is to establish, based on testing a minimum of three batches of the drug substance or product, a retest period or shelf life and label storage instructions applicable to all future batches manufactured and packaged under similar circumstances. The degree of variability of individual batches affects the confidence that a future production batch will remain within acceptance criteria throughout its retest period or shelf life. Although normal manufacturing and analytical variations are to be expected, it is important that the drug product be formulated with the intent to provide 100 percent of the labeled amount of the drug substance at the time of batch release. If the assay values of the batches used to support the registration application are higher than 100 percent of label claim at the time of batch release, after taking into account manufacturing and analytical variations, the shelf life proposed in the application can be overestimated. On the other hand, if the assay value of a batch is lower than 100% of label claim at the time of batch release, it might fall below the lower acceptance criterion before the end of the proposed shelf life. A systematic approach should be adopted in the presentation and evaluation of the stability information. The stability information includes the results from the physical, chemical, biological, and microbiological tests, including those related to particular attributes of the dosage form (for example, dissolution rate for solid oral dosage forms). The adequacy of the mass balance should be assessed. Factors that can cause an apparent lack of mass balance should be considered, including, for example, the mechanisms of degradation and the stability-indicating capability and inherent variability of the analytical procedures. The basic concepts of evaluation of stability data are the same for single- versus multi-factor studies and for full- versus reduced-design studies. Data from formal stability studies and, as appropriate, supporting data should be evaluated to determine the critical quality attributes likely to influence the quality and performance of the drug substance or product. Each attribute should be assessed separately, and an overall assessment should be made of the findings for the purpose of proposing a retest period or shelf life. The retest period or shelf life proposed should not exceed for any single attribute. The decision tree in Appendix A outlines a stepwise approach to stability data evaluation and much extrapolation can be considered for a proposed retest period or shelf life. Appendix B provides-

(1) information on how to analyse long-term data for appropriate quantitative test attributes from a study with a multi-factor, full or reduced design,
(2) information on how to use regression analysis for retest period or shelf life estimation, and
(3) examples of statistical procedures to determine poolability of data from different batches or other factors.

Additional guidance can be found in the references listed; the examples and references do not cover all applicable statistical approaches. Generally, certain quantitative chemical attributes (assay, degradation products, preservative content) for a drug substance or product can be assumed to follow zero-order kinetics during long-term storage. Data for these attributes are therefore amenable to the type of statistical analysis described in Appendix B, including linear regression and poolability testing. Although the kinetics of other quantitative attributes (pH, dissolution) is generally not known, the same statistical analysis can be applied, if appropriate. Qualitative attributes and microbiological attributes are not amenable to this kind of statistical analysis. The recommendations on statistical approaches in this guideline are not intended to imply that use of statistical evaluation is preferred when it can be justified to be unnecessary. The statistical analysis can be useful in supporting the extrapolation of retest periods or shelf lives in certain situations and can be called for to verify the proposed retest periods or shelf lives in other cases.

Data Presentation

Data for all attributes should be presented in an appropriate format (tabular, graphical, narrative) and an evaluation of such data should be included in the application. The values of quantitative attributes at all time points should be reported as measured (assay as percent of label claim). If a statistical analysis is performed, the procedure used and the assumptions underlying the model should be stated and justified. A tabulated summary of the outcome of statistical analysis and/or graphical presentation of the long-term data should be included.

Extrapolation

Extrapolation is the practice of using a known data set to infer information about future data. Extrapolation to extend the retest period or shelf life beyond the period covered by long-term data can be proposed in the application, particularly if no significant change is observed at the accelerated condition. Whether extrapolation of stability data is appropriate or not, this depends on the extent of knowledge about the change pattern, the goodness of fit of any mathematical model, and the existence of relevant supporting data. Any extrapolation should be done in such a way that the extended retest period or shelf life would be valid for a future batch released with test results close to the release acceptance criteria. An extrapolation of stability data assumes that the same change pattern will continue to apply beyond the period covered by long-term data. The correctness of the assumed change pattern is critical when extrapolation is considered. When estimating a regression line or curve to fit the long-term data, the data themselves provide a check on the correctness of the assumed change pattern, and statistical methods can be applied to test the goodness of fit of the data to the assumed line or curve. No such internal check is possible beyond the period covered by long-term data. Thus, a retest period or shelf life granted on the basis of extrapolation should always be verified by additional long-term stability data as soon as these data become available. Sufficient care must be taken to include in the protocol for commitment batches a time point that corresponds to the end of the extrapolated retest period or shelf life[49].

Data Evaluation for Retest Period or Shelf-Life Estimation for Drug Substances or Products Intended for Room Temperature Storage

A systematic evaluation of the data from formal stability studies should be performed. Stability data for each attribute should be assessed sequentially. For drug substances or products intended for storage at room temperature, the assessment should start with any significant change at the accelerated condition and, if appropriate, at the intermediate condition, and progress through the trends and variability of the long-term data. The circumstances are delineated under which extrapolation of retest period or shelf life beyond the period covered by long-term data can be appropriate. A decision tree is provided in Appendix A as an aid.

No significant change at Accelerated Condition

Where no significant change occurs at the accelerated condition, the retest period or shelf life would depend on the nature of the long-term and accelerated data.

Long-term and accelerated data showing little or no change over time and little or no variability

Where the long-term data and accelerated data for an attribute show little or no change over time and little or no variability, it might be apparent that the drug substance or product will remain well within the acceptance criteria for that attribute during the proposed retest period or shelf life. In these circumstances, a statistical analysis is normally considered unnecessary. Justification for the omission should be provided. Justification can include a discussion of the change pattern or lack of change, relevance of the accelerated data, mass balance, and/or other supporting data as described in the parent guideline. Extrapolation of the retest period or shelf life beyond the period covered by long-term data can be proposed. The proposed retest period or shelf life can be up to twice, but should not be more than 12 months beyond, the period covered by long-term data.

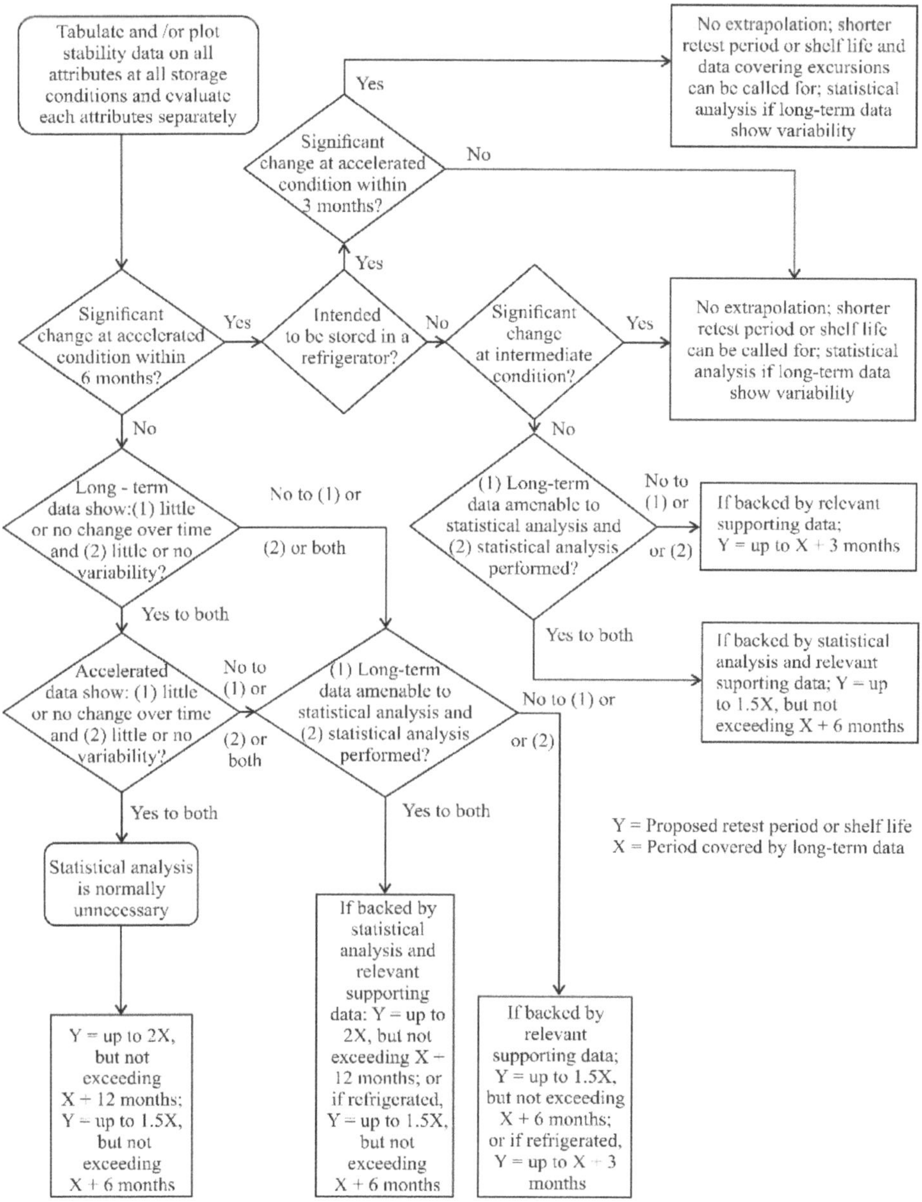
Tabulate and /or plot stability data on all attributes at all storage conditions and evaluate each attributes separately
Significant change at accelerated condition within 6 months?
Yes
Intended to be stored in a refrigerator?
Yes
Significant change at accelerated condition within 3 months?
Yes
No extrapolation; shorter retest period or shelf life and data covering excursions can be called for; statistical analysis if long-term data show variability
No
No
Significant change at intermediate condition?
Yes
No extrapolation; shorter retest period or shelf life can be called for; statistical analysis if long-term data show variability
No
(1) Long-term data amenable to statistical analysis and (2) statistical analysis performed?
No to (1) or (2)
If backed by relevant supporting data; Y = up to X + 3 months
Yes to both
If backed by statistical analysis and relevant suporting data; Y = up to 1.5X, but not exceeding X + 6 months
No
Long - term data show:(1) little or no change over time and (2) little or no variability?
No to (1) or (2) or both
Yes to both
Accelerated data show: (1) little or no change over time and (2) little or no variability?
No to (1) or (2) or both
(1) Long-term data amenable to statistical analysis and (2) statistical analysis performed?
No to (1) or or (2)
Yes to both
Yes to both
Statistical analysis is normally unnecessary
Y = up to 2X, but not exceeding X + 12 months; Y = up to 1.5X, but not exceeding X + 6 months
If backed by statistical analysis and relevant supporting data: Y = up to 2X, but not exceeding X + 12 months; or if refrigerated, Y = up to 1.5X, but not exceeding X + 6 months
If backed by relevant supporting data; Y = up to 1.5X, but not exceeding X + 6 months; or if refrigerated, Y = up to X + 3 months
Y = Proposed retest period or shelf life
X = Period covered by long-term data

Long-term or accelerated data showing change over time and/or variability

If the long-term or accelerated data for an attribute show change over time and/or variability within a factor or among factors, statistical analysis of the long-term data can be useful in establishing a retest period or shelf life. Where there are differences in stability observed among batches or among other factors (strength, container size and/or fill) or factor combinations (strength-by-container size and/or fill) that preclude the combining of data, the proposed retest period or shelf life should not exceed the shortest period supported by any batch, other factor, or factor combination. Alternatively, where the differences are readily attributed to a particular factor (strength), different shelf lives can be assigned to different levels within the factor (different strengths). A discussion should be provided to address the cause for the differences and the overall significance of such differences on the product. Extrapolation beyond the period covered by long-term data can be proposed; however, the extent of extrapolation would depend on whether long-term data for the attribute are amenable to statistical analysis.

Significant change at Accelerated Condition

Where significant change occurs at the accelerated condition, the retest period or shelf life would depend on the outcome of stability testing at the intermediate condition, as well as at the long-term condition.

**Note:* The following physical changes can be expected to occur at the accelerated condition and would not be considered significant change that calls for intermediate testing if there is no other significant change: softening of a suppository that is designed to melt at 37°C, if the melting point is clearly demonstrated, failure to meet acceptance criteria for dissolution for 12 units of a gelatine capsule or gel coated tablet if the failure can be unequivocally attributed to cross-linking. However, if phase separation of a semi-solid dosage form occurs at the accelerated condition, testing at the intermediate condition should be performed. Potential interaction effects should also be considered in establishing that there is no other significant change[50].

No significant change at Intermediate Condition

If there is no significant change at the intermediate condition, extrapolation beyond the period covered by long-term data can be proposed; however, the extent of extrapolation would depend on whether long-term data for the attribute are amenable to statistical analysis.

- Data not amenable to statistical analysis

  When the long-term data for an attribute are not amenable to statistical analysis, the proposed retest period or shelf life can be up to 3 months beyond the period covered by long-term data, if backed by relevant supporting data.

- Data amenable to statistical analysis

  When the long-term data for an attribute are amenable to statistical analysis but no analysis is performed, the extent of extrapolation should be the same as when data are not amenable to statistical analysis. However, if a statistical analysis is performed, the proposed retest period or shelf life can be up to one-and-half times, but should not be more than 6 months beyond, the period covered by long-term data, when backed by statistical analysis and relevant supporting data.

Significant change at Intermediate Condition

Where significant change occurs at the intermediate condition, the proposed retest period or shelf life should not exceed the period covered by long-term data. In addition, a retest period or shelf life shorter than the period covered by long-term data could be called for.

Data Evaluation for Retest Period or Shelf-Life Estimation for Drug Substances or Products Intended for Storage Below Room Temperature

Drug substances or products intended for storage in a refrigerator

Data from drug substances or products intended to be stored in a refrigerator should be assessed according to the same principles for drug substances or products intended for room temperature storage, except where explicitly noted in the section below. The decision tree can be used as an aid.

No significant change at Accelerated Condition

Where no significant change occurs at the accelerated condition, extrapolation of retest period or shelf life beyond the period covered by long-term data can be proposed based on the principles outlined, except that the extent of extrapolation should be more limited. If the long-term and accelerated data show little change over time and little variability, the proposed retest period or shelf life can be up to one-and-a-half times, but should not be more than 6 months beyond, the period covered by long-term data normally without the support of statistical analysis. Where the long-term or accelerated data show change over time and/or variability, the proposed retest period or shelf life can be up to 3 months beyond the period covered by longterm data if (1) the long-term data are amenable to statistical analysis but a statistical analysis is not performed, or (2) the long-term data are not amenable to statistical analysis but relevant supporting data are provided. Where the long-term or accelerated data show change over time and/or variability, the proposed retest period or shelf life can be up to one-and-a-half times, but should not be more than 6 months beyond, the period covered by long-term data if (1) the long-term data are amenable to statistical analysis and a statistical analysis is performed, and (2) the proposal is backed by the result of the analysis and relevant supporting data.

Significant change at Accelerated Condition

If significant change occurs between 3 and 6 months 'testing at the accelerated storage condition, the proposed retest period or shelf life should be based on the long-term data. Moreover, a retest period or shelf life shorter than the period covered by long-term data could be called for. If the long-term data show variability, verification of the proposed retest period or shelf life by statistical analysis can be appropriate. If significant change occurs within the first 3 months 'testing at the accelerated storage condition, the proposed retest period or shelf life should be based on long-term data. Extrapolation is not considered appropriate. A retest period or shelf life shorter than the period covered by long-term data could be called for. If the long-term data show variability, verification of the proposed retest period or shelf life by statistical analysis can be appropriate. Moreover, a discussion should be provided to address the effect of short-term excursions outside the label storage condition (during shipping or handling). This discussion can be supported, if appropriate, by further testing on a single batch of the drug substance or product at the accelerated condition for a period shorter than 3 months.

Drug substances or Products Intended for Storage in a Freezer

For drug substances or products intended for storage in a freezer, the retest period or shelf life should be based on long-term data. In the absence of an accelerated storage condition for drug substances or products intended to be stored in a freezer, testing on a single batch at an elevated temperature (5°C ±3°C or 25°C ±2°C) for an appropriate time period should be conducted to address the effect of short-term excursions outside the proposed label storage condition (during shipping or handling).

SOLID STATE STABILITY

The breakdown of drugs in the solid state is an important topic, but it has not been studied extensively in pharmacy. The subject has been reviewed by Garrett, Lachman, and Carstensen, and is discussed here briefly.

Pure Solids

The decomposition of pure solids, as contrasted with the more complex mixture of ingredients in a dosage form, has been studied. A number of theories have been proposed to explain the shapes of the curves obtained when decomposition of the compound is plotted against time. Carstensen and Musa described the decomposition of solid benzoic acid derivatives, such as aminobenzoic acid, which broke down into a liquid, aniline, and a gas, carbon dioxide. The plot of concentration of decomposed drug versus time yielded a sigmoidal curve. After liquid begins to form, the decomposition becomes a first-order reaction in the solution. Such single-component pharmaceutical systems can degrade by either zero-order or first-order reaction. It is often difficult to determine which pattern is being followed when the reaction cannot be carried through a sufficient number of half-lives to differentiate between zero and first order.

Solid Dosage Forms

The decomposition of drugs in solid dosage forms is more complex than decay occurring in the pure state of the individual compound. The reactions may be zero or first order, but in some cases, as with pure compounds, it is difficult to distinguish between the two. Tardif observed that ascorbic acid decomposed in tablets by a pseudo–first-order reaction.

In tablets and other solid dosage forms, the possibility exists for solid–solid interaction. Carstensen et al. devised a program to test for possible incompatibilities of the drug with excipients present in the solid mixture. The drug is blended with various excipients in the presence and absence of 5% moisture, sealed in vials, and stored for 2 weeks at 55°C. Visual observation is done and the samples are tested for chemical interaction by thin-layer chromatography. The method is qualitative but, in industrial preformulation, provides a useful screening technique for uncovering possible incompatibilities between active ingredient and pharmaceutical additives before deciding on a suitable dosage form. Lach and associates used diffuse reflectance spectroscopy to measure interactions of additives and drugs in solid dosage forms. Blaug and Huang used this spectroscopic technique to study the interaction of spray-dried lactose with dextroamphetamine sulfate. Goodhart and associates studied the fading of coloured tablets by light (photolysis reaction) and plotted the results as colour difference at various light-energy values expressed in foot-candle hours. Lachman, Cooper, and their associates conducted a series of studies on the decomposition of FD&C colours in tablets and established a pattern of three separate stages of breakdown. The photolysis was found to be a surface phenomenon, causing fading of the tablet colour to a depth of about 0.03 cm. Interestingly, fading did not occur further into the coating with continued light exposure, and the protected contents of the color-coated tablets were not adversely affected by exposure to light. The quantitative and theoretical approaches to the study of solid-state kinetics are at their frontier, which, when opened, will probably reveal a new and fruitful area of chemistry and drug science. The authors classify solid-state reactions as addition when two solids, A and B, interact to form the new solid, AB. For example, picric acid reacts with naphthols to form what are referred to as picrates. A second kind of solid-state reaction is an exchange process, in which solid A reacts with solid BC to form solid AB and release solid C. Solid–gas reactions constitute another class, of which the oxidation of solid ascorbic acid and solid fumagillin are notable examples. Other types of solid-state processes include polymorphic transitions, sublimation, dehydration, and thermal decomposition. Monk house and Van

Campen reviewed the experimental methods used in solid-state kinetics, including reflectance spectroscopy, x-ray diffraction, thermal analysis, microscopy[51], dilatometry, and gas pressure–volume analysis. Their review closes with sections on handling solid-state reaction data, temperature effects, application of the Arrhenius plot, equilibria expressions involved in solid-state degradation, and use of the van Hoff equation for, say, a solid drug hydrate in equilibrium with its dehydrated form.

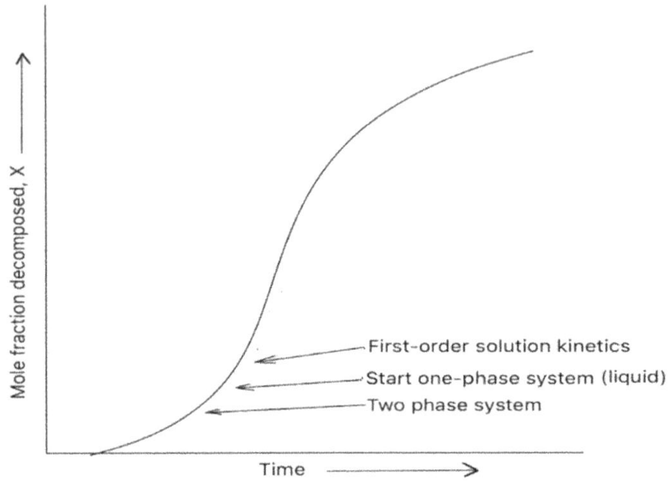

Fig.5.4 Decomposition of a pure crystalline solid such as potassium permanganate, which involves gaseous reaction products.

SELF-LIFE ASSIGNMENT

The continued integrity of products in multi-dose containers after the first opening is an important quality issue. While this principle is acknowledged in various Guidelines, no specific guidance is available on defining test design and conduct of studies to be undertaken to define in-use shelf life in a uniform fashion. Stability of products is the length of time that they retain their properties and functionality while stored or handled as defined by the manufacture's specifications. During their life span, products may change as they age but they are considered to be stable as long as their characteristics remain with the specifications. The change of the performance as products age is called degradation and is usually defined in terms of loss of activity or/and decrease of performance. Stability includes several stages of product life; that is, time and events during transportation of products from manufacturer to the end user, the length of time that products are stored at recommended conditions without being used, time and events while products are being used. The last stage is referred to as in-use stability. The above stages may not be all inclusive and all products may not go through all of them. There are products that are designed for a single use while others are stored in containers that can be used for a period of time after it is opened. The absence of a detailed and authoritative guideline for the human pharmaceutical sector does not assist in the design and conduct of such studies, and when manufacturers design their own studies it is by no means certain that the regulatory agencies will find the data to be completely acceptable. Moreover, there are circumstances when the generation of data from specific in-use simulations may not add significantly to the data already generated from International Conference on Harmonisation of Technical Requirements for Registration of Pharmaceuticals for Human Use (1CH)-compliant stability studies. There are also situations (when small multi-dose containers are involved) where it is difficult to conduct meaningful studies due to the limited quantities of residual product on which to perform chemical or microbiological testing[52].

Modified Approach for the assessment of In-use shelf life for multi dose container after first opening: Selection of batches

A minimum of two batches, at least pilot scale batches, should be subjected to the test. At least one of the batches should be chosen towards the end of its shelf life. If such results are not available, one batch should be tested at the final stage of the submitted stability studies. The batch number, date of manufacture and size of each batch should be stated. The container and closure of the product and, if present, the medicinal device should be equivalent to that proposed for marketing. Study can also be conducted by bracketing the study design on same batch i.e. study should be initiated at beginning and at the end of shelf life of the product.

In use period (Design of study)

As far as possible the period to which the stability study is to be performed should be design in such a way that it will simulate the use of the product in practice taking into consideration the filling volume of the container and any dilution/reconstitution before use. The appropriate physical, chemical and microbial properties of the product susceptible to change during storage should be determined over the period of the proposed in-use shelf life. As per board of pharmacy regulation once dispense the product is given a shelf life of 1 year and if it is approaching its expiry than the number of days reaming for expiration is mentioned. In various guidelines the stability study for 28 days is recommended for bulk packs but the quantity of units in bulk pack may change, and the pack may be used for more than 28 days, so it is also necessary to design the study in such a way that it will simulate the use of product in practise. The following study was carried out to determine the effect of shelf-life period on in use stability of product, vials of the reagent were stored at recommended storage conditions and tested on a haematology analyser in 5 replicates at 34, 48, 62, 77, 90, 105, 120, 133, and 146 days after manufacturing. A new vial is opened at each testing time point. This constitutes real time closed container stability testing of the product. The in-use stability testing was performed at three different time points of product's life, 36, 77, and 120 days after manufacturing. Let us denote with t_c time of closed container stability, to is time of in-use open container stability, and e events (n is the number of instances that the same vial/container is used). Vials were open at these time points and tested 20 times in duplicates for a maximum of 35 days. Number of platelets ×103 cells/ Lt is the measuring parameter in the tests. Estimated degradation patterns of PLT (platelet cells/Lt × 103) closed container and in-use open container at three closed times are shown in Fig. 5.5.

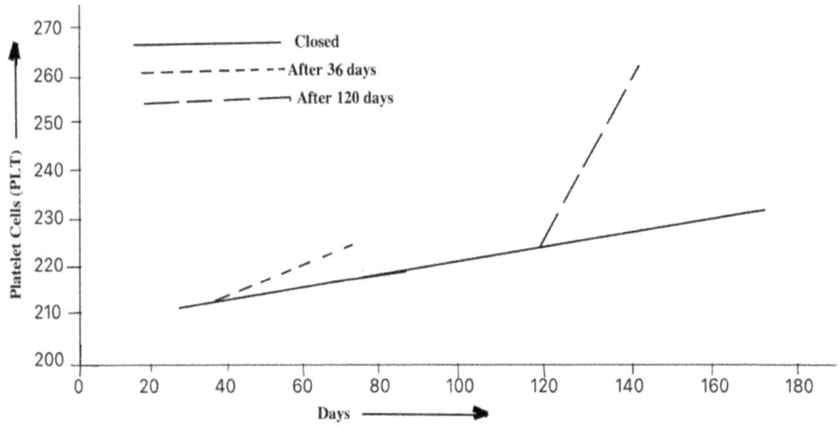

Fig.5.5 Degradation pattern of closed container and in-use open container.

Degradation statistics for in-use open container for the three scenarios, time, events, and both time and events are defining parameter. Drift of in-use stability depends on the age of closed container. Regardless of the way (time, events, time & events) drift is estimated, its magnitude increases as closed container product gets older. Drift of in-use open container for t_{ot} = 35 days and et = 20 events is 15.32 × 103 cells/Lt at t_{ct} = 36 in comparison to 34.56 ×103 cells/Lt at t_{ct} = 77 and 50.81 × 103 cells/Lt at t_{ct} = 120. The 95% confidence intervals of these three drift estimates do not overlap providing additional evidence that they are statistically different from each other. Drift estimate for the time of open container (tot = 35 days) is greater than the drift estimate for the number of events (et = 20 events) when they are considered independently. This indicates that the length of time of open container contributes more to the in-use degradation in comparison to the number of events. Time of open container and events are highly correlated with each other but when considered together multiplicatively the degradation accelerated in comparison to their separate effects. The estimated platelet drift for the multiple effects of time and events is 50.81 × 103 cells/Lt at tot = 120 days. This drift is 8.04 × 103 cells/Lt greater than the drift for the effect of time of open container and 11.99 × 103 cells/Lt greater than the drift of the effect of number of events. In-use degradation drift of open container for 35 days and 20 events is greater that the drift of closed container for 120 days. This evidenced the fact that the majority of degradation occurs during the period that the product is in use. From the following article we can say that the duration to which the container is open for use and the age of container are determining factor for its degradation i.e its stability. So, it is necessary to determine the period to carry out in use stability study for different packs as the period may vary as per the pack size[53].

Number of Counts in each container

If the product is to be supplied in more than one container size or in different strengths, in use stability test should be applied to the product which presents the greatest susceptibility to change. The choice of the tested product should always be justified.

1. ***Selection of pack Size***

   The question remains the same on which pack the study to be carried out. As there are multiple packs with different pack design which makes each pack individual entity. So is it necessary to carry out study on each pack or to use bracketing. There is no such guideline which sheds light on pack size selection and also each product may act differently as compared to other. In this case we can use bracketing for various pack size available, it will cover the entire range of pack size.

2. ***How to determine susceptibility of a pack***

   Susceptibility is defined in terms of microenvironment present in the container after first opening of container which increases the degradation rate of product in container. Change in head space due to sampling also accelerates the degradation of product. Presence or absence of canister also affects the microenvironment. We need to consider this condition while selection of pack in term of susceptibility.

3. ***Dispensing***

   Frequency of dispensing and duration to dispense the total medicament need to be considered. There are chances that after tampering the seal the pharmacist may keep the pack till end of its shelf life. There are also chances that pharmacist can open the bulk pack container at the end of its shelf life, as we know that the shelf life is provided only for sealed container and not for open container. So it is necessary to complete the in use study till its shelf life and determine the period to which the product is stable for safe use.

4. ***Desiccants, Canisters and oxygen scavengers Evaluation***

   We need to evaluate wither the canister incorporated in given pack is suitable to withstand the microenvironment after the pack is open at least it should keep the product stable for the duration for which it was evaluated under in use study condition.

5. ***If we consider 30's pack and 90's packs and further***

   If we consider 30's and 90's pack, the quantity of tablets will fall short for complete analysis as per finished product specifications. Is it feasible to keep 2 bottles during whole study and pooled sample to be used for analysis purpose? Also, what time point to be selected for the study, can it be 15, 30, 60, 90 days for 90's count or it should be directly 90 days. Similar is for 30's count can it be 15, 30 days or directly 30 days. What would be the time point for 250's count, 500's count, 1000's count and so on? We can perform in use study for 90 days and if results are within specification, it can be stated on label that once open it should be utilise within 90 days or the date till the pack is safe to dispense and consume.

6. ***Use of controlled sample along with test samples and the condition for controlled samples***

   Control samples are sample kept along with test sample at similar condition. Is there any need to keep control sample? Is there any need to open the seal of control sample when the study is initiated? Is there any need to withdraw same amount of sample as that of test at given time point? We usually face these questions when we keep control sample along with test sample, and we don't have any guideline regarding same. What could be done is to break the seal of container when the study is initiated and then to keep the sample as it is till the end of study. It can act as control sample.

7. ***Fish bone Blister pack***

   If we consider fish bone blister pack, once if taken out one tablet from the given pack, the canister present starts saturating and at some time point it will be no use and degradation of product accelerates. So, it is necessary to determine for what duration the following pack can be utilise after first tablet is taken out from the pack, and also it is necessary to mention it on the label the duration for which the tablet is safe to consume after first tablet is taken out.

8. ***Storage condition for test product***

   The product should be stored under conditions as recommended in the product literature (PIL) throughout the in-use stability test period. Any other storage conditions should be justified.

1. **Sample susceptible to light**

   Mostly light sensitive products are coated which acts as a barrier, but in use stability of such products to be performed to evaluate the stability of product once the seal is broken.

2. ***Sample highly susceptible to moisture***

   Most of the moisture sensitive drug products are coated which acts as an barrier, but in use stability of such products to be performed to evaluate the stability of product once the seal is broken. e.g OROS product are considered to be more susceptible to moisture as they contain salts which may absorb moisture during its storage[54].

Test to be performed

The appropriate physical, chemical and microbial properties of the product susceptible to change during use should be monitored. The tests used must be appropriate to individual dosage forms, for example, parameter types which may need to be studied are given below:

Physical

Description, colour, clarity, closure integrity, particulate matter, particle size, dissolution.

Chemical

Assay of active substance, degradation product level (impurities), antimicrobial preservative and antioxidant content(s), pH, Water by Karl fisher's method.

Microbial

Total viable count, sterility.

Labelling

Labelling of primary container

The in-use shelf life should be stated on the label. Manufacture can also provide a space for the user to write the date of opening or the "use-by" date.

Labelling of secondary container

The in-use shelf life should be stated on the label of secondary container.

STABILITY PROTOCOLS

Pharmaceutical product stability is a complex process collection that requires considerable time, expense, use, and scientific expertise to develop pharmaceutical formulation effectiveness, quality, and safety. Any alteration that occurs after its preparation in a pharmaceutical product that adversely affects a patient's fitness for use in the quality of the product is of interest in the stability screening of pharmaceutical researchers and regulators. The pharmaceutical stability test is defined according to the International Conference of Harmonization (ICH) guidelines as a systemic test conducted in pharmaceutical products to demonstrate that drug quality is subject to various environmental factors such as temperature, humidity, and light for setting a drug test period or a pharmaceuticals shelf life and to recommend a good storage condition. The USP defines the stability of the pharmaceutical product as "extension within certain limits" and uses the same characteristics and attributes as it had when its products were made. The stability of active drugs and formulation is determined at an early phase of the drug development process. The identity, strength, and pureness of components, as well as the stability and pharmaceutical analysis of manufactured products, are essential in determining and ensuring product quality. The stability of chemical products plays an essential role in reactions to chemical degradation such as oxidation, reduction, hydrolysis, and racemisation. The pharmaceutical product stability also influences factors such as the concentration of reactants, pH, radiation, catalysts, raw materials, and the period between development and use of the product. Physical changes due to impacts, abrasion and temperature fluctuations such as freezing or shearing can also impact drug stability, leading to the loss of the active pharmaceutical components. Forced degradation, including degradation of drug products and drug substances under conditions greater than accelerated conditions, assess the stability of the molecules and therefore produce degradation products. The stability test of a drug product is designed to ensure the effectiveness, safety, and quality of the active drug substances and type of dose and to assess shelf life or date of expiration to support branded claims. Studies on stability must be carefully performed in compliance with legislation regulated by ICH, World Health Organisation (WHO), and similar bodies[54].

Types of Stability of Drug Substances

Physical stability

Physical stability is important for safety and efficacy as it affects drug uniformity and release rate. Physical characteristics include size, palatability, homogeneity, dissolution, and suspension.

Chemical stability

Chemical stability of drugs is less active as deterioration takes place. The chemical quality and the labeled strength of each active ingredient remain within the specific limits.

Microbiological stability

Antimicrobial agents retain their effect within specified limits, also sterilisation or resistance to microbial growth as per the requirements stated.

Therapeutic stability

The therapeutic effect will remain unchanged. Toxicological stability Enhanced toxicity significantly does not occurs.

STABILITY TESTING METHOD

Stability tests are a routine operation used in the various phases of product development for drug substances and products. Early stages use accelerated stability tests to measure the type of degraded products found following long-term storage. The main objectives of the pharmaceutical stability test are to ensure that products remain on the market for the duration of their acceptable fitness or quality and are fit for consumption until the last pharmaceutical unit is used. Stability testing procedures are divided into four groups.

1. Real-time stability testing
2. Accelerated stability testing
3. Retained sample stability testing
4. Cyclic temperature stress testing.

Real-Time Stability Testing

It is conducted to allow substantial product degradation for a longer length of the trial period under storage circumstances. The test period relies on product stability which must remain sufficiently long to clearly show that no observable degradations occur and that degradation must be separated from the variability of the inter-assay. Trend analysis can differentiate instability from day-to-day ambiguity during the test by gathering information at an appropriate frequency. Reference material stability involves reagent stability and instrument quality consistency to be used during the stability studies. However, process efficiency and regulation of drift and irregularity arising from reaction and instrument modifications need to be controlled.

Guidelines for Stability Testing

In 1980, these guidelines were issued, and later the ICH harmonized (made uniform) to solve the bottleneck for marketing and registration in other nations. In the drug regulation, the regulatory authority in several nations has created regulations for the producers to submit stability information to ensure that molecules and products are generated with optimum stability, circulated, and provided to the patient. These guidelines aimed to introduce consistency in testing from supplier to supplier and also involve fundamental problems linked to stability, stability information for application dossier requirements, and implementation steps. In 1991, ICH was established which was a consortium created by the European Commission, Japan, and the USA with inputs from both regulatory and business. These guidelines are referred to as guidelines for quality, safety, efficacy, and multidisciplinary (also referred to as QSEM). In 1996, these guidelines were modified by the WHO because ICH guidelines did not address the extreme climatic conditions in many nations, but only new drug substances and products were covered and not the product already in use which was circulated in the entire nations by the WHO. In June 1997, the United States Food and Drug Administration (USFDA) also issued guidance documents entitled "Expiration dating of solid oral dosage form containing Iron." In 2004, WHO also issued guidelines for worldwide environment stability research. These ICH guidelines for veterinary products were subsequently expanded. The Indian Drug Manufacturers Association also published a technical monograph on drug and product stability testing in India. In the guidance documents, various test conditions and requirements for active pharmaceutical ingredients (APIs), drug products, or formulation and excipients have been established. The codes and titles for stability research covered by the ICH guidelines were presented in Table 5.4.

Q1A (R2): Stability Testing of New Drug Substances And Products

These guidelines address that new molecular entities and associated applications. Stability testing aims to provide evidence on how the quality of the drug substances or drug product changes over time under the influence of multiple environmental factors such as temperature, light, humidity, and also to establish a retest or shelf life for drug substance or drug product and recommend the storage conditions.

Q1B: Photostability Testing of New Drug Substances and Products

The ICH Harmonised tripartite guideline on new drug substances and stability testing for products (referred to as parent guidelines) states that light testing should be an essential component of stress testing. This document is an appendix to the parent guideline and discusses the guidelines for photostability evaluation. Photostability testing is performed on one batch of selected materials in compliance with the parent guidelines.

Q1C: Stability Testing for New Dosage Forms

These guidelines address a recommendation made by the original applicant on the stability of new dosage forms following the original application for new drug substances and products. The new dosage form is defined as a pharmaceutical product containing the same active substance as the existing drug product approved by the regulatory authority differing in the route of administration (e.g., oral to parental), new delivery system (e.g., tablet to modified tablet immediate release), and different dosage forms of the same dosage route (e.g., capsule to tablet, a solution to suspension). The parent stability guideline should be the concept of stability for a new dosage.

Q1D: Bracketing and Matrixing Design

This guideline proposes the use of bracketing and matrixing instability research. This guideline proposes the use of bracketing and matrixing instability research. Bracketing is described as designing a timetable for stability where only specimens are always tested to the extreme layout variables such as strength, container size, or complete design filling. The structure also presumes that any intermediate level of stability is the stability of the test ends. Matrixing is defined as the development of a stability schedule in which selected subsets of the total number of samples should be tested for all combinations of factors at a specified time point and specific sample subsets should be checked later. The design assumes that each sample's stability at a given time is the strength of all samples.

Q1E: Evaluation of Stability Data

This guideline defines when and how to consider extrapolation when recommending a re-assessment duration for the drug substance or drug product shelf life that goes beyond the period covered by "long-term storage conditions information accessible from the stability research." The design and performance of the official stabilisation research should follow the parent guideline values. The stability research aims to develop standards for the retest or shelf life and storage of all future batches produced and packaged under comparable conditions based on the minimum testing of three batches of drug substances or products. The degree of variability on individual batches also impacts the assurance that a future production batch will remain within acceptance requirements during its retest or shelf life[55].

Table 5.4 Codes and titles used in ICH guidelines.

ICH Codes	Guideline titles
Q1A	Stability testing of new drug substances and products (second revision)
Q1B	Photostability testing of new drug substances and products
Q1C	Stability testing of new dosage forms
Q1D	Bracketing and matrixing designs for stability testing of drug substances and product
Q1E	Evaluation of stability data
Q1F	Stability data package for registration applications in climatic Zones 3 and 4
Q5C	Stability testing of biotechnological/ biological products

Q1F: Stability Data Package for Registration Applications in Climatic Zone III and IV

In February 2003, these documents were accepted by the ICH Steering Committee and then enforced in the ICH regions. This guideline sets the storage requirements for stability testing in climatic zone III (hot and dry) and IV (hot and humid). To promote access to medicinal products by reducing the number of storage conditions, it specifies harmonized international stability testing requirements. In general cases, accelerated and long-term storage conditions recommended for climatic zone III and IV are shown in Table 2 (described in the parent guideline). Long-term and accelerated storage conditions for aqueous material packed in semi-permeable containers recommended storage conditions for climatic zone III and IV (described in parent guideline).

Q5C: Stability Testing of Biotechnological/Biological Products

This guidance refers to well-defined polypeptides and proteins, their products, and derivatives that are isolated from body fluids, tissues, cell cultures, or developed using r-DNA technology. The document thus includes the development and submission of stability information for products such as cytokines (interferons, interleukins, colony-stimulating factors, tumour necrosis factors), erythropoietin's, plasminogen activators, blood plasma factors, growth hormones and growth factors, insulin's, monoclonal antibodies, and vaccines consisting of well-characterized proteins or polypeptides.

Table 5.5 Long-term and accelerated storage conditions for climatic zone III and IV.

Study	Storage condition	The minimum time covered by data at submission
Long-term	30°C±2°C/65% RH±5% RH	12 months
Accelerated	40°C±2°C/75% RH±5% RH	6 months

Q6: Good Manufacturing Practice (GMP) Guide for APIs

This document (Guide) provides guidance on GMP for APIs manufacturing under a suitable quality management framework. It guarantees that APIs meet the requirements of consistency and purity criteria that they possess. This guide describes "manufacturing" as relating to all operations involving product receipt, manufacture, labelling, re-labelling, packaging, repackaging, quality control, shipment, storage, and distribution of APIs and related control. As a whole, this document does not address the safety aspects of production workers or environmental protection issues. Such checks are the manufacturer's intrinsic obligations and are regulated by national laws. This guide does not define pharmacopeia requirements for registration, filling, or adjustment. This guide refers to the production of APIs for human drug products. It also includes APIs generated through chemical synthesis, extraction, cell culture/fermentation, recovery from natural sources, or any combination of these processes.

Table 5.6 Long-term and accelerated storage conditions for a queous material.

Study	Storage conditions	The minimum time covered by data at submission
Long-term	30°C±2°C/35% RH±5% RH	12 months
Accelerated.	40°C±2°C/not more than 25% RH±5% RH	6 months

The committee for Proprietary Medicinal Products (CPMP)

In the framework of the European Agency for the Evaluation of Medicinal Products (EMEA), CPMP has issued a set of stability testing recommendations to assist those seeking authorisation to sell medicinal products in the European Union. The CPMP stability guidelines are shown in Table 5.4. Stability testing for climatic zone. In 1972, Futscher and Schumacher suggested the possibility of dividing the earth into four temperature and humidity-based zones, namely Zone I (temperature climate), Zone II (subtropical and Mediterranean climates), Zone III (hot and dry climate), and Zone IV (hot and humid climate). The WHO guidelines for stability monitoring, including four climatic zones storage conditions, outline guidelines for stability monitoring. The guidelines for stability testing assessments are based on the parent guidelines and guidelines for WHO. In climatic Zones I and II and climatic Zone III and IV, the parent guideline outlines the stability information package for tripartite ICH regions (European Union, Japan, and the United States). The world has been divided into four climate zones to harmonise and simplify worldwide stability testing. The Current Climatic Zone III and IV were recommended for long term 30°C/65% RH for 12 months and accelerated conditions for 40°C 75% RH for 6 months. The climatic zones for long-term testing and accelerated condition are shown in Table 5.5. Based on this long-term stability data, stability in real-time and accelerated conditions for stability testing have been derived. Protocol for stability testing Stability testing protocol is a pre-condition for initiation of stability tests and is essentially a written document describing the main components of a well-controlled and regulated stability test. The protocol relies on the type of drug substance or the product because, it depends on the compound's intrinsic stability, dosage form, and process of closing the container implied. It is also possible to determine whether the drug is new or already on the market. Stability tests are designed to determine a pharmaceutical product expiry date and shelf life. The protocol should also include the areas where the product is expected to be put on the market, for example, where it is planned for use in climatic Zones I-IV.

The following information should be included in the stability protocol:

- Number of batches
- Containers and closures
- The orientation of storage of containers
- Sampling time points
- Sampling plan
- Test storage conditions
- Test parameters
- Test methodology
- Acceptance criteria

Table 5.7 The CPMP stability guidelines.

CPMP code	Guideline title
CPMP/QWP/576/96 Rev.1	Guideline on stability testing for applications f or variations to a marketing authorization
CPMP/QWP/6142/03	Guideline on stability testing for active substances and medicinal products manufactured in climatic zones III and IV to be marketed in the EU
CPMP/QWP/609/96 Rev.1	Note for guidance on a declaration of storage conditions for medicinal products particulars and active substances
CPMP/QWP/122/02 Rev.1	Note for guidance on stability testing of existing active substances and related finished products
CPMP/QWP/072/96	Note for guidance on the start of shelf life of the finished dosage form
CPMP/QWP/2934/99	Note for guidance for in-use stability testing of human medicinal products
CPMP/QWP/576/96	Note for guidance on stability testing for a type 2 variation to a marketing authorization
CPMP/QWP/159/96	Note for guidance on maximum shelf life for sterile products after first opening or the following reconstitution

REPORTS

Impurity content of batches analytical results provided in the application for all batches of the new drug substance used for clinical, safety, and stability testing, as well as for batches representative of the proposed commercial process have been reported. Quantitative results should be presented numerically, and not in general terms such as "complies"," meets limit" etc. Any impurity at a level greater than (>) the reporting threshold and total impurities observed in these batches of the new drug substance should be reported with the analytical procedures indicated. Below 1.0%, the results should be reported to two decimal places (0.06%, 0.13%); at and above 1.0%, the results should be reported to one decimal place (1.3%). Results should be rounded using conventional rules. Tabulation (spreadsheet) of the data is recommended. Impurities should be designated by code number or by an appropriate descriptor, for example, retention time. If a higher reporting threshold is proposed, it should be fully justified. All impurities at a level greater than (>) the reporting threshold should be summed and reported as total impurities. When analytical procedures change during development, reported results should be linked to the procedure used, with appropriate validation information. Representative chromatograms should be provided. Chromatograms of representative batches from analytical validation studies showing separation and detect ability of impurities (on spiked samples), along with any other impurity tests routinely performed. These can serve as the representative impurity profiles. The applicant should ensure that complete impurity profiles (chromatograms) of individual batches are available. Tabulation should be provided that must link the specific batch of new drug substance to[55] each safety study and each clinical study in which the new drug substance has been used. For each batch of the new drug substance, the report should include:

* Batch identity and size
* Date of manufacture
* Site of manufacture
* Manufacturing process
* Impurity content, individual and total
* Use of batches
* Reference to analytical procedure used
* Listing of impurities in specification

In other words, the new drug substance specification should include, where applicable, the following list of impurities:

* Organic impurities
* Each specified identified impurity
* Each specified unidentified impurity

Any unspecified impurity with an acceptance criterion of not more than the total impurities identification threshold.

ICH GUIDELINES

Q1A Stability testing of new drugs substances and products

The guideline seeks to exemplify the core stability data package for new drug substances and products but leaves sufficient flexibility to encompass the variety of different practical situations. This may be experienced due to specific scientific considerations and characteristics of the materials being evaluated. Alternative approaches can be used when there are scientifically justifiable reasons. The guideline speaks the submitted in registration applications for new information which may be molecular entities and associated drug products. This guideline does not currently cover the information to be submitted for abbreviated or abridged applications, variations, clinical trial applications, etc. Specific details of the sampling and testing for particular dosage forms in their proposed container closures are not covered in this guideline. Further guidance on new dosage forms and on biotechnological/biological products can be found in ICH guidelines Q1C and Q5C, respectively. The purpose of stability testing is to provide evidence on how the quality of a drug substance or drug product varies with time under the influence of a variety of environmental factors such as temperature, humidity, and light, and to establish a re-test period for the drug substance or a shelf life for the drug product and recommended storage conditions.

The choice of test conditions defined in this guideline is based on an analysis of the effects of climatic conditions in the three regions of the EC, Japan and the United States. The mean kinetic temperature in any part of the world can be obtained from climatic data, and the world can be divided into four climatic zones, I - IV. The principle is based on the stability information generated in any one of the four regions. This is obtained from the information, consistent with this guideline. The labelling is according to the national/regional requirements[56].

Guidelines

Drug substances

Based on the information on the stability of the drug substance, an integral part of the systematic approach to stability evaluation includes

1) Stress testing.
2) Selection of batches
3) Container closure system
4) Specification
5) Testing frequency
6) Storage condition
7) Stability commitment

8) Evaluation
9) Statements / labelling

Drug product

The design of the formal stability studies for the drug product should be made on the basis of knowledge of the behaviour and properties of the drug substance and on the basis of stability studies on the drug substance and on the experience gained from clinical formulation studies. The possible changes on storage and the reason for the selection of attributes should be tested in the formal stability studies. This includes-

* Photo stability testing.
* Selection of batches.
* Container closure system.
* Specification.
* Testing frequency.
* Storage conditions.
* Stability commitment.
* Evaluation.
* Statements/ labeling.

The function of this is to outline the changes mentioned in Q1A(R), this is resulted from adoption of ICH Q1F "Stability Data Package for Registration Applications in Climatic Zones III and IV". These changes are:

1. The intermediate storage condition has been changed from 30 °C±2 °C/60% RH±5% RH to 30°C±2°C/65% RH±5% RH in the following sections:
   * Drug Substance - Storage Conditions - General Case
   * Drug Product - Storage Conditions - General Case
   * Drug products packaged in semi-permeable containers
2. 30 °C±2 °C/65% RH±5% RH can be a suitable alternative long-term storage condition to 25 °C±2°C/60% RH±5% in the following sections:
   * Drug Substance - Storage Conditions - General Case
   * Drug Product - Storage Conditions - General Case
3. 30 °C±2 °C/35% RH±5% RH has been added as a suitable alternative long-term storage condition to 25 °C±2 °C/40% RH±5% and the corresponding example for the ratio of water-loss rates has been included in the following section:
   * Drug products packed in semi-permeable containers

4. Mid-stream switch of the intermediate storage condition from 30 °C±2 °C/60% RH±5% RH to 30°C±2 °C/65% RH±5% RH can be appropriate provided that the respective storage conditions and the date of the switch are clearly documented and stated in the registration application.

It is recommended that the registration applications must contain the data from complete studies at the intermediate storage condition, 30°C±2°C/65% RH±5% RH, if applicable, by three years after the date of publication of this revised guideline in the respective ICH tripartite region.

Q1B Stability Testing

Photo-stability testing of new drug substances and products

The ICH harmonised tripartite guideline covers the stability testing of new drug substances and Products, and notes that light testing is an integral part of stress testing. This document is an annex to the Parent Guideline and mentions the recommendations for photo stability testing. Drug substances and drug product.

* Presentation of samples
* Analysis of samples
* Judgment of results

Primary pack is that constituent of the packaging that is in direct contact with the drug substance or drug product and is mentioned on any appropriate label. Marketing pack is the combination of primary pack and other secondary packaging such as a carton. Forced gradation testing studies are those performed to degrade the sample deliberately. The studies may be carried out in the development phase normally on the drug substances. These studies are used to evaluate the overall photosensitivity of the material for the method development purposes and/or elucidation of degradation pathway. Confirmatory studies are those performed to determine the photo-stability characteristics under standardised conditions. These studies are used to identify precautionary measures required in manufacturing or formulation and whether light resistant packaging and/or special labelling would be required to mitigate exposure to light. For confirmation, the batches should be selected according to the selection of batch for long-term and accelerated testing which is described in the Parent Guideline[57].

Q1C Stability Testing for New Dosage Form

The ICH harmonised tripartite guideline on stability testing of new drug substances and products was issued on October 27, 1993. This document is annexed to the ICH parent stability guideline and mentions the recommendations on what should be submitted in support of the stability of new dosage forms by the owner of the original application, after the original submission for new drug substances and products. A New dosage form is defined as a drug product which is a different pharmaceutical product type, but contains the same active substance as mentioned in the existing drug product approved by the pertinent regulatory authority. Such pharmaceutical product types include the products to be administered through different routes (oral to parenteral), new specific functionality/delivery systems (immediate release tablet to modified release tablet), and different dosage forms of the same route of administration (capsule to tablet, solution to suspension).

Q1D Bracketing and matrixing designs for stability testing of new drug substances and products

This guideline mentions the recommendations on the application of bracketing and matrixing to stability studies conducted according to the principles outlined in the ICH Q1A(R). Harmonised Tripartite guideline on Stability Testing of New Drug Substances and Products is also called the parent guideline. This document gives the guidance on bracketing and matrixing study designs. Specific principles are defined in this guideline for situations in which bracketing or matrixing can be applied. A full study design is one in which the samples for every combination of all design factors are tested at all times points. A reduced design is one in which the samples for every combination of factors is not all tested at all times point. A reduced design can be a suitable alternative to a full design when multiple design factors are involved. Any reduced design should have the ability to adequately predict the retest period or shelf life. Before a reduced design is considered, certain assumptions should be assessed and justified. The potential risk should be considered of establishing a shorter retest period or shelf life than could be derived from a full design due to the reduced amount of data collected.

Bracketing

As defined in the glossary to the parent guideline, bracketing is the design of a stability schedule such that only samples on the extremes of certain design factors (strength, container size and/or fill) are tested at all times point as in a full design. The design is made in such a way that the stability of any intermediate levels is represented by the stability of the extremes tested. The use of a bracketing design would not be considered appropriate if it fails to demonstrate the strengths or container sizes and/or fills selected for testing are required the extremes. Bracketing can be applied to study the multiple strengths of identical or closely related formulations, for example, capsules of different strengths made with different fill plug sizes from the same powder blend, tablets of different strengths prepared by compressing varying amounts of the same granulation, or oral solutions of different strengths with formulations that differ only in minor excipients, such as colorants, flavourings. With proper justification, bracketing can be applied to studies with multiple strengths where the relative amounts of drug substance and excipients change in a formulation. Such justification can include a demonstration of comparable stability profiles among the different strengths of clinical or development batches. In cases where different excipients are used among strengths, bracketing generally should not be applied.

Matrixing

As defined in the glossary of the parent guideline, matrixing is the design of a stability schedule. A selected subset of the total number of possible samples for all combinations of factors would be tested at a specified time point. At a subsequent time point, another subset of samples for all combinations of factors would be tested. The design also assumes that the stability of each subset of samples tested represents the stability of all samples at a given time point. The differences in the samples for the same drug product should be identified. In other words, this covers different batches, different strengths, different sizes of the same container closure system, and possibly, in some cases, different container closure systems. When a secondary packaging system contributes to the stability of the drug product, matrixing can be carried out across the packaging systems. Each storage condition should be treated separately under its own matrixing design. Matrixing should not be performed across test attributes. However, alternative matrixing designs for different test attributes can be applied if found satisfactory. Matrixing designs can be applied to strengths with identical or closely related formulations, for example, this is not limited to

(1) capsules of different strengths made with different fill plug sizes from the same powder blend,

(2) tablets of different strengths manufactured by compressing varying amounts of the same granulation, and

(3) oral solutions of different strengths with formulations that differ only in minor excipients (colorants or flavourings).

Other examples of design factors that can be matrixes include batches made by using the same process and equipment, and container sizes and/or fills in the same container closure system. With justification, matrixing designs can be applied, for example, to different strengths where the relative amounts of drug substance and excipients change or where different excipients are used or to different container closure systems. Justification should generally be based on supporting data. For example, to matrix across two different closures or container closure systems, supporting data could be supplied showing relative moisture vapour transmission rates or similar protection against light. Alternatively, supporting data could be supplied to show that the drug product is not affected by oxygen, moisture, or light[58].

Q1E Evaluation of Stability Data

This guideline is intended to provide recommendations on how to use stability data generated in accordance with the principles detailed in the ICH guideline

"Q1A(R) Stability Testing of New Drug Substances and Products" (hereafter referred to as the parent guideline) to propose a retest period or shelf life in a registration application. This guideline states when and how extrapolation can be considered when proposing a retest period for a drug substance or a shelf life for a drug product that extends beyond the period covered by "available data from the stability study under the longterm storage condition" (hereafter referred to as long-term data). The guidance on the evaluation and statistical analysis of stability data provided in the parent guideline is brief in nature and limited in scope. The parent guideline states that regression analysis is an appropriate approach to analyse quantitative stability data for retest period or shelf-life estimation and recommends that a statistical test for batch pool ability be performed using a level of significance of 0.25. However, the parent guideline contains few details and does not cover situations where multiple factors are involved in a full- or reduced-design study. This guideline is an expansion of the guidance presented in the Evaluation sections of the parent guideline. This guideline states the evaluation of stability data that should be submitted in registration applications for new molecular entities and associated drug products. The guideline provides recommendations on establishing retest periods and shelf lives for drug substances and drug products intended for storage at or below "room temperature"*. It covers stability studies using single- or multi-factor designs and full or reduced designs.

***Note:** The term "room temperature" refers to the general customary environment and should not be inferred to be the storage statement for labelling. ICH Q6A and Q6B should be consulted for recommendations on the setting and justification of acceptance criteria and ICH Q1D should be referenced for recommendations on the use of full- versus reduced-design studies. The design and execution of formal stability studies should follow the principles outlined in the parent guideline. The purpose of a stability study is to establish, based on testing a minimum of three batches of the drug substance or product, a retest period or shelf life and label storage instructions applicable to all future batches manufactured and packaged under similar circumstances. The degree of variability of individual batches affects the confidence that a future production batch will remain within acceptance criteria throughout its retest period or shelf life.

Q2 (R1) Validation of analytical procedures

The objective of validation of an analytical procedure is to demonstrate that it is suitable for its intended purpose. A tabular summation of the characteristics applicable to identification, control of impurities and assay procedures is included. Other analytical procedures may be considered in future additions to this document. Types of analytical procedures to be validated.

1) The discussion of the validation of analytical procedures is directed to the four most common types of analytical procedure: Identification tests;
2) Quantitative tests for impurities' content;
3) Limit tests for the control of impurities;
4) Quantitative tests of the active moiety in Samples of drug substance or drug product or other selected component(s) in the drug product.

Although there are many other analytical procedures, such as dissolution testing for drug products or particle size determination for drug substance, these have not been addressed in the initial text on validation of analytical procedures. Validation of these additional analytical procedures are equally important to those listed herein and may be addressed in subsequent documents. A brief description of the types of tests considered in this document is provided below.

* Identification tests are intended to ensure the identity of an analyte in a sample. This is normally achieved by comparison of a property of the sample (spectrum, chromatographic behaviour, chemical reactivity, etc) to that of a reference standard;
* Testing for impurities can be either a quantitative test or a limit test for the impurity in a sample. Either test is intended to accurately reflect the purity characteristics of the sample. Different validation characteristics are required for a quantitative test than for a limit test;
* Assay procedures are intended to measure the analyte present in a given sample. In the context of this document, the assay represents a quantitative measurement of the major component(s) in the drug substance.

For the drug product, similar validation characteristics also apply when assaying for the active or other selected component(s). The same validation characteristics may also apply to assays associated with other analytical procedures (dissolution).

The objective of the analytical procedure should be clearly understood since this will govern the validation characteristics which need to be evaluated. Typical validation characteristics which should be considered are listed below:

* Accuracy
* Precision
* Repeatability
* Intermediate Precision
* Specificity
* Detection Limit
* Quantisation Limit

* Linearity
* Range

The revalidation may be necessary in the following circumstances:

* Changes in the synthesis of the drug substance;
* Changes in the composition of the finished product;
* Changes in the analytical procedure.

The degree of revalidation required depends on the nature of the changes. Certain other changes may require validation as well[59].

Q3A (R2) Impurities in new drug substances

This document is intended to provide guidance for registration applications on the content and qualification of impurities in new drug substances produced by chemical syntheses and not previously registered in a region or member state. It is not intended to apply to new drug substances used during the clinical research stage of development. The following types of drug substances are not covered in this guideline: biological/biotechnological, peptide, oligo-nucleotide, radiopharmaceutical, fermentation product and semi-synthetic products derived there from, herbal products, and crude products of animal or plant origin. Impurities in new drug substances are addressed from two perspectives:

1) Chemistry aspects contain classification and identification of impurities, report generation, listing of impurities in specifications, and a brief discussion of analytical procedures; and

2) Safety aspects include specific guidance for qualifying those impurities that were not present,or were present at substantially lower levels, in batches of a new drug substance used in safety and clinical studies.

Classification of impurities Impurities can be classified into the following categories:

* Organic impurities (process- and drug-related)
* Inorganic impurities
* Residual solvents Organic impurities can arise during the manufacturing process and/or storage of the new drug substance.

They can be identified or unidentified, volatile or non-volatile, and include:

* Starting materials
* By-products
* Intermediates
* Degradation products

* Reagents, ligands and catalysts Inorganic impurities can result from the manufacturing process.

They are normally known and identified and include:

* Reagents, ligands and catalysts
* Heavy metals or other residual metals
* Inorganic salts
* Other materials (filter aids, charcoal)

Solvents are inorganic or organic liquids used as vehicles for the preparation of solutions or suspensions in the synthesis of a new drug substance. Since these solvents have generally known toxicity, the selection of appropriate solvents and controls is easily done (ICH Guideline Q3C on Residual Solvents). From this document excluded solvent are:

(1) extraneous contaminants that should not occur in new drug substances and are more appropriately addressed as Good Manufacturing Practice (GMP) issues,

(2) polymorphic forms, and

(3) enantiomeric impurities.

Q3B (R2) Impurities in new drug products

This document provides guidance for registration applications on the content and qualification of impurities in new drug products produced from chemically synthesised new drug substances not previously registered in a region or member state. This guideline addresses only those impurities in new drug products classified as degradation products of the drug substance or reaction products of the drug substance with an excipient and/or immediate container closure system (collectively referred to as "degradation products" in this guideline). Generally, impurities present in the new drug substance need not be monitored or specified in the new drug product unless they are also degradation products. Impurities derived from these excipients present in the new drug product or extracted or leached from the container-closure system are not covered by this guideline. This guideline also does not apply to new drug products used during the clinical research stages of development. The following types of products are not covered in this guideline:

Biological/biotechnological products, peptide, oligonucleotides, radio-pharmaceuticals, fermentation products and semi-synthetic products derived there from, herbal products, and crude products of animal or plant origin. Also excluded from this document are:

(1) extraneous contaminants that should not occur in new drug products and are more appropriately addressed as good manufacturing practice (GMP) issues,

(2) polymorphic forms, and

(3) enantiomeric impurities.

The applicant summarises that

1) the degradation products observed during manufacture and/or

2) stability studies of the new drug product.

This summary is based on sound scientific appraisal of potential degradation pathways in the new drug product and impurities arising from the interaction with excipients and/or the immediate container closure system. In addition, the applicant should summarise any laboratory studies conducted to detect degradation products in the new drug product. This summary also includes test results of batches manufactured during the development process and batches representative of the proposed commercial process. A rationale should be provided for exclusion of those impurities that are not degradation products (process impurities from the drug substance and impurities arising from excipients). The impurity profiles of the batches representative of the proposed commercial process should be compared with the profiles of batches used in development and any differences discussed. Any degradation product observed in stability studies conducted at the recommended storage condition should be identified when present at a level greater than (>) the identification thresholds. When identification of a degradation product is not possible, a summary of the laboratory studies stating the unsuccessful efforts to identify, it should be included in the registration application. Degradation products present at a level of not more than (1) the identification threshold generally would not be identified. The analytical procedures should be developed for those degradation products that are suspected to be unusually potent, producing toxic or significant pharmacological effects at levels not more than (2) the identification threshold. In unusual circumstances, technical factors (manufacturing capability, a low drug substance to excipient ratio, or the use of excipients that are crude products of animal or plant origin) can be considered as part of the justification for selection of alternative thresholds based upon manufacturing experience with the proposed commercial process.

For each batch of the new drug product described in the registration application, the documentation should include:

* Batch identity, strength, and size
* Date of manufacture
* Site of manufacture
* Manufacturing process
* Immediate container closure
* Degradation product content, individual and total
* Use of batch (e.g., clinical studies, stability studies)

* Reference to analytical procedure used
* Batch number of the drug substance used in the new drug product
* Storage conditions for stability studies

In summary, the new drug product specification should include, where applicable, the following list of degradation products:

* Each specified identified degradation product
* Each specified unidentified degradation product
* Any unspecified degradation product with an acceptance criterion of not more than the identification threshold
* Total degradation products[60].

Q3C (R5) Residual Solvents

The objective of this guideline is to recommend acceptable amounts for residual solvents in pharmaceuticals for the safety of the patient. The guideline recommends use of less toxic solvents and describes levels considered to be toxicologically acceptable for some residual solvents.

Residual solvents in pharmaceuticals are defined here. Organic volatile chemicals that are used or produced in the manufacture of drug substances or excipients, or in the preparation of drug products. The solvents are not completely removed by practical manufacturing techniques. Appropriate selection of the solvent for the synthesis of drug substance may increase the yield, or determine characteristics such as crystal form, purity, and solubility. Therefore, the solvent may sometimes be a critical parameter in the synthetic process. This guideline does not address solvents deliberately used as excipients nor does it address solvates. The content of solvents in such products should be evaluated and justified. Since there is no therapeutic benefit from residual solvents, all residual solvents should be removed to the extent possible to meet product specifications, good manufacturing practices, or other quality-based requirements. Drug products should contain no higher levels of residual solvents than can be supported by safety data. Some solvents are known to cause unacceptable toxicities (Class 1). These solvents should be avoided in the production of drug substances, excipients, or drug products unless their use can be strongly justified in a risk-benefit assessment. Some solvents associated with less severe toxicity (Class 2) should be limited to protect patients from potential adverse effects. Ideally, less toxic solvents (Class 3) should be used where practical.

The lists are not exhaustive and other solvents can be used and later added to the lists. Recommended limits of Class 1 and 2 solvents or classification of solvents may change as new safety data becomes available. Supporting safety data in a marketing application for a new drug product containing a new solvent may be based on concepts in this guideline or the concept of qualification of impurities as expressed in the guideline for drug substance (Q3A, Impurities in New Drug Substances) or drug product (Q3B, Impurities in New Drug Products), or all three guidelines. Therefore, testing should be carried out for residual solvents when production or purification processes are known to result in the presence of such solvents. It is necessary to test for solvents that are used or produced in the manufacture or purification of drug substances, excipients, or drug product. The manufacturers may choose to test the drug product, a cumulative method may be used to calculate the residual solvent levels in the drug product from the levels in the ingredients used to produce the drug product. If the calculation results in a level equal to or below that recommended in this guideline, no testing of the drug product for residual solvents need be considered. If, however, the calculated level is above the recommended level, the drug product should be tested to ascertain whether the formulation process has reduced the relevant solvent level to within the acceptable amount. Drug product should be tested, if a solvent is used during its manufacture. This guideline does not apply to potential new drug substances, excipients, or drug products used during the clinical research stages of development, nor does it apply to existing marketed drug products. The guideline applies to all dosage forms and routes of administration. Higher levels of residual solvents may be acceptable in certain cases such as short term (30 days or less) or topical application. Justification for these levels should be made on case by case basis. Classification of residual solvents can be done by risk assessment. The term "tolerable daily intake" (TDI) is used by the International Program on Chemical Safety (IPCS) to describe exposure limits of toxic chemicals and "acceptable daily intake" (ADI) is used by the World Health Organisation (WHO) and other national and international health authorities and institutes. The new term "permitted daily exposure" (PDE) is defined in the present guideline as a pharmaceutically acceptable intake of residual solvents to avoid confusion of differing values for ADI's of the same substance. Residual solvents have been evaluated for their possible risk to human health and placed into one of three classes as follows:

Class 1 solvents: Solvents to be avoided are known human carcinogens, strongly suspected human carcinogens, and environmental hazards.

Class 2 solvents: Solvents to be limited Non-genotoxic animal carcinogens or possible causative agents of other irreversible toxicity such as neurotoxicity or teratogenicity. Solvents suspected of other significant but reversible toxicities.

Class 3 solvents: Solvents with low toxic potential solvents with low toxic potential to man; no health-based exposure limit is needed. Class 3 solvents have PDEs of 50 mg or more per day[61].

Q3D Guidelines for elemental impurities

Elemental impurities in drug products may come from several sources; they may be residual catalysts that had been added intentionally in synthesis or may be present as impurities (through interactions with processing equipment or container/closure systems or by being present in components of the drug product). Because elemental impurities do not provide any therapeutic benefit to the patient, their levels in the drug product should be controlled within acceptable limits. There are three parts of this guideline: (1) the evaluation of the toxicity data for potential elemental impurities; (2) the establishment of a Permitted Daily Exposure (PDE) for each element of toxicological concern; and (3) application of a risk-based approach to control elemental impurities in drug products.

An applicant is not expected to tighten the limits based on process capability, provided that the elemental impurities in drug products do not exceed the PDEs. The PDEs established in this guideline are considered to be protective of public health for all patient populations. In some cases, lower levels of elemental impurities may be warranted when levels below toxicity thresholds have been shown to have an impact on other quality attributes of the drug product (element catalysed degradation of drug substances). In addition, for elements with high PDEs, other limits may have to be considered from a pharmaceutical quality perspective and other guidelines should be consulted (ICH Q3A). This guideline gives a process for assessment and control of elemental impurities in the drug product using the principles of risk management as described in ICH Q9. This process gives a platform for developing a risk-based control strategy to limit elemental impurities in the drug product. The guideline applies to new finished drug products (as defined in ICH Q6A and Q6B) and new drug products containing existing drug substances. The drug products containing purified proteins and polypeptides (proteins and polypeptides produced from recombinant or non-recombinant origins), their derivatives, and products of which they are components (conjugates) are within the scope of this guideline, as are drug products containing synthetically produced polypeptides, polynucleotide, and oligosaccharides. This guideline does not apply to herbal products, radio-pharmaceuticals, vaccines, cell metabolites, DNA products, allergenic extracts, cells, whole blood, cellular blood components or blood derivatives including plasma and plasma derivatives, dialyses solutions not intended for systemic circulation, and elements that are intentionally included in the drug product for therapeutic benefit. This guideline does not apply to products based on genes (gene therapy), cells (cell therapy) and tissue (tissue engineering). In some regions, these products are known as advanced therapy medicinal products. This guideline does not apply to drug products used during clinical research stages of development. As the commercial process is developed, the principles contained in this guideline can be useful in evaluating elemental impurities that may be present in a new drug product. Application of Q3D to existing products is not expected prior to 36 months after publication of the guideline by ICH. The factors considered in the safety assessment for establishing the PDE are listed below in approximate order of relevance:

1) The likely oxidation state of the element in the drug product;
2) Human exposure and safety data when it provided applicable information;
3) The most relevant animal study;
4) Route of administration;
5) The relevant endpoint(s).

Classification of elements

* Class:1
* Class:2
* Class :2A
* Class:2B
*. Class: 3

Q4B Evaluation and recommendation of pharmacopeia texts for use in "ICH" regions

This document describes a process for the evaluation and recommendation by the Q4B Expert Working Group (EWG) of selected pharmacopoeia texts to facilitate their recognition by regulatory authorities for use as interchangeable in the ICH regions[62].

Q5A (R1) Viral safety evaluation of biotechnology products derived from cell lines of human or animal origin

This document is concerned with testing and evaluation of the viral safety of biotechnology products derived from characterized cell lines of human or animal origin (i.e., mammalian, avian, insect) and outlines data that should be submitted in the marketing application/registration package. For the purposes of this document the term virus excludes nonconventional transmissible agents like those associated with Bovine Spongiform Encephalopathy (BSE) and scrape. Applicants are encouraged to discuss issues associated with BSE with the regulatory authorities. The scope of the document covers products derived from cell cultures initiated from characterized cell banks. It covers products obtained from *in vitro* cell culture, such as interferon's, monoclonal antibodies and recombinant DNA-derived products including recombinant subunit vaccines, and also includes products derived from hybridoma cells grown in vivo as ascites. In this latter case, special considerations apply and additional information on testing cells propagated in vivo. Inactivated vaccines, all live vaccines containing self-replicating agents, and genetically engineered live vectors are excluded from the scope of this document. The risk of viral contamination is a feature, common to all biotechnology products derived from cell lines. Such contamination could have serious clinical consequences and can arise from the contamination of the source cell lines themselves (cell substrates) or from adventitious introduction of virus during production. Till date, biotechnology products derived from cell lines have not been implicated in the transmission of viruses. Nevertheless, it is expected that the safety of these products with respect to viral contamination can be reasonably assured. This is possible by the application of a virus testing program and assessment of virus removal and inactivation achieved by the manufacturing process, as outlined below. Three principal, complementary approaches have evolved to control the potential viral contamination of biotechnology products:

* Selecting and testing of cell lines and other raw materials, including media components, for the absence of undesirable viruses which may be infectious and/or pathogenic for human;
* Assessing the capacity of the production processes to clear infectious viruses;
* Testing the product at appropriate steps of production for absence of contaminating infectious viruses.

All testing suffers from the inherent limitation of quantitative virus assays, that is, the ability to detect low viral concentrations depends for statistical reasons on the size of the sample. Therefore, no single approach will establish the safety of a product. The infectious virus is absent from the final product in many instances may not be derived solely from direct testing for their presence. Also, from a demonstration that the purification regimen is capable of removing and/or inactivating the viruses. The type and extent of viral tests and viral clearance studies required at different steps of production will depend on various factors and should be considered on a case-by-case and step-by-step basis. The factors that should be taken into account include the extent of cell bank characterisation and qualification, the nature of any viruses detected, culture medium constituents, culture methods, facility and equipment design, the results of viral tests after cell culture, the ability of the process to clear viruses, and the type of product and its intended clinical use.

The manufacturers should adjust the recommendations presented here to their specific product and its production process. The approach used by manufacturers in their overall strategy for ensuring viral safety should be explained and justified. This should contain a brief description of all aspects of the viral safety studies and strategies used to prevent virus contamination as they pertain to this document.

Q5B Quality of biotechnological products

This document presents guidance regarding the characterisation of the expression construct for the production of recombinant DNA protein products in eukaryotic and prokaryotic cells. This document is intended to describe the types of information that are considered valuable in assessing the structure of the expression construct used to produce recombinant DNA derived proteins. This document is not intended to cover the whole quality aspect of rDNA derived medicinal products. Segments of the expression construct should be analysed using nucleic acid techniques in conjunction with other tests performed on the purified recombinant protein for assuring the quality and consistency of the final product. Analysis of the expression construct at the nucleic acid level should be considered as part of the overall evaluation of quality, taking into account that this testing only evaluates neither the coding sequence of a recombinant gene and not the translational fidelity nor other characteristics of the recombinant protein, such as secondary structure, tertiary structure, and post-translational modifications[63].

Q5C Quality of Biotechnological Products

Stability testing of Biotechnological/Biological Products

The guidance stated in this annex applies to well-characterized proteins and polypeptides, their derivatives and products of which they are components, and which are isolated from tissues, body fluids, cell cultures, or produced using rDNA technology. The document covers the generation and submission of stability data for products such as cytokines (interferons, interleukins, colony-stimulating factors and tumour necrosis factors), erythropoietin's, plasminogen activators, blood plasma factors, growth hormones and growth factors, insulin, monoclonal antibodies, and vaccines consisting of well-characterized proteins or polypeptides. In addition, the guidance outlined in the following sections may apply to other types of products, such as conventional vaccines, after consultation with the appropriate regulatory authorities. The document does not cover antibiotics, allergenic extracts, heparins, vitamins, whole blood, or cellular blood components.

Q5D Derivation and characterisation of cell substrates

This guideline covers cell substrates having a cell banking system. In this document, "cell substrate" refers to microbial cells or cell lines derived from human or animal sources that possess the full potential for generation of the desired biotechnological/biological products for human in vivo or ex vivo use. Reagents for in vitro diagnostic use are outside the scope of this document. Animal sources of cell lines include all those of metazoan origin. Both continuous cell lines of indefinite in vitro lifespan and diploid cells of finite in vitro lifespan are included. Microbial sources include bacteria, fungi, yeast, and other unicellular life forms. "Biotechnological/biological products" refers to any products prepared from cells cultivated from cell banks with the exception of microbial metabolites such as, for example, antibiotics, amino acids, carbohydrates, and other low molecular weight substances. Cell banks used to prepare gene therapy products or vaccines should follow the recommendations presented in this document. Some biological products, such as certain viral vaccines, are prepared in primary cell cultures derived directly from animal tissues or organs. Primary cells are not banked and therefore are not addressed by this document. It is important to provide supportive documentation which describes the history of the cell substrate that is used in the manufacture of a biotechnological/biological product, as well as any parental cell line from which it was totally or partially derived. Events during the research and development phases of the cell substrate may contribute significantly to assessment of the risks associated with the use of that particular cell substrate for production. The information supplied in this regard is meant to facilitate an overall evaluation which will ensure the quality and safety of the product.

Careful records of the manipulation of the cell substrate should be maintained throughout its development. Description of cell history is only one tool of many used for cell substrate characterisation. In general, deficiencies in documented history may not, by itself, be an impediment to product approval, but extensive deficiencies will result in increased reliance on other methods to characterise the cell substrate.

Q5E Comparability of biotechnological/biological products subject to changes in their manufacturing process

The objective of this document is to provide principles for assessing the comparability of biotechnological/biological products before and after changes are made in the manufacturing process for the drug substance or drug product. Therefore, this guideline is intended to assist in the collection of relevant technical information which serves as evidence that the manufacturing process changes will not have an adverse impact on the quality, safety and efficacy of the drug product. The document does not prescribe any particular analytical, nonclinical or clinical strategy. The main emphasis of the document is on quality aspects[64].

Q6A Specifications: test procedures and acceptance criteria, for new drug substances and new drug products

This guideline is intended to assist to the extent possible, in the establishment of a single set of global specifications for new drug substances and new drug products. It provides guidance on the setting and justification of acceptance criteria and the selection of test procedures for new drug substances of synthetic chemical origin, and new drug products produced from them, which have not been registered previously in the United States, the European Union, or Japan. The quality of drug substances and drug products is determined by their design, development, in-process controls, GMP controls, and process validation, and by specifications applied to them throughout development and manufacture. This guideline addresses specifications, that is, those tests, procedures, and acceptance criteria which play a major role in assuring the quality of the new drug substance and new drug product at release and during shelf life. Specifications are an important component of quality assurance but are not it only Component. All of the considerations listed above are necessary to ensure consistent production of drug substances and drug products of high quality. This guideline addresses only the marketing approval of new drug products (including combination products) and, where applicable, new drug substances; it does not address drug substances or drug products during the clinical research stages of drug development. This guideline may be applicable to synthetic and semi-synthetic antibiotics and synthetic peptides of low molecular weight; however, it is not sufficient to adequately describe specifications of higher molecular weight peptides and polypeptides, and biotechnological/biological products. The ICH Guideline Specifications:

Test Procedures and Acceptance Criteria for Biotechnological/Biological Products address guideline specifications, tests and procedures for biotechnological/biological products. Radio-pharmaceuticals, products of fermentation, oligonucleotides, herbal products and crude products of animal or plant origin are similarly not covered. Guidance is provided with regard to acceptance criteria which should be established for all new drug substances and new drug products, i.e. universal acceptance criteria, and those that are considered specific to individual drug substances and/or dosage forms. This guideline should not be considered all encompassing. New analytical technologies, and modifications to existing technology, are continually being developed. Such technologies should be used when justified. Dosage forms addressed in this guideline include solid oral dosage forms, liquid oral dosage forms, and parenterals (small and large volume). This is not meant to be an all-inclusive list, or to limit the number of dosage forms to which this guideline applies. The dosage forms presented serve as models, which may be applicable to other dosage forms which have not been discussed. The extended application of the concepts in this guideline to other dosage forms, e.g., to inhalation dosage forms (powders, solutions, etc.), to topical formulations (creams, ointments, gels), and to transdermal systems, is encouraged[65].

Q6B Specifications: Test procedures and acceptance criteria for biotechnological/biological products

The principles adopted and explained in this document apply to proteins and polypeptides, their derivatives, and products of which they are components (conjugates). These proteins and polypeptides are produced from recombinant or non-recombinant cell-culture expression systems and can be highly purified and characterized using an appropriate set of analytical procedures. The principles outlined in this document may also apply to other product types such as proteins and polypeptides isolated from tissues and body fluids. To determine applicability, manufacturers should consult with the appropriate regulatory authorities. This document does not cover antibiotics, synthetic peptides and polypeptides, heparins, vitamins, cell metabolites, DNA products, allergenic extracts, conventional vaccines, cells, whole blood, and cellular blood components. A separate ICH Guideline, "Specifications: Test Procedures and Acceptance Criteria for New Drugs Substances and New Drug Products: Chemical Substances" addresses specifications, and other criteria for chemical substances. This document does not recommend specific test procedures or specific acceptance criteria nor does it apply to the regulation of preclinical and/or clinical research material.

Q7 Good manufacturing practice guide for active pharmaceutical ingredients

This document (Guide) is intended to provide guidance regarding good manufacturing practice (GMP) for the manufacturing of active pharmaceutical ingredients (APIs) under an appropriate system for managing quality. It is also intended to help ensure that APIs meet the requirements for quality and purity that they purport or are represented to possess. In this Guide "manufacturing" is defined to include all operations of receipt of materials, production, packaging, repackaging, labelling, relabelling, quality control, release, storage and distribution of APIs and the related controls. In this Guide the term "should" indicates recommendations that are expected to apply unless shown to be inapplicable or replaced by an alternative demonstrated to provide at least an equivalent level of quality assurance. For the purposes of this Guide, the terms "current good manufacturing practices" and "good manufacturing practices" are equivalent. The Guide as a whole does not cover safety aspects for the personnel engaged in the manufacture, or aspects of protection of the environment. These controls are inherent responsibilities of the manufacturer and are governed by national laws. This Guide is not intended to define registration/filing requirements or modify pharmacopoeia requirements. This Guide does not affect the ability of the responsible regulatory agency to establish specific registration/filing requirements regarding APIs within the context of marketing/manufacturing authorisations or drug applications. All commitments in registration/filing documents must be met.

Q8 (R2) Pharmaceutical development

This guideline is intended to provide guidance on the contents of section 3.2.P.2 (pharmaceutical development) for drug products as defined in the scope of module 3 of the common technical document (ICH guideline). The guideline does not apply to contents of submissions for drug products during the clinical research stages of drug development. However, the principles in this guideline are important to consider during those stages as well. This guideline might also be appropriate for other types of products. To determine the applicability of this guideline to a particular type of product, applicants can consult with the appropriate regulatory authorities.

Q9 Quality risk management

This guideline provides principles and examples of tools for quality risk management that can be applied to different aspects of pharmaceutical quality. These aspects include development, manufacturing, distribution, and the inspection and submission/review processes throughout the lifecycle of drug substances, drug (medicinal) products, biological and biotechnological products (including the use of raw materials, solvents, excipients, packaging and labelling materials in drug (medicinal) products, biological and biotechnological products).

Two primary principles of quality risk management are:

* The evaluation of the risk to quality should be based on scientific knowledge and ultimately link to the protection of the patient; and
* The level of effort, formality and documentation of the quality risk management process should be commensurate with the level of risk[66].

Q10 Pharmaceutical quality system

This guideline applies to the systems supporting the development and manufacture of pharmaceutical drug substances (API) and drug products, including biotechnology and biological products, throughout the product lifecycle. The elements of ICH Q10 should be applied in a manner that is appropriate and proportionate to each of the product lifecycle stages, recognising the differences among, and the different goals of each stage. For the purposes of this guideline, the product lifecycle includes the following technical activities for new and existing products:

Pharmaceutical development

* Drug substance development;
* Formulation development;
* Manufacture of investigational products;
* Delivery system development;
* Manufacturing process development and scale-up;
* Analytical method development. Technology transfer
* New product transfers during Development through Manufacturing;
* Transfers within or between manufacturing and testing sites for marketed products.

Commercial manufacturing

* Acquisition and control of materials;

* Provision of facilities, utilities, and equipment;
* Production (including packaging and labelling);
* Quality control and assurance;
* Release;
* Storage;
* Distribution (excluding wholesaler activities).

Product discontinuation

* Retention of documentation;
* Sample retention;
* Continued product assessment and reporting.

Q11 Development and manufacture of drug substances (chemical entities and biotechnological/biological entities)

It addresses aspects of development and manufacture that pertain to drug substance, including the presence of steps designed to reduce impurities. In addition, ICH Q11 provides further clarification on the principles and concepts described in ICH Guidelines on Pharmaceutical Development (Q8), Quality Risk Management (Q9) and Pharmaceutical Quality System (Q10) as they pertain to the development and manufacture of drug substance.

A company can choose to follow different approaches in developing a drug substance. For the purpose of this guideline, the terms "traditional" and "enhanced" are used to differentiate two possible approaches. In a traditional approach, set points and operating ranges for process parameters are defined and the drug substance control strategy is typically based on demonstration of process reproducibility and testing to meet established acceptance criteria. In an enhanced approach, risk management and scientific knowledge are used more extensively to identify and understand process parameters and unit operations that impact critical quality attributes (CQAs) and develop appropriate control strategies applicable over the lifecycle of the drug substance which may include the establishment of design space(s). As discussed in ICH Q8 for drug product, a greater understanding of the drug substance and its manufacturing process can create the basis for more flexible regulatory approaches. The degree of regulatory flexibility is generally predicated on the level of relevant scientific knowledge provided in the application for marketing authorisation. Traditional and enhanced approaches are not mutually exclusive. A company can use either a traditional approach or an enhanced approach to drug substance development, or a combination of both. This guideline is applicable to drug substances as defined in the Scope sections of ICH Guidelines Q6A and Q6B but might also be appropriate for other types of products following consultation with the appropriate regulatory authorities. The guideline does not apply to contents of submissions during the clinical research stages of drug development. Nevertheless, the development principles presented in this guideline are important to consider during the investigational stages. Regional requirements for post-approval changes are not covered by this guideline.

Q12 Technical and regulatory considerations for pharmaceutical product lifecycle management

This guideline provides a framework to facilitate the management of post-approval CMC changes in a more predictable and efficient manner. It is also intended to demonstrate how increased product and process knowledge can contribute to a reduction in the number of regulatory submissions. Effective implementation of the tools and enablers described in this guideline should enhance industry's ability to manage many CMC changes effectively under the firm's Pharmaceutical Quality System (PQS) with less need for extensive regulatory oversight prior to implementation[67].

Q13 Continuous manufacturing of drug substances and drug products

The new ICH guideline will establish harmonised scientific and technical requirements needed to fulfil regulatory expectations for the implementation and assessment of CM to improve access to medicines. An ICH guideline would facilitate international harmonization and could reduce barriers to the adoption of CM technology.

Q14 Analytical procedure development

The new guideline is proposed to harmonise the scientific approaches of Analytical Procedure Development, and to provide the principles relating to the description of Analytical Procedure Development process. This new guideline is intended to improve regulatory communication between industry and regulators and facilitate more efficient, sound scientific and risk-based approval as well as post-approval change management of analytical procedures.

Exercises

Multiple Choice Questions

1. Fill in the blank with the following words given below.

   Evaluation of degradation rate under different stress conditions reveals the .... of drug stability.

   a) CQAs b) QCAs

   c) ACQs d) AQCs

2. Fill in the blank with the following words given below.

   Physicochemical properties of drug substances and drug products can get altered during their use, ..., and transport.

   a) Dissolution, b) Test
   c) Storage d) Purchase

3. Fill in the blank with the following words given below.

   The significance of .... that occur in drug products are primarily described by stability of drug products.

   a) Stabilities b) Instabilities
   c) Disintegration d) Dissolution

4. Fill in the blank with the following words given below.

   The degradation rate constants are mostly independent of concentration and sometimes depend on other factors, such as ....

   a) Pressure b) Impurities
   c) pH d) Temperature

5. Which of the following statement is correct?

   a) A 1°C increase in temperature can double the reaction rate with the same activation energy.
   b) A 10°C increase in temperature can double the reaction rate with the same activation energy.
   c) A 20°C increase in temperature can double the reaction rate with the same activation energy.
   d) A 0.5°C increase in temperature can double the reaction rate with the same activation energy.

6. Which of the following statements is correct?

   a) Advanced oxidative degradation uses reducing agents with UV exposure for degradation of the system.
   b) Advanced reductive degradation uses oxidising agents with UV exposure for degradation of the system.
   c) Advanced oxidative degradation uses oxidising agents with UV exposure for degradation of the system.
   d) None of the above.

7. Which of the following statements is correct?

   a) HPLC can be used to track oxidative degradation experiments by using TiO_2 as a stressor.
   b) HPLC can be used to track hydrolytic degradation experiments by using TiO_2 as a stressor.

c) HPLC can be used to track any type of degradation experiments by using TiO_2 as a stressor.

d) HPLC can be used to track photocatalytic degradation experiments by using TiO_2 as a stressor.

8. Which of the following statements is correct?

a) Most pharmaceutical products are found to get degrade through first-order reactions.

b) Most pharmaceutical products are found to get degrade through pseudo zero-order reactions.

c) Most pharmaceutical products are found to get degrade through pseudo first-order reactions.

d) Most pharmaceutical products are found to get degrade through zero order reactions.

9. Which of the following statements is correct?

a) Photodegradation of formamethylflavin in acidic solution in alkaline solution follows zero-order degradation reaction.

b) Photodegradation of formamethylflavin in acidic solution in alkaline solution follows pseudo first-order degradation reaction.

c) Photodegradation of formamethylflavin in acidic solution in alkaline solution follows first-order degradation reaction.

d) Photodegradation of formamethylflavin in acidic solution in alkaline solution follows second-order degradation reaction.

10. Which of the following statements is correct?

a) In zero-order kinetic, degradation reactions do not depend on the concentration of the drug and stressor.

b) In first-order kinetic, degradation reactions do not depend on the concentration of the drug and stressor.

c) In zero-order kinetic, degradation reactions depend on the concentration of the drug and stressor.

d) In pseudo zero-order kinetic, degradation reactions do not depend on the concentration of the drug and stressor.

11. Which of the following statements is correct?

a) The main principle of zero-order kinetics is that the drug concentration is kept constant throughout course of reaction.

b) The main principle of pseudo-zero-order kinetics is that the drug concentration is kept constant throughout course of reaction.

c) The main principle of pseudo-zero-order kinetics is that the drug concentration is not kept constant throughout course of reaction.

d) The main principle of zero-order kinetics is that the drug concentration is not kept constant throughout course of reaction.

12. Which of the following statements is correct?

a) Stability of a pharmaceutical product may be defined as the ability of a particular formulation in a specific container/closure system to remain within its physical, chemical, microbiological specifications.

b) Stability of a pharmaceutical product may be defined as the ability of a particular formulation in a specific container/closure system to remain within its physical, chemical, microbiological, toxicological, protective, and informational specifications.

c) Stability of a pharmaceutical product may be defined as the ability of a particular formulation in a non-specific container/closure system to remain within its physical, chemical, microbiological, specifications.

d) Stability of a pharmaceutical product may be defined as the ability of a particular formulation in a non-specific container/closure system to remain within its physical, chemical, microbiological, toxicological, protective, and informational specifications.

13. Which of the following statements is correct?

a) The rate of reaction in the case non-ionic reaction strongly depends on the nature of the solvent used and ionic strength.

b) The rate of reaction in the case ionic reaction strongly depends on the nature of the solvent used.

c) The rate of reaction in the case ionic reaction strongly depends on the nature of the ionic strength.

d) The rate of reaction in the case ionic reaction strongly depends on the nature of the solvent used and ionic strength.

14. Fill the blank with the appropriate word given below.

The logarithm of the rate constant will .... with the reciprocal of the dielectric constant of the solvent.

a) vary

b) not vary,

c) be constant,

d) none of the above

15. Fill the blank with the appropriate words given below.

    The period of the real-time test depends upon the stability of the product which should .... enough to indicate clearly that no measurable degradation occurs.

    a) not be long
    b) be long
    c) be short
    d) not be short

16. Fill the blank with the appropriate words given below.

    Stability testing is .... procedure performed on drug substances and products and is employed at various stages of the product development.

    a) a special
    b) not a special
    c) not a routine
    d) a routine

17. Fill the blank with the appropriate words given below.

    Stability chambers are .... environmental chambers that can simulate the storage condition and enable evaluation of product stability based on real-time, accelerated, and long-term protocols.

    a) normal
    b) specialised
    c) All the above
    d) None of the above

18. Fill the blank with the appropriate words given below.

    The extrapolation of retest period or .... beyond the period covered by long-term data can be appropriate.

    a) real time
    b) limited time
    c) time
    d) shelf life

19. Fill the blank with the appropriate words given below.

    The .... of the product and, if present, the medicinal device should be equivalent to that proposed for marketing.

    a) Container and closure
    b) Packing materials
    c) All the above
    d) None of the above

20. Fill the blank with the appropriate words given below.

    Physical stability is important for .... as it affects drug uniformity and release rate.

    a) therapeutic efficacy
    b) safety and efficacy
    c) dose of the drug
    d) none of the above

Short Questions

1. What is meant by autocatalytic kinetics of hydrolysis?
2. What do you mean Oxidation by using Fe (II) activated bisulphate?
3. What do you know about 'Quality risk management'?
4. Explain Q10 and Q8 (R2) as per ICH guidelines.
5. What is Q7 and discuss it as per ICH guidelines.
6. What is meant by Q5E? Write about stability of biotechnological/ biological products (Q5C).
7. Explain the term, Q5B, 'Quality of biotechnological products '.
8. What is meant by Q3C(R5)? Define the term 'residual solvent.'
9. What is Q1E as per ICH guidelines? How do you evaluate the stability data?
10. What is Q1B as per ICH guidelines? What do you know about Photo-stability testing of new drug substances and products?

Long Questions

1. 'Stability of pharmaceuticals is a critical quality attribute (CQA) and an integral part of the pharmaceutical drug development program. – ' justify the statement.
2. 'Physicochemical properties of drug substances and drug products can get altered during their use, storage, and transport. – 'justify the statement.
3. Explain pseudo-zero-order reaction. What do you understand by zero-order reaction and pseudo-zero-order reaction?
4. How can you determine stability of drugs and pharmaceuticals?
5. Describe the effect of solvent.
6. What do you by 'accelerated stability testing'?
7. Describe what do you understand by 'stability testing of new drug substances and guidelines 'as per ICH guidelines.
8. Define the term, matrixing. Describe how can matrixing is done.
9. Discuss about 'Development manufacture of drug substance (chemical entities and biotechnological/biological entities)
10. What do you know about Good manufacturing practice guide for active pharmaceutical ingredients.

Answers

1	2	3	4	5	6	7	8	9	10	11	12	13	14	15	16	17	18	19	20
a	c	b	d	b	c	d	a	d	a	b	c	d	a	b	d	b	d	a	b

References

1. Jain G, Khar RK, Ahmad FJ. Kinetics, degradation and stability. In: Theory and practice of physical pharmacy-E-book. Elsevier Health Sciences; 2011. p. 285–330.
2. Tapkir N, Soni F, Sahu AK, Jadav T, Tekade RK, Sengupta P. A comprehensive review on assessment and key control strategies for impurities in drug development with a special emphasis on post-marketing surveillance. J Pharm Innov. 2021.
3. Sahu AK, Goswami A, Kate AS, Sengupta P. Identification and structural characterization of potential degraded impurities of ribociclib by time of fight-tandem mass spectrometry, and their toxicity prediction. J Pharm Biomed Anal. 2021;197:113933.
4. Sharma MK, Pandey K, Shah RP, Kumar D, Sengupta P. A mechanistic explanation on degradation behavior of fibanserin for identifcation and characterization of its potential degradants using LC-DAD/ESI/APCI-Q-TOF-MS/ MS. Microchem J. 2021;167:106281.
5. Pokar D, Rajput N, Sengupta P. Industrial approaches and consideration of clinical relevance in setting impurity level specifcation for drug substances and drug products. Int J Pharm. 2020a;576:1–10.
6. Zhou D, Porter WR, Zhang GG. Drug stability and degradation studies: developing solid oral dosage forms. Cambridge: Academic press; 2017. p. 113–49.
7. Oliveira MA, Yoshida MI, Belinelo VJ, Valotto RS. Degradation kinetics of atorvastatin under stress conditions and chemical analysis by HPLC. Molecules. 2013;18:1447–56.
8. Yoshioka S, Stella VJ. Physical stability of drug substances. In: Stability of drugs and dosage forms. Berlin: Springer; 2000. p. 139–150.
9. Rehman Q, Akash MS, Imran I, Rehman K. Stability of pharmaceutical products. In: Drug stability and chemical kinetics. Singapore: Springer; 2020. p. 147–54.
10. Bajaj S, Singla D, Sakhuja N. Stability testing of pharmaceutical products. J Appl Pharm Sci. 2012;2:129–38
11. Barbosa F, Pezzi L, Sorrentino J, Steppe M, Volpato N, Mendez ASL. pH efect on stability and kinetics degradation of nitazoxanide in solution. Drug Anal Res. 2020;4:12–7.

12. Djordjević Filijović N, Antonijević MD, Pavlović A, Vučković I, Nikolić K, Agbaba D. The stress stability of olanzapine: studies of interactions with excipients in solid state pharmaceutical formulations. Drug Dev Ind Pharm. 2015;41:502–14.

13. Ahmad I, Anwar Z, Ahmed S, Sheraz MA, Bano R, Hafeez A. Solvent effect on the photolysis of ribofavin. AAPS PharmSciTech. 2015;16:1122–8.

14. Shubha JP, Sushma N. Kinetics of oxidation of benzocaine hydrochloride by N-Halo-P-toluene sulfonamides in acid medium: a mechanistic approach. IOSR J Appl Chem. 2015;8:20–8.

15. Zhao J, Sun Y, Wu F, Shi M, Liu X. Oxidative degradation of amoxicillin in aqueous solution by thermally activated persulfate. J Chem. 2019;2019:1–10.

16. Wang H, Wang S, Liu Y, Fu Y, Wu P, Zhou G. Degradation of diclofenac by Fe (II)-activated bisulfte: kinetics, mechanism and transformation products. Chemosphere. 2019;237:124518.

17. Lu X, Shao Y, Gao N, Chen J, Zhang Y, Xiang H, Guo Y. Degradation of diclofenac by UV-activated persulfate process: Kinetic studies, degradation pathways and toxicity assessments.Ecotoxicol Environ Saf. 2017;141:139–47.

18. Shestakova M, Vinatoru M, Mason TJ, Iakovleva E, Sillanpää M. Sonoelectro - chemical degradation of formic acid using Ti/Ta2O5-SnO2 electrodes. J Mol Liq. 2016;223:388–94.

19. Kušić H, Koprivanac N, Božić AL, Selanec I. Photo-assisted Fenton type processes for the degradation of phenol: a kinetic study. J Hazard Mater. 2006;136:632–44.

20. Kwiecień A, Krzek J, Żmudzki P, Matoga U, Długosz M, Szczubiałka K, Nowakowska M. Roxithromycin degradation by acidic hydrolysis and photocatalysis. Anal Methods. 2014;6:6414–23.

21. Mao Y, Liang J, Ji F, Dong H, Jiang L, Shen Q, Zhang Q. Accelerated degradation of pharmaceuticals by ferrous ion/chlorine process: roles of Fe (IV) and reactive chlorine species. Sci Total Environ. 2021;787:147584.

22. Loos G, Scheers T, Van Eyck K, Van Schepdael A, Adams E, Van der Bruggen B, Cabooter D, Dewil R. Electrochemical oxidation of key pharmaceuticals using a boron doped diamond electrode. Sep Purif Technol. 2018;195:184–91.

23. Robnik, B., Likozar, B, Wang, B, Stanić Ljubin, T, Časar, Z; Understanding and kinetic modeling of complex degradation pathways in the solid dosage form: the case of saxagliptin.; Pharmaceutics;. 2019;11:452

24. Denisov ET, Denisov E, Sarkisov O, Likhtenshtein G. General ideas of chemical kinetics. In: Chemical kinetics: fundamentals and recent developments. Elsevier; 2003. p. 1–15

25. Stanisz B, Regulska K. Kinetics of degradation of imidapril hydrochloride in finished dosage formulations. Acta Pol Pharm. 2013;70:737–42.

26. Ahmad I, Vaid FH. Thermal degradation of 7, 8-dimethyl-10-formylmethylisoal- loxazine in acid solution: a kinetic study. J Chem Soc Pak. 2011;30:688.

27. Mendez AS, Dalomo J, Steppe M, Schapoval EE. Stability and degradation kinetics of meropenem in powder for injection and reconstituted sample. J Pharm Biomed Anal. 2006;41:1363–6.

28. Aulton ME, Taylor KM. Aulton's pharmaceutics. Des Manuf Med. 2007;3:176–8.

29. Song J-F, Li D-J, Pang H-L, Liu C-Q. Effect of ultrasonic waves on the stability of all-trans lutein and its degradation kinetics. Ultrason Sonochem. 2015;27:602–8.

30. Oliveira MA, Yoshida MI, Belinelo VJ, Valotto RS. Degradation kinetics of atorvas- tatin under stress conditions and chemical analysis by HPLC. Molecules. 2013;18:1447–56.

31. Shetty BV, Schowen RL, Slavik M, Riley CM. Degradation of dacarbazine in aqueous solution. J Pharm Biomed Anal. 1992;10:675–83.

32. Hawe A, Poole R, Romeijn S, Kasper P, Van Der Heijden R, Jiskoot W. Towards heat-stable oxytocin formulations: analysis of degradation kinetics and identification of degradation products. Pharm Res. 2009; 26:1679–88.

33. Singh S., Bakshi M. Guidance on conduct of stress test to determine inherent stability of drugs. Pharm Technol Asia, Special Issue, Sep./Oct. 2000; 24-36.

34. Carstensen JT. Drug Stability, Principles and Practices, Marcel Dekker, New York (2000)

35. Matthews RB. Regulatory Aspects of Stability Testing in Europe. Drug Dev. Ind. Pharm. 1999;25:831-856.

36. Kommanaboyina B., Rhodes CT. Trends in stability Testing , with Emphasis on Stability During Distribution and Storage. Drug Dev. Ind. Pharm. 1999;25:857-867

37. Anderson G., Scott M. Determination of product shelf life and activation energy for five drugs of abuse. Clin. Chem. 1991;37:398-402

38. Bott RF., Oliveira WP. Storage conditions for stability testing of pharmaceuticals in hot and humid regions. Drug Dev. and Indus. Pharm. 2007;33:393-401.
39. Carstensen JT., Rhodes CT. Clin. Res. Drug Reg. Affairs. 1993;10:177-185
40. WHO. Stability studies in a global environment. Geneva meeting working document QAS/05.146 with comments, (2004).
41. ICH Q1A(R2). Stability testing guidelines: Stability testing of new drug substances and products. ICH Steering Committee, 2003.
42. Ali J., Khar RK., Ahuja A. Dosage form and design.3rd ed. Delhi. Birla Publications Pvt. Ltd (2008) 100-123
43. Cha J., Gilmor T., Lane P., Ranweiler JS. Stability studies in Handbook of modern pharmaceutical analysis. Separation Science and Technology. Elsevier (2001) 459-505
44. ICH Q1A (R2) - stability testing of new drug substances and products.
45. ICH Q1C- stability testing for new dosage forms.
46. ICH Q1D- bracketing and matrixing design for stability testing of new drug substances and products.
47. ICH Q1E- evaluation of stability data.
48. ICH Q2 (R1)-validation of analytical procedures: text and methodology.
49. ICHQ3A (R2)-impurities in new drug substances.
50. ICHQ3B (R2)-impurities in new drug products.
51. ICHQ3C (R5)-impurities: guidelines for residual solvents.
52. ICHQ3D-guidelines for elemental impurities.
53. ICHQ4B-pharmacopeias
54. ICHQ5A (R1)-viral safety evaluation of biotechnology products derived from cell lines of human or animal origin.
55. ICHQ5b- analysis of the expression construct in cells used for production of R-DNA derived protein products.
56. ICHQ5C-stability testing of biotechnological/biological products.
57. ICHQ5D- derivation and characterisation of cell subtracts used for production of biotechnological/biological products.
58. ICHQ5E-comparability of biotechnological/biological products subject to changes in their manufacturing process.
59. ICHQ6A-specifications: test procedure and acceptance criteria for new drug substances and new drug products: chemical substances.
60. ICHQ6B-specification: test procedures and acceptance criteria for biotechnological/biological products.